*"First they ignore you,*

*then they laugh at you,*

*then they fight you,*

*…then you win."*

…Mahatma Gandhi

# RECAGING the BEAST

## The Disease Behind Disease:
## The Yeast–Fungal Connection

By

Jane Remington

## Disclaimer

The material and diet guidelines described (herein) in *Recaging the Beast* are for informative purposes only and are not intended to replace the advice of a medical doctor or trained healthcare professional. Neither the publisher nor the author shall be liable or legally responsible for any loss or damage allegedly arising from the use of any information or suggestions contained in this book. The author strongly recommends if you suspect you have a medical problem, please seek medical help immediately.

## Recaging the Beast

ISBN: 978-1-479-31847-6

Published By: Aerie LLC

Portrait of lion and photograph by William C. Remington

# Table of Contents

REVIEW
By
TRACY ROBERTS


Recaging The Beast
The Disease Behind Disease: The Yeast-Fungal Connection
By
Jane Remington

In the 1980s, author Jane Remington developed a systemic yeast infection after taking several courses of antibiotics prescribed after dental surgeries. While looking for a way to eliminate the Candida overgrowth, she found a naturopath by the name of Dr. Sylvia Flesner who put her on a yeast-free diet. Several weeks later, her immune system was restored and she regained her energy and health. In her book, *Recaging the Beast, the Disease Behind Disease: The Yeast-Fungal Connection,* Jane Remington shares her knowledge about how the rise of diseases is directly linked to the overgrowth of the fungus Candida albicans. She contends there is a direct relationship between the yeast levels in our body and disease. Each health condition is a different but distinct manifestation of the same etiology or cause–fungus.

Remington explains that Candida albicans is a naturally occurring tiny one celled organism that normally resides in our gastrointestinal tract. When there is a fungal overgrowth that escapes from the gastrointestinal tract, the fungus goes on a rampage throughout the body and wreaks havoc on every system right down to the cellular level. The chemicals released from the yeast are toxic which leaves the body susceptible to a broad range of diseases such as cancer, diabetes, and even childhood conditions such as autism. Remington goes into much detail in explaining what yeasts are, their affects on the body and its systems, and the damage that results from the proliferation of yeast throughout he body. She highlights her own experiences working with renowned naturopath, Dr. Sylvia Flesner, and the astonishing results when patients embraced a yeast-free diet. As well, she cites many health studies to support her claims. She provides a detailed guide on adopting a yeast-free diet in order to contain the yeast in the gastrointestinal tract. She also outlines what should be avoided to eliminate yeast overgrowth and prevent future infestation, such as certain foods and beverages, antifungal supplements, antibiotics, and more. As well, Remington takes on the controversial issues surrounding vaccines, antibiotics, and the role Big Pharma plays in treating illness, not curing it.

One of the most impressive features of the book is the research. Remington does not just provide information on the importance of adopting a yeast-free lifestyle, but she has a done an incredible amount of research to support her arguments. She is able to deliver an honest account of where our future is going regarding the food and pharmaceuticals we put in our bodies. The book is a wake-up call about the health of our society and what we as individuals can do to take control of our own health. Remington makes a compelling case supported by studies that show that the yeast-fungal connection is directly linked to most of the disease and health conditions we see today, and that things will only get worse if we do not take control of our own bodies instead of relying on a multibillion dollar pharmaceutical industry to treat our illnesses. *Recaging The Beast* is an easy to understand, comprehensive study of the multiple causes of disease today. The book is highly recommended to readers who want to embrace a healthier lifestyle and combat disease.

Tracy Roberts<br>
Write Field Services<br>
August, 2010

~~Dedication~~

This book is dedicated to

SYLVIA

Whose love and wisdom shine through

these pages to make all our lives better

## ACKNOWLEDGEMENTS

There is no way I can express my gratitude fully to all who have been the "wind beneath my sails." Thank you, many friends, who made it clear to me that there was a real need for a book about Candida written by a layperson for laypeople. Suffice it to say, I couldn't have undertaken this project without your encouragement and faith.

Special hugs to my husband, Bill, for your long hours of editing, many insightful suggestions, and especially for your patience in helping me with this project of so many years. Thank you for putting up with my attempts to achieve this goal in the midst of our home and sometimes chaotic daily life. It wasn't all smooth sailing. Thank you also for being so tolerant of my grand kitchen experiments, some of which bypassed the dinner table and went straight to the dogs' dishes.

Thank you, daughter Laura, for reviewing thirty chapters in the midst of your hectic life. You helped me clarify my manuscript. Thank you son, Craig, and wife Carrie, for all your good ideas, for your long distance calls made mainly from your car, to see how the project was coming and generally cheering me on. Thank you, daughter Mary, for the list of helpful comments and suggestions you so lovingly prepared for the book. Thank you, sons-in-law Dave and Chris, for giving me so generously of your time and expertise on the computer to help this novice unravel the mysteries of such a frustrating and mystifying machine.

Thank you, Dr. Douglas M. Cox, D.C., for your support and most of all your friendship of many years. You will never know how much I appreciate the time you took to read and review my book in spite of your heavy schedule.

Sincere thanks also to Dr. Harold E. Buttram, M.D. for proofing the book for any medical errors or misconceptions, and again to Dr. Buttram for your wonderful foreword and the essay on Volatile Organic Compounds.

Kudos also to Susannah Nagle, my yeast-free buddy, for the final read through, legal expertise, and incredible editing work. I'll always be in your debt.

More heartfelt thanks to my husband, Bill, artist and photographer extraordinaire, for your excellent illustration on the cover. I am so pleased to have your beautiful lion looking back at me and my readers.

Special thanks to my adopted family member and friend, Vicki Griffin, who spent special weeks with me critiquing and formatting both the original and final layouts. I couldn't have done it without you.

Huge hugs to my farm manager/housekeeper/secretary/dog sitter/best neighbor and dear friend, Barbara Colvin, who lovingly kept the home fires burning so I could devote as much of my time as possible to this project. It would have been impossible without you.

Loving thanks to Dolores Ruybal for the countless hours you spent creating the original layout and formatting from a computer draft that looked like it had been written by a four-year-old. It was tedious and painstaking work, which was more than vindicated by the superb results. I so appreciate your dogged determination to make everything "perfect."

I am also very grateful for the invaluable contributions to the book by Catherine J. Frompovich, my "Book Doctor", book consultant and editor, who so skillfully guided me through the intricacies of creating a book and the minefields of self publishing. You were heaven-sent. Your advice and editing skills were indispensable to me. Thank you.

And to Sylvia–words cannot express how grateful I am to you and for you. You are our teacher.

*Gracias, hermanita mia, madre de muchos.*

# Foreword
By
Harold E. Buttram, M.D.


As background for this text, I must point out the critical needs for its messages.  It is important to review the adverse health trends that have been taking place among American children in the past several decades.

Many years ago in my medical practice, I observed increasing numbers of children with learning and behavioral problems.  My staff and I began asking school teachers if they had observed any health changes in children. Without exception they reported that there had been dramatic changes since the 1980s. Steadily increasing numbers, they said, were showing autistic-like behaviors; were restless, impulsive, less focused, less able to concentrate, and therefore less able to learn.

It has been documented that a sharp and persisting rise in the incidence of childhood autism commenced following the 1978 introduction of the MMR vaccine in the U.S.A.(1-2) This occurred at the same time mercury-laced Hepatitis B and Hemophilus influenza vaccines were also introduced.  For many years up to this time, the live measles, mumps, and rubella vaccines had been administered separately with negligible increases in autism. It was only after they were combined in the MMR vaccine that the incidence of autism began soaring with 1 in 150 children being affected, according to a U.S. multisite study in 2000.(3)  This is to be compared with 1 in 10,000 several generations ago. Considering that the incidence of autism in boys is approximately four times greater than in girls, the relative incidence of autism in just boys would be far greater than 1 in 150.

In a bulletin sponsored by the American Academy of Pediatrics, January, 2004, entitled "AUTISM A.L.A.R.M.," in addition to an announcement about the increasing prevalence of autism at that time, it was announced that *one in six American children were diagnosed with a learning and/or significant behavioral disorder.*(Emphasis added)

In similar fashion the incidence of asthma has increased from roughly two and a half million children, ages 0-17 years in 1979, to nine million children in 2004,(4) (roughly 12 percent of that age-group). This represents a 360 percent increase in asthma during a time period in which this age-group population increased only114 percent.

Autoimmune diseases are also increasing, including juvenile diabetes, multiple sclerosis, Guillain-Barre Syndrome, and Crohn's inflammatory bowel disease. Based on the work of Vijendra Singh, who demonstrated marked elevations of brain antibodies in the form of myelin basic protein antibodies in autistic children,(5-6) autism can also be considered an autoimmune disease.

As one of today's senior citizens who grew up in a mid-western state in the 1930s, and as a doctor who treated many autistic children, I may have a special advantage of time and experience in regard to the changes that have taken place in American children since the relatively innocent days of the 1930s.

At a summer camp in the New Mexico mountains, which I was fortunate to attend, no boy had allergies, none were on mediation, and none were sick with the common ailments of today. It was much the same in the schools. I don't recall ever seeing a child with the easily recognized behaviors now described as the attention deficit hyperactivity disorder (ADHD) and autism. I don't recall seeing a single child or adolescent whose health was significantly compromised by asthma. Today, in stark contrast, one-third of our youngsters are afflicted with the 4-A disorders (Autism, ADHD, Asthma, Allergies), as described and documented by Dr. Kenneth Bock.(7)

Turning next to the controversies surrounding current childhood vaccine programs, relatively few today are aware of the series of U.S. Congressional Hearings that were held from 1999 to December, 2004 on issues of vaccine safety. The hearings were called and chaired by Congressman Dan Burton who had two grandchildren whom he believed to have been damaged by vaccines, one of whom was autistic. As chronicled by reporter David Kirby in his book, *Evidence of Harm*,(8) it was during these hearings that gross deficiencies in vaccine safety testing were disclosed, with none of the federal government health agencies (FDA, CDC, NIH) able to produce a single vaccine safety test which would meet with current scientific standards. By way of explanation, valid vaccine safety tests are those in which before-and-after vaccine tests are performed that are specifically designed to test for possible adverse effects of vaccines on the neurologic, immunologic, hematologic, genetic, and other systems of the body, with sufficient numbers of test patients and (when applicable) control patients to be statistically significant.

As an example, in a little noted 1984 study from Germany by Eibl et al,(9) a significant though temporary drop in T-helper lymphocytes was found in 11 healthy adults following tetanus booster vaccinations. Special concern rests in the fact that, in four of the subjects, T-helper lymphocytes (a class of white blood cells that govern the immune system), temporarily fell to levels seen in active AIDS patients. If this was the result of a single vaccine in healthy adults, one must wonder what the results would be from today's mandatory childhood vaccine programs (over 36 vaccines before school age). The above-study was too small to carry statistical significance, but it did provide important clues which should have had follow-up. However, after a lapse of 26 years, to the best of my knowledge this test has never been repeated. Someone with proper authority should be looking into this.

If we consider only surface appearances, take a graph of the steadily increasing incidence of childhood autism since 1980(10) and project the graph into an unknown future, the dangers of our present situation would become very clear: It is questionable if any people or society could continue to prosper or even survive with the current rate of health attrition that is taking place among our children. The situation does indeed appear quite grim, but take heart! There are many indications that the pendulum is beginning to swing the other way.

Regarding the premise proposed by this text, that virtually all diseases conditions are complicated by fungal infections, it appears that this is one of the basic truisms (laws) of nature, which does not tolerate weakness in any of its species. If one thinks about it, every life-form has a predator, with the possible exception of the multiple fungi species themselves, which appear to be at the end of the line of the survival process.

Under present circumstances, *Recaging the Beast* may prove to be a Godsend to the families of America, somewhat like a literary Noah's Ark. Written in a fluent and readable fashion, the book probes deeply into the multiple causes that are contributing to today's adverse health trends, along with suggested guidelines for their correction.

Harold E Buttram, MD

## *Introduction*

---

*"Never, no, never did nature say one thing and Wisdom say another."*
                                        *...Edmund Burke (1728–1797)*

Every farmer will tell you that his number one enemy in raising crops is FUNGUS.  It is a constant battle to keep this enemy from consuming and destroying the fruits of his labor and livelihood.

This pesky organism masquerades in many different guises.  We know them as: scabs, mildews, molds, smuts, rusts, spots, cankers, sac fungi, blights, wilts, root rots, ergots, etc.  Each is a different but distinct manifestation of one etiology or cause: fungus.  Each disease name is simply another name for fungus.

It is my contention that almost all diseases of humankind, major and minor, ancient and modern, are intimately connected to, and also may have as their root cause, this same basic organism–fungus.  We call these fungal guises: cancer, heart disease, arthritis, rheumatoid arthritis, allergies, asthma, COPD, diabetes, lupus, fibromyalgia, multiple sclerosis, ALS, chronic fatigue syndrome, high blood pressure, high cholesterol, digestive problems, vitiligo, psoriasis, cystitis, Alzheimer's, hypothyroidism, all autoimmune diseases, autism, ADHD, and countless others.  I believe that each is a different but distinct manifestation of the same etiology or cause: fungus. Each disease name is just another name for fungus. So far, this lowly little microbe has been completely ignored and overlooked as the cause of these–and many other–diseases.

We humans and plants live on the same planet.  We occupy the same environments.  We share the same variables of nutrition, heat, humidity, rain, sunlight, and seasons. Why should humans be immune to fungal attacks when plants are not?  The answer is, *we are not.*

I came to this conclusion honestly–by working with a remarkable naturopath and her patients for over twenty-five years. I took notice as the yeast-free diet and anti-fungal protocols worked their magic on patients who presented with all the diseases listed above–and more. Not one or two diseases, *but almost all diseases.* I watched in awe as almost everyone seemed to get well following the same nourishing diet and taking special fungus-killing supplements–*no matter what the ailment.*

Many sages through the ages have implored us to study nature to find the answers to our questions. I believe that when we do, we will start connecting the dots between fungus and disease. Then many answers will be found that will lead to finding cures for many of the diseases that have plagued humankind through the centuries.

As I watched nature for clues and began connecting the dots, I gradually began to see the links that existed between overgrowths of fungus and the manifestation of so many diseases in the human body. Fungus continuously appeared to be the common denominator. It was undeniable. As people followed the protocols set out in this book, they seemed to be able to tap into their own innate restorative powers and get well. It was miraculous. What a thrilling and humbling experience it has been for me to witness so many people regain control of their health and lives.

Leading pathologists now estimate that a minimum of *eighty percent* of our population has been significantly affected by yeast, and it seems that almost every week new books or cookbooks on yeast infection or *Candida albicans* appear. Unfortunately, all the authors are not in agreement as to what is acceptable–or not acceptable–to eat and drink while on their programs. Some allow a few dairy products, and beef and pork, while others severely restrict fruits and grains. I even ran across one recipe in a yeast-free cookbook that called for brewer's yeast!

That, of course, is very confusing, especially to someone who is not feeling well, and at the same time is trying to sort out conflicting points of view and decide which version of the "yeast-free" diet to follow.

Which brings me to why I am here, writing a book for the first time in my life.

For over twenty-five years I have been privileged to work closely with an exceptionally gifted woman named Dr. Sylvia Flesner. After my family and I moved to Houston from Nashville, Tennessee, in 1985, I heard about Sylvia through a local health food store. I was told she was an extraordinary healer and naturopathic physician who worked very much in the same manner as Edgar Cayce. I was thrilled, not knowing someone living now could be compared with Edgar Cayce.

For those of you who are unfamiliar with Cayce, he was an American medical intuitive whose phenomenal "readings" are still being studied by thousands of people, including many doctors, who are interested in holistic healing. At a very young age Cayce discovered he was psychically gifted, and as a young man he developed the ability to "see" into the body. His diagnoses were astoundingly accurate. In describing the workings and malfunctions of the body, he used precise and correct medical terminology, even though he had only a grade school education. Although he died in 1945, his prescriptions for healing, using only natural methods and easily available substances, are still used to this day. Today anyone can have access to his readings through books or by going to The Association for Research and Enlightenment, (the A.R.E.) in Virginia Beach, Virginia, where all of his readings are archived.

Public interest in his life and work has virtually exploded in the last few years, and there are many books and pamphlets about Cayce's life and work available in book stores for your further reading. Cayce's two best known biographies are, *There Is a River*, by Thomas Sugrue, and *The Sleeping Prophet*, by Jess Stearn. Both are excellent, and describe well the battle Cayce went through trying to understand his baffling gift, and how this humble Christian man learned to use this gift for the highest good of his fellow human beings.

I personally had been an avid "Cayce reader," having collected almost every book ever published about him.  My husband, three children and I were "treated" with Cayce remedies through the years whenever needed, and they always worked.  They worked so well, that aside from a few baby shots and childhood check-ups, only four doctor's appointments were necessary for the entire family during our children's growing up years.

Many times I wished I had known Edgar Cayce, or at least someone who was close to him.  I kept thinking how wonderful it would be to be able to ask him questions and benefit from his incredible knowledge...and the universe must have heard. The old saying "when the student is ready, the teacher will appear," kept running through my mind.  My years of studying Cayce must have been preparing me for my association and work with Sylvia, because I truly was ready for "the teacher" who appeared.  The universe literally dropped her into my lap.

Sylvia was born in Quito, Ecuador, and had intuitive abilities from an early age. She lived in the Houston area for twelve years before moving to Denver, Colorado, where she opened a small office.  She regularly flew back to Houston, usually one week out of the month, to see her patients. With a mixture of hesitation and excitement I made my first appointment with her.

At that time I was struggling with fatigue and headaches, which I attributed to the stress from a complicated and difficult move that came on the heels of my having five gum surgeries and five courses of antibiotics.  I knew I wasn't my usual self, and I needed help.  I counted the days until I saw her.

Finally the day of my appointment arrived and I went to her office. At that time her patients were asked to lie on a gurney, and after a centering prayer Sylvia would start her reading. Without any prompting or clues, she told me that I had a sluggish thyroid, a congested liver, and a hormone imbalance, and that all these conditions were caused by the same condition–a systemic infection of yeast. She carefully and lovingly explained what it was–even drawing a picture of the yeast colonizing–and gave me a copy of the diet which would rid my body of yeast overgrowth. She also suggested certain herbs for my liver and ovaries, a homeopathic for my thyroid, and a special bath that would speed up the healing overall.

I went home, cleaned out my cabinets and refrigerator, restocked my shelves with acceptable food, and embarked on my very personal journey of self-healing. Slowly but surely (after a short and uncomfortable "healing crisis", which I will alert you to later in the book), my headaches faded away and my energy returned in leaps and bounds.

I was ecstatic. My old self was back. The diet worked, and now all my body systems were functioning in a balanced manner. I felt reborn, renewed, even resurrected!

Then, about a week before Sylvia was scheduled to return, I mysteriously developed a severe case of diarrhea. It occurred every morning within minutes of eating breakfast. I couldn't figure out what was wrong–my lunch was fine, dinner was fine, I felt fine. *What was happening to my breakfast?*

I made an appointment with Sylvia and anxiously awaited my turn. Again I gave her no symptoms or clues. I simply asked her how the yeast was looking since I had been faithfully following the diet for three weeks. She said the yeast was very low, and congratulated me for doing such a good job of "cleaning house."

Then she "looked" again, and proclaimed, "My dear, what you have now is a protozoan infestation."

My brain began whirring, trying to remember my college biology days when we were studying protozoa and one-celled amoeba...oh, no, amoebic dysentery?

Sylvia then suggested I eat one tablespoon of raw pumpkin seeds before breakfast every morning for several weeks, and asked me to purchase a special homeopathic remedy to combat protozoa. And then, as I was about to get down from the gurney, just as an aside, she said, "Oh, by the way, my dear, this particular little protozoa only eats once a day. *It eats your breakfast.*"

Instantly I knew I had found a very gifted, special person. With absolutely no clues she "read" me twice, this time not only identifying a protozoa, but a specific *kind* of protozoa, and at that moment I made a silent vow to do everything I could to help Sylvia help others. Shortly after that I began keeping her appointments book and working side by side with her and her patients when she came to Houston.

It was a fascinating and rewarding nine-year experience for me. We worked with thousands of people during that time and I saw more miracles than I could count. I could fill a book with testimonials alone. Sylvia's beautiful gift has wrought healings in every disease imaginable, and she has the profound respect of many doctors all over the world, many of whom make appointments for themselves and their families. She was even a guest lecturer at the University of Colorado Medical School (Denver) for two years (2003–2004), teaching doctors how to access their own intuitive abilities. At a later date I intend to write a personal book just about Sylvia and her work. But for now, my mission is to impart much of what I have witnessed and experienced as to the miraculous healing power of her diet.

On any normal day when we were working in Houston, we saw between fifteen and twenty people. They came with every disease and condition imaginable. But the one common denominator that seems to affect most of her patients is a *systemic overgrowth of fungus named Candida albicans.*

It is very clear to Sylvia–she can "see" it with her clairvoyant eyes. Like Cayce, with her inner vision she can see it growing all over organs and glands, on top of and inside tissue, lining the mucous membranes of the intestinal tract, in the brain, etc., wherever the yeast has set up housekeeping in the body. She has no doubt as to why this body is sick. How can any organ, or gland, or immune system function correctly if its very life force is being drained by a parasite? How can anyone feel well, have lots of energy and stamina, or look forward to tackling the problems and challenges of life when his or her body systems are struggling and straining to work, but can't because they are too busy fighting an invasive army of yeast?

It became obvious to me very early that the more yeast the patient had growing in his body, the more serious the symptoms of illness and disease. *There seemed to be a direct relationship between yeast levels and disease.* I watched closely as person after person committed to, persevered, and completed the diet. Something miraculous seemed to be happening to almost all of them–as it had happened to me.

Each month as patients returned, they reported changes for the better. It seemed that as they started on the diet and the yeast began to die, symptoms of disease seemed to slowly die with them. Many times several conditions improved. For example, a diabetic's need for insulin would be lowered and at the same time his prostate numbers lowered *and* his psoriasis cleared up! As yeast levels fell, immune systems strengthened. Organs and glands began to wake up as if from a deep sleep and function as our Creator intended them to function. I heard and continue to hear the words "miracle" and "miraculous" a lot. You will never know how thrilling, rewarding, and humbling it is for me to be a part of these miracles.

While Sylvia was out of town, I worked with many of her patients, helping them to find the correct foods and good recipes to keep them "on the path." I started holding cooking classes in my kitchen, which everyone seemed to enjoy. Then requests started for my writing a book and cookbook so others could be helped. Patients began calling and coming to my house to get copies of recipes and many trips were made to Kinko's to satisfy the growing demand. *The Yeast-Free Kitchen*, the cookbook portion of the project, was published in 1992 in response to that demand. It has been updated and expanded twice since then and will be updated again in 2011.

Over the years I have received many inquiries and requests for the "big" book on yeast to be written. At first I resisted, fearing that it would be too big a job with too much responsibility. I am well aware that I have no medical or scientific degrees, just a degree in English and a "gift of gab," coupled with a love of healing and the privilege of witnessing thousands of people get well. But as the requests for the book kept coming, I realized the need was greater than my fear, and I neither should–nor could–keep silent. The feeling kept growing inside me that perhaps it was time for a book on the subject of yeast to be written *by* a layperson *for* the layperson. I knew that what I wrote might require a leap of faith on the part of the reader. But remembering that faith is the opposite of fear, I began to write.

Using the lion as my metaphor for the yeast/beast, I hope to illustrate that humans and plants do, indeed, have a common over-arching enemy. It is known to biologists as The Third Kingdom–the kingdom of mold, mildew, and fungus. It is our enemy only because it is out of control. This out of control kingdom now constitutes the "disease behind disease."

*Just as fungus is the plant world's ever-present adversary, so it is ours.*

I truly believe that it is the only logical conclusion there is.

*Recaging the Beast* is an attempt to add my work and thoughts into the marketplace of ideas. In doing so I hope to educate and motivate readers to follow easy guidelines to both create and maintain health. By recognizing diseases for what they truly are–mainly yeast or fungus in disguise–we can draw up a battle plan to thwart and eradicate our common enemy. The cornerstone of our battle plan is called "the yeast-free diet."

So it is with faith, and wonder, and love that I offer to you my years of research and experience with one of the world's most remarkable and gifted healers, and her diet that heals.

Jane Remington
Gordonsville, Virginia
Summer 2010

**Chapter 1**

---

# What Are Yeasts?

*"It is a mistake to consider candidiasis a simple yeast infection. It is not. It is a fungus that may have originated as a yeast, but has become a fungus and learned how to attack cells. As a fungus it does not behave like yeast or yeast infection."*

...Jack Tips, N.D., Ph.D.

I don't think anyone in this country can get through twenty-four hours these days without hearing the words "yeast" or "fungus." All you have to do is turn on the television or open a newspaper or magazine and someone is trying to sell you something to treat some form of them.

Since 1985 over-the-counter sales have skyrocketed for preparations that treat everything from vaginal yeast infections, to nail fungus, to athlete's foot, to "jock itch," which should alert us that something now is different about our human bodies. Some basic, underlying flaw seems to be working its way to the surface.

In recent years there has been a tremendous increase in research about this enigmatic organism, due to the undeniable evidence that we are now in the midst of a potentially cataclysmic epidemic of yeast and yeast-related illnesses. Much more research needs to be done, but to date we have a pretty good idea of what it is, how it grows, and what its ultimate goal is.

The word yeast comes from the Old English word *gist,* or *gyst,* and from the Indo-European root word *yes*–meaning to **boil, foam, or bubble**. Remember these descriptive terms as we explore their relationship to disease in the coming chapters.

Reduced to the fewest words, (this is the only technical part of the book, so bear with me), basically yeast is a microbe, a member of a subgroup of the family of plants known as fungi or molds. (The word fungus is Latin, meaning mushroom, and I use the words yeast, fungus, and fungi interchangeably.) Most fungal species are multi-cellular. However, yeast is a *single* cell organism whose *cell structure is nearly identical to that of a human cell.*

This tiny micro-flora literally inundates the earth. A single teaspoon of topsoil contains about 120,000 fungi. There are about a million spores nestled in your pillow alone. Fungi can range in size from single-celled organisms to giant puffballs that can grow up to six feet in diameter.

The honey mushroom (*Armillaria ostoyae*), or the "humongous fungus," can grow to unbelievable proportions. The largest growth to date was found in an Oregon forest in 2000. Living mostly underground, it covers 3.4 square miles, weighs 6,000 tons, and is estimated to be between 2,400 and 7,200 years old, giving it the dubious distinction of being the largest and oldest living organism on earth. Talk about tenacious.

Fungi have learned to adapt to the most extreme conditions and a wide range of habitats, from salt water to the deep sea, to Arctic tundra, to living on rocks. They have been found in burning desert sand and some have survived even the intense ultraviolet and cosmic radiation encountered in space travel. They are hardy and ubiquitous to say the least.

We live in *their* world, not the other way around. There are over 100,000 species of fungi (with estimates of over one million to be found in the future), of which only five percent have been formally classified. About 400 of these species can cause diseases in humans. We recognize their different strains in damp, musty basements, in our refrigerators and between our toes, but the strain called *Candida albicans* is the one that gives us so much grief.

Yeasts are part of the natural order of things. They are in every breath of air we breathe, on our skin, in our food, and inside our bodies, living in the warm moist recesses of the digestive tract and other organs. (98.6 ° F is *Candida's* favorite temperature.) Anything that is alive, or has ever been alive, is capable of supporting yeast and fungi.

Not quite plant and not quite animal, molds, mildews, puffballs, and yeasts have been assigned by scientists to a kingdom all their own: The Third Kingdom. Many scientists classify them as plants because they have plant-like features. For instance, they grow by sprouting roots or filaments called *hyphae*. But unlike plants, yeasts contain no chlorophyll and do not synthesize sunlight in order to live. Like animals, they have a cell nucleus and burn food with oxygen and store their food as glycogen. In fact, fungal cells are so much like animal cells that much about the basics of human life has been extrapolated from studies of baker's yeast! But unlike animals, they respire or breathe anaerobically, without oxygen. In other words, *they ferment.* Even so, scientists have determined that fungi are more closely related to human beings than other plants. Keep that in mind as you read.

Fungi reproduce by fission or sprouting from spores. They grow as hyphae, or filaments. These hyphae branch continuously with the hyphae of other fungi to form one larger mass called a *mycelium.* Hyphae grow from their tips in search of new food supplies, and can penetrate hard surfaces such as your nails or wood. They also burrow into their food sources, where they intertwine with tissue. (That's why you can't scrape away athlete's foot or ringworm. Their roots are too deeply entrenched.)

The Candida yeast is the yeast that this book addresses in particular. It is a form of mold or fungus and is characterized as an *ascomycete,* or a *sac fungus.* Sac fungi grow by sending out spores that are encased in hard protective coatings. These coatings enable them to lie dormant in an *ascus* (sac) for indefinite periods of time. There they survive intact and bide their time until conditions are ideal for them to grow. Once they are stimulated to grow and change from their yeast (benign) form to their fungal (malignant) form in your body, their ultimate goal is your destruction and eventual disposal.

Basically, yeast is a *unicellular* fungus, and fungi are almost entirely *multicellular*. Some fungi (called *dimorphic* fungi) can mutate and change their own DNA, alter their appearance and *alternate* between two body forms–depending on environmental conditions. These fungi may produce a mycelium (the mass of thread-like branching hyphae) while in the soil, but also have the ability to convert to single cell fungal spores (called *conidia)* at body temperature if necessary to elude the immune system's attempts to destroy it. The microscopic conidia form allows the fungus to spread via the bloodstream and lymphatic channels and infect organs, glands, and tissues throughout the body.

Once inside the body, conidia shed their protective shells and become what is called a "deficient form," now free to invade a human cell. Once this "deficient form" invades or hijacks a human cell it can lie dormant or it can reproduce more fungal cells, using the human cell as an *incubating sac*. But the scariest fact is that the fungus, now inside a human cell, can incorporate its DNA with that of the host cell, creating a *hybrid* cell–a fungal/human hybrid cell. Squamous and basal cell cancer cells are fungal/human hybrid cells. (How creepy is that!) *The fungal DNA then becomes dominant and trumps the human DNA.* The fungal DNA is now in charge. This has devastating and far-reaching repercussions for all living things, as you will see.

Yeast and fungi do not feed by ingesting their food. Their cell walls are so rigid that even microscopic particles cannot enter. In order to feed they secrete potent enzymes that break down the material or tissue from which they extract their nutrients. *They digest their way into food!* In other words, we eat our food and then digest it, but fungi digest their food and then *absorb* it. Their enzymes are so powerful that they can turn the hardest, densest wood into a soft pulpy mass. Ascomycetes digest cellulose (found in plant cell walls), lignan (found in wood), and collagen (found in connective tissue in humans and animals.) In our bodies yeast lives by fermenting (digesting) sugars and carbohydrates, and if allowed to spread uncontrolled, *it can literally break our human bodies down into a soft pulpy mass as well.*

As a single-celled plant–called a *saprophyte*–it remains a benign parasite, living peacefully, feeding on dead or decaying matter. Then, for a variety of reasons we will explore later, the yeast saprophyte alters its own DNA and transforms itself into a *pathogen*–a substance or organism that is capable of producing infection or disease. The docile yeast becomes a dangerous multi-cellular fungus, and instead of living on *dead or dying tissue only,* it is capable of feeding on *living* tissue. From the pathogenic state it can move easily into an invasive (tumoral) state.

Candida yeast is particularly wily, obstinate, and devious. It can morph and mutate quickly to whatever form is necessary for its survival. In the event it is attacked by the immune system of the host or with conventional anti-mycotic treatments or therapies, it can transform itself into smaller and undifferentiated elements to elude both the host's immune system and the doctor's diagnostic evaluations. If need be, it can even revert to its even smaller and more benign form–the spore–which cannot be attacked, hiding until the danger passes. In histoplasmosis, a fungal infection of the lungs, fungal spores actually get inside white blood cells or macrophages, the very cells that are supposed to be destroying them. Pretty crafty little organisms, wouldn't you say?

It is this feature, the ability to change its shape and activity that makes it so elusive and difficult to identify. But more importantly, that is what makes it so dangerous. The yeast/fungus goes from living quietly on DEAD tissue, to living aggressively on LIVE tissue, and in the process has learned how to ATTACK. Its armies then begin to marshal their forces–proliferate–send out mercenaries, ("buds" that shoot out spores to create more colonies), and declare war on and invade neighboring cells. In the body this has devastating effects. *Candida albicans* has been shown to have the ability to invade VIRTUALLY EVERY TISSUE IN THE BODY except the enamel in teeth.

To illustrate this devastation I like to use the analogy of the bowl of leftovers in the refrigerator. After a few days, mold starts growing all over the food, and if left long enough, the leftover will be entirely consumed, and you will have a bowl empty of food but full of hairy mold. The fungus will have digested all the nutrients it needed to live, and its numbers will have increased a million fold. Another good example is a peach bruise. If you watch a bruise on a peach (or any fruit or vegetable), you will see that yeast from the air is attracted to and starts colonizing on the *bruised area first–the area of damage.* From there it spreads to the surrounding tissue and eventually consumes the whole peach, most of which had been healthy.

In nature, molds, fungi, and yeast are the great recyclers, the garbage disposals of the planet. *They are the principle decomposers of every ecosystem.* Planet earth would be uninhabitable without them. They are attracted to diseased, decayed, and dying tissue. It is their function to keep the planet clean, and they are just doing their job, constantly breaking down, digesting, and eliminating debris, making room for the growth of new plants. By speeding up the rate of decay, vital minerals and organic matter are returned to the soil quickly so life can begin anew.

Years ago I watched as a magnificent old tree in our back yard died. Near the end, a third of the way up the trunk, several layers of a large mushroom-like fungus began to grow in rings around the tree. I knew this was a signal from Mother Nature that the rate of decay was being sped up, and the end was near. A few months later we had to have the dead tree removed.

In the human body, we don't fully understand yeast's role. It seems we all harbor small colonies that live peacefully both on and in the body– mainly in the colon–with no harm done. Our bodies have accepted them as harmless tenants, and they seem to have no obvious purpose, aside from assisting in digestion–until the end of our lives.

That is when yeast swings into action and performs the one major job we know it has–*that of decomposing and recycling our bodies back into the earth. Dust to dust.* (The embalming of bodies has interrupted this natural process.)

Because we have strayed far from the more natural life and the way we were designed to live, the yeast/beast has been artificially and prematurely stimulated to escape from the intestines (where it was meant to stay until our death), and has instead gotten into the bloodstream–the body's highway of life. This highway goes everywhere there is blood and tissue, which means it leads to *all the cells of our bodies, spreading and growing more colonies, and doing its foreordained job, that of decomposing us, only doing it prematurely...BEFORE we die.*

It is literally ***TRYING TO DECOMPOSE AND RECYCLE US WHILE WE ARE STILL LIVING!*** In other words, it is perversely attempting to decompose a living body instead of a dead one. This is a critical point to understand as we attempt to uncover the true causes of diseases in the pages that follow.

In some ways, our bodies are like that bowl of leftovers in the refrigerator. The only reason we don't get eaten alive and disappear is that our bodies are constantly struggling to make new cells to replace the old ones. But how well do you think a liver or a pancreas or any organ or gland would function with a crop of fungus growing all over it, consuming its life force?

And it makes perfectly logical sense, that anyone who is loaded with yeast, which is feeding on and digesting his cells and organs, and wreaking havoc with his immune system, *simply cannot be healthy.*

**Chapter 2**

---

# How Did This Happen?

*"If you give careful attention to the voice of the Lord Your God, do what is right in his sight, give ear to his commandments, and keep all his statutes, I will put none of these diseases upon you which I have brought upon the Egyptians, for I am the Lord who heals you."*

...Exodus 15:26

My purpose in writing this book is both to alert and alarm you as to the gravity of the situation unfolding before us. One tiny little organism run amuck has the potential to prematurely recycle us right back into the earth, and also has the potential to bankrupt us both personally and nationally if we don't take action soon.

How did we get to this state? Why have we become so weak? What have we been doing to allow a quiet, mild-mannered yeast to turn into a raging beast? Why are the very foundations of our defenses–our immune systems–crumbling and allowing armies of yeast to send their storm troopers over the wall, hell bent on missions of annihilation? Does God really want mankind to be disease-ridden and miserable?

There is a simple answer that involves a complex explanation.

The simple answer is that we have strayed far from the way our Creator intended us to live, and we are neither living nor healing in accord with His specific prescriptions we call Natural Law, the precepts of which are universally knowable through the observation of nature.

The complex explanation involves the abuse of our physical, mental, and spiritual selves–our bodies, minds, and souls. We are finding that when we don't follow the laws of nature, they do their own enforcing, and when not obeyed, they do their own punishing. It has always been so.

There is no doubt we are living in a scientific age, which may be only in the earliest stages of its evolution. Even so, the state of our medical technology is astounding, and there are many benefits from living in such a time. I don't think many of us would want to turn back the clock to even fifty years ago. But we all are paying a price for this marvelous technology and science. Our miracles of science have tended to distract us from our true natural selves and the natural methods of cure that bring about true healing.

There is also no doubt that we are living in one of the most stressful periods in recorded history. Most of us run from morning to night, juggling schedules and responsibilities, eating on the run, not getting enough rest or sleep, many times taking drugs to pep us up, and more drugs to calm us down. We take synthetic prescriptions or street drugs. We eat processed, chemically-laden and denatured food, and swill down soft drinks full of more chemicals. We consume quantities of junk food, caffeine and alcohol, breathe polluted air, and watch or read material that harms our psyches. And through all this we expect our bodies, minds, and souls to remain balanced and whole. We are beginning to realize it just is not possible.

Three thousand five hundred years ago, God gave Moses and the ancient Hebrews the astounding promise that heads this chapter. What a beautiful compact. They were guaranteed that *not one* disease would befall them if they kept His guidelines for living, diet, sex and marriage, mental and physical health, and worship. Not one! Those guidelines were followed carefully by the early Jews, and the promise was fulfilled as, indeed, the Jews were much healthier and hardier than the many tribes around them. All in all, Moses recorded hundreds of health care regulations, and so far no medical misconceptions have been found. You can read many of them in the book of law, Leviticus. It is time to revisit these age-old prescriptions for living long, healthy, and fulfilling lives.

Because we have not kept so many of God's precepts but have gone our own way, our bodies, our minds, and our lives have become unbalanced and full of disease. The tipping point for the rise of *Candida albicans*, the major contributor to this imbalance, came with the explosion in the use of man-made, synthetic chemicals called prescription drugs, during and after World War II.

Every day in the United States, *seventy-five million people take one or more drugs.* Every year in the United States, three billion prescriptions are filled, costing patients, the government, and insurance companies $70.3 billion. Add to that the incalculable number of over-the-counter drugs being sold and it is safe to say we have become a nation of junkies, hooked on various chemicals to help us cope.

The annual death rate resulting from improper use of prescription drugs equals that of breast cancer! And even used properly, many suffer adverse reactions, uncomfortable side effects, and dependency addictions.

For every adverse drug reaction that is reported, many more go unreported. Doctors and hospitals usually don't even keep track of incidences as they occur. Hospitals themselves are one of the primary sources for the spread of Candida. Aside from the drugs and awful food, yeast organisms can be placed *directly* into the body and bloodstream through any catheterization procedure, such as bladder catheterizations, intravenous feedings and dialysis instruments, or during surgery. Mycotic (yeast) endocarditis is seen frequently after heart valve surgery because of this problem.

It is important to remember that drugs *do not heal.* We rarely hear the word "healing" in the medical profession anymore. We hear words like "symptomatic relief," "management of symptoms," or "remission" instead. Drugs only mask symptoms, suppress disease, and harm other areas of the body.

Drugs *do* cause changes in the body, but at what price? We are beginning to see now that the price exacted from using most drugs is too

high, and in many, many cases, people are paying the ultimate price with
their lives.

The four most harmful classes of prescription drugs as far as the
proliferation of Candida and Candida-related illnesses is concerned, include:
**antibiotics, birth control pills, immune-suppressive drugs such as
steroids and cortisone, and hormones.**

## Antibiotics

Antibiotics were hailed as the wonder drug of the century when they were
first marketed.  There is no doubt they have saved many lives and they hold
a prominent position in any physician's medical bag.  There are times they
are appropriate and times we need them–and need them in a hurry.

But where we have gone wrong is in their over-use.  Instead of being
used for emergencies or life-threatening situations, we take them for
everything from the sniffles to itchy ears. (Especially little children.) Many
dentists prescribe them for precautionary or preventive measures, even when
no infection is present.

Before antibiotics were so widely prescribed, Candida infections
were rarely, if ever, seen.  However, after the introduction of each new type
of antibiotic from the 1940s on, major increases of vaginal and intestinal
yeast infections began to be reported in medical journals.

When an antibiotic reaches the intestines, it kills indiscriminately
both the good or beneficial bacteria along with the bad bacteria that caused
the infection. Antibiotics don't know the difference between the two. (One
doctor described antibiotics as "the pharmaceutical equivalent of a
*thermonuclear bomb*," wiping out everything in its path.)  This
indiscriminate killing disrupts the natural balance of intestinal flora, and
once the bacteria are out of the way, the yeast takes off like a rocket.
Bacteria, yeast's natural enemy that for centuries kept yeast colonies from
exploding, have been killed off, enabling the yeast to head for the wide open

spaces. They quickly start proliferating to fill up the empty intestinal real estate and claim more territory.

Yeast cannot harm or cause disease in a healthy host. However, when we become ill with a bacterial infection, we take antibiotics to kill the bad bacteria. Since antibiotics are mold–or yeast–based, they thrive on the diseased, decaying material inside *us*. So, antibiotics not only kill the bacteria that keep the yeast in bounds, they *provide additional food for the yeast.* As yeast eats the antibiotics, they stimulate the growth of *more yeast*! Even decomposing bacteria become fodder for the yeast! What an orgy.

Recent research into antibiotics shows that antibiotics actually *suppress* the immune system by damaging cells, making it easier for viruses and bacteria to enter. Damaged cells are more vulnerable to future infections. Many people report picking up another infection within days or weeks of completing a course of antibiotics. The poor host, dragging himself around, is trying to recover from a disease with drugs that have created more disease. How can he ever get well?

Today we are fortunate that we are getting away from the old broad-spectrum antibiotics, and developing antibiotics that are more selective, targeting specific bacteria, thereby not upsetting the intestinal flora as much. But all are still destructive to the immune system, and the reason that new and more resistant strains of bacteria are evolving.

*Never forget that an antibiotic is the waste product of a live fungus colony. Most antibiotics are, in fact, fungal metabolites or mycotoxins!*

In addition, antibiotics deplete the body's stores of B vitamins, calcium, zinc, potassium, magnesium, vitamin K, and vitamin C. The bottom line is that even though they are needed at times, they end up harming the body and *do not* work with the body's natural law of cure. Truly, today's Candidiasis is the legacy of antibiotics introduced in the 1940s and '50s.

**Birth Control Pills**

The scary thing about birth control pills is that doctors are beginning to think they are worse than antibiotics for stimulating yeast! Candida became pandemic after they were introduced in the 1960s.

Normally a woman has two hormones, estrogen and progesterone, which regulate her menstrual cycles. Estrogen is produced daily, while progesterone kicks in mid-cycle, causing changes in the mucous membranes of the vagina, which in turn makes a more hospitable environment for yeast to grow. Many women complain of vaginitis at this time of month due to the progesterone.

When a woman is on the birth control pill (or pregnant), progesterone is supplied to her tissues *constantly*. If she is taking birth control pills, she is being fed a hormone that stimulates the overgrowth of yeast–*constantly*.

Doctors have known for a long time that oral contraceptives create deficiencies in vitamin $B_6$ and folic acid. (Spina bifida and other birth defects can be traced back to deficiencies of folic acid in the mother's body). Oral contraceptives interfere with the endocrine system of the entire body. All in all a bad idea.

**Hormones**

During menopause many women are prescribed synthetic hormones that promise to help alleviate some of its more annoying symptoms such as hot flashes, mood swings, bone loss, heart disease, etc. Our grandmothers and great-grandmothers rarely had any of these problems! Known as Hormone Replacement Therapy, or HRT, it is a *synthetic* combination of the hormones estrogen and progestin. Unfortunately synthetic hormones are different from natural hormones. *They have been changed structurally so they can be patented.*

One of the best known of the synthetic hormones is a drug called Premarin®. It is made synthetically from the urine of pregnant horses. (Pre:_preg_nant, mar:_mar_e, in:ur_ine_.)Why would any woman want to put THAT into her body?

A major federally funded study in 1992 by the Women's Health Institute was halted when it was discovered that HRT increased the rate of breast cancer and provided no benefit against heart attack and stroke. The study found that women on the HRT drug Prempro® experienced:

1. 41% increase in stroke
2. 29% increase in heart attacks
3. 100% increase in the rate of blood clots
4. 22% increase in total cardiovascular disease
5. 24% increase in breast cancer
6. 100% increase in the rate of Alzheimer's disease in women over 65

Clearly the risks outweigh any benefits that may be derived from HRT use.

Hormone replacement therapy upsets the intestinal flora, just as antibiotics do. The symptoms of hot flashes, vaginal dryness, mood swings and depression, so common to menopause, are caused mainly by hormonal imbalances *caused by yeast*. So why take a drug that will just exacerbate the original problem? Also, today many men who have prostate cancer are put on female hormones as part of their treatment. Such treatment is asking for trouble. Here again, hormones will only create *more* yeast, and eventually *MORE* symptoms and disease.

### Immuno–suppressive drugs, steroids, and cortisone

In the battle against disease, medical science has developed some high tech drugs that have far-reaching consequences and negative side effects. They suppress the immune system and even shut down the body's defense mechanisms. Steroids, such as cortisone and prednisone, are two of the best known. Cancer chemotherapies are notorious for immune system suppression, as are certain drugs used in the treatment of arthritis. Remember:

*Any drug that suppresses the immune response encourages yeast to multiply!*

Steroids, cortisone, and so-called "anti-inflammatory" drugs stimulate the adrenals to pump out more adrenalin. *Adrenalin then stimulates the growth of yeast.* Anything that primes or over-stimulates the body, e.g., prednisone, also stimulates the growth of yeast. (That is why caffeine is so harmful.) Even over-the-counter cortisone cream is absorbed into the body through the skin, and feeds yeast.

**Other Contributors to Candidiasis**

**1. Failure to breastfeed.**

The most important meal a baby will ever get is the first one he or she receives from the mother's breast. In that wonderful, rich, forerunner of milk called *colostrum* is the beneficial bacteria put there by our Creator to "seed" the newborn's large and small intestines. Babies pick up yeast from the normal colonies of yeast that live in the vagina as they make their entries into the world. Yeast also enters their bodies with the first breaths they take. Colostrum quickly balances the yeast with "friendly" bacteria and also contains antibodies that help establish immunity to disease.

Those first nurslings become part of a child's ecological system for life, and it is entirely possible to wipe it *all out with one round of antibiotics.* By age six months, ninety percent of American babies test positive for Candida.[1]

It is very hard to re-seed the human intestinal tract once the good bacteria have been destroyed. Human colostrum is sticky, and adheres to the walls of the baby's intestines, allowing the bacteria to stay in place. Cultures of *acidophilus, lactobacillus, bifidus, bulgaricus,* etc. are not sticky, and as such are hard to "plant." Also, cow's milk is not hospitable to *lactobacillus bacteria,* so all the cow's-milk based baby formulas actually encourage yeast to grow.

All babies who start life without the benefit of being breast-fed have two big strikes against them: Lowered immunity and unhealthy, imbalanced intestinal flora compromise their health from the beginning. Both invite an overgrowth of yeast with the ensuing predispositions to allergies, hay fever, asthma, and a lifetime of health problems. There are at least 400 nutrients found in breast milk that are not found in infant formulas. Breastfeeding offers lifelong health benefits to a baby. It cuts the risk of Sudden Infant Death Syndrome (SIDS) in *half* and provides protection against heart disease, bowel diseases, asthma, allergies, respiratory infections, diabetes, and eczema.

A study in the *Archives of Internal Medicine,* Aug. 10, 2009, reported that a long-term study on more than 60,000 mothers found that women with a close family history of breast cancer had significantly lower risks of developing breast cancer before menopause if they breastfed, compared with women who did not breastfeed. Breastfeeding is good for babies and mama too!

Failure to breastfeed is one of the most glaring reflections of our falling away from Natural Law. Please encourage all new mothers to give their newborns the best chance at life by starting them out healthy–on God's formula.

## 2. Eating the Standard American Diet, or SAD.

The Standard American Diet (SAD) consists mainly of foods from the yeast-free diet's "no-no" list of foods. All either feed yeast or cause allergic responses. *Have you seen the FDA's new food pyramid?* Still way too heavy on grains and milk products. But the yeast approve, though.

We are eating more carbohydrates than ever before in our history. Complex carbohydrates in the form of starches, such as potatoes, pastas, rice, beans, grains and whole grain breads, and highly refined carbohydrates, in the form of cakes, cookies, white flour, candies, chips, and junk food in general, have become major parts of our diets. The number one industry in the United States I believe is most responsible for the decline in the health of our nation is the *soft drink industry*. Loaded with sugar, high fructose corn syrup, artificial sweeteners, dyes, and chemicals of all kinds, soft drinks are the perfect "quick fix" for yeast.

### 3. Ingesting antibiotics, hormones, herbicides, pesticides, GMOs and additives from our food.

Our national food supply is fast becoming lethal. Most of our commercially raised meat and poultry is chock full of antibiotics, hormones, steroids, plus residues of herbicides and pesticides.

The discovery in 1949 that sub-therapeutic doses of antibiotics added to animal feed *caused the animals to gain weight at a rate of ten to twenty percent faster*, has led to a commercial bonanza for the pharmaceutical companies. The antibiotics market is the gift that keeps on giving to U.S. drug makers. In 1985 over eleven million pounds, or one-third of the approximately *thirty-five million pounds of antibiotics made in the United States, were sold to manufacturers of animal feed. Today, seventy percent of our antibiotics go into animal feed.*[2]

By promoting abnormal growth, farmers can use less feed to produce more meat. Juicier meat means juicier profits. The "economics of antibiotics" has proved irresistible to the beef, poultry, and pork industries. While they are reaping the profits, we are reaping disease. The terrible rise of obesity–especially in children–is directly linked to the combination of antibiotics and grains. They fatten up just like cattle when given lots of antibiotics plus lots of grains!

These hidden drugs slowly take their toll on our health. The constant, low-level bombardment of our bodies with steroids and antibiotics every day from our food is one of the major reasons yeast infection has gone from *an acute, self-limiting condition* (such as thrush), to becoming *a simmering, chronic condition* (such as asthma). Many diseases produce vague and seemingly unrelated symptoms, making it all too easy to remain unrecognized, undiagnosed, and unfortunately, untreated.

England outlawed antibiotics in the feed of livestock in 1971, as did many other European countries. In 1977, the FDA recommended a similar ban in the United States, but Congress refused, saying more proof was needed that tetracycline added to animal feed posed problems for the nation's health. And so it goes on to this very day.

There is much evidence accumulating now that documents the harmful effects of herbicides and pesticides. In babies and young children the damage is even more profound. Why? Because they ingest more of them. Non-nursing infants consume fifteen times more pears and apple juice per pound of body weight than an adult. That means they are exposed to any pesticide or herbicide that might have been sprayed on those foods at a rate fifteen times higher than the average adult. A young child's "detoxification" systems are immature, and therefore unable to break down and excrete toxins from their bodies very efficiently. Unfortunately, those toxins remain in their tissues, carrying the potential for disease with them.

Bovine Growth Hormone, used to stimulate the production of more milk, also stimulates Candida to grow. Thankfully the dairy industry is bowing to pressure from the public and some hormones are being discontinued.

**4. Immunizations.**

This is an extremely controversial area, but the evidence that immunizations have dealt our immune systems a serious blow is very compelling. (See chapter 19 on vaccines.) Many books have been and are being written about the subject. I hope you will take time to find and read them. Immunizations, or vaccinations (which are actual "pieces" of disease put inside the body), work by stimulating the immune system to make antibodies to diseases, so that if the person is ever exposed to a disease, the body will be prepared to fight it quickly. Thus immunity is supposedly established. Both live and dead viruses are used.

However, we are now beginning to see that there is a downside to immunizations, especially the live vaccines. There is growing evidence that live viruses continue to live in the body–hidden–in a *smoldering* state, waiting to be activated at a later time when the immune system is low. The smallpox vaccine is suspected of nesting in the pancreas, and may be responsible for diabetes in later years.

Latent chronic diseases are going to be a big issue in coming years. Doctors are seeing more and more adverse reactions and *deaths* associated with immunizations. (Remember the swine flu debacle in 1976 when 25 people died from the vaccine and the program was halted?) There has to be a better way.

In Europe progressive medical doctors have started giving a biological antidote, called a homeopathic nosode, to stimulate the body to get rid of the toxic virus being injected into it. Then only the antibodies remain to keep their vigils. I hope more mothers will find homeopathics for their children who have received immunizations in order to detoxify their little bodies.

In the USA, the American Medical Association and assorted government agencies such as the Food and Drug Administration, have done everything in their power to suppress the informed consent movement against vaccines. (Much of this movement is being led by doctors themselves.) They have banned books and even had them forcibly removed from the shelves of health food stores. But, the story is still being written, and the truth will eventually be revealed.

We know that immunizations strengthen one small area of the immune system, *but weaken it overall.* Yeast gets going when the immune system is down or suppressed. Doesn't it make more sense simply to do everything possible to *strengthen* an immune system and create a healthy body so that it can battle microorganisms the way it was designed to?

## 5. Silver/mercury amalgam fillings.

Mercury is a heavy metal, known to be extremely toxic. In the 1950s, 121 people died in Japan from eating fish that had been contaminated with methyl mercury. Iraq has recorded three major incidents of mercury poisoning from seed grains that had been treated with a mercury-based fungicide. In 1969 a family of nine in the United States nearly died from eating their newly-butchered hogs that had eaten mercury-treated seed grain.

Symptoms of mercury toxicity are numbness and tingling of extremities, hand tremors, unsteady gait, and derangement of the spinal cord and brain–same as the symptoms of multiple sclerosis and Parkinson's disease. The amalgam that fills the holes in our teeth is *fifty percent mercury!*

In 1833, when mercury was introduced by dental salesmen as a cheaper alternative to gold, dentist were outraged, called the compound dangerous, and warned it would lead to gum disease and other dental problems. The American Society of Dental Surgeons denounced the use of silver/mercury fillings and pledged not to use them. But soon, cheaper won out over better. Silver/mercury amalgams slowly became acceptable, and the old fears were soon forgotten.

There is mounting and impressive evidence that the dentists of 1833 were right. Scientific evidence is becoming irrefutable that mercury in dental fillings leaks out of the fillings into the teeth and gums, and into the mouth in the form of vapors, where it is swallowed, inhaled, and absorbed into the bloodstream. Once in the bloodstream, it goes everywhere in the body, and is especially damaging to the brain, kidneys, and all endocrine glands. All of this damage compromises our immune systems and makes yeast flourish.

Many animal studies confirm that mercury damages blood cells that normally would have provided immunity, and recent human studies have shown the same effect. One test, run by a dentist named David W. Eggleston in *The Journal of Prosthetic Dentistry*, showed a fascinating correlation between T-lymphocyte cells before and after using mercury amalgam fillings.

T-lymphocytes, or T-cells, are one of the best indicators of how our immune systems are functioning. They are made in the bone marrow and mature in the thymus to become a crucial part of our body's defense forces. Their function is to destroy bad bacteria and kill foreign antigens in the blood. If their numbers are within normal blood test parameters, we know our immunity is high. If their numbers are low, the immune system is stressed.

After Dr. Eggleston removed the silver/mercury fillings from his patients, their T-cell counts went up a whopping 55.5 percent. When he reinserted them, the T-cell count immediately dropped to their former levels. Mercury, which stressed the spleen, damaged lymphocytes, crippled the immune system, and stimulated more yeast–where will it end?—was the obvious culprit.

Every day dentists are removing silver/mercury amalgam fillings and replacing them with composites. Many people are finding new levels of health as a result–especially those suffering from autoimmune diseases.

**6. Toxin accumulation in tissue.**

When the liver is sluggish and kidneys are malfunctioning, the body can't detoxify according to its natural pathways. Toxins from industrial chemicals, pesticides, auto exhaust, cigarettes, drugs, heavy metals, and aluminum from pans and antiperspirants, etc., as well as air pollution, are stored in body tissue since the kidneys and liver are too weak to eliminate them. *Candida always goes to the toxic or damaged tissue first*. So toxic areas invite the colonizing of yeast.

## 7. Fluoride in our drinking water and dental care.

 Sodium fluoride is a protoplasmic poison.  It is as lethal and as potent as cyanide and arsenic, and is a toxic by-product of the manufacture of the *aluminum and fertilizer industries.*  Scientifically it has been established that instead of helping the teeth, fluoride starts an insidious process of degeneration in the entire body because it tends to cripple enzyme activity, thus interfering with calcium metabolism.  Fluoride poisoning is the result, making teeth weak and prone to early deterioration and fluorosis.

Court documents attest to fluoride causing at least 10,000 deaths annually[3], and damage to the brain, kidneys, thyroid, eyes, hearing, and other medical problems is incalculable.  There are very strong links to birth defects and mental problems from ingesting it.

Fluoride also interferes with the utilization of B vitamins, disturbs the chromosome repair enzyme, interrupts the amino acid chain in collagen, (contributing to aging), and turns thought processes into *slow motion.*

*Fluoride is tasteless and so toxic that if a small child ate a tube of fluoridated tooth paste it could kill him.*  Even the CDC has warned mothers not to give babies under twelve months fluoridated water, and Gerber has removed it from its baby food products.

In small doses, we know fluoride stops the function of enzymes and damages all cells in the body, including our helper white cells.  There goes another blow to our immune system!  And guess who is coming to dinner!

So much damning evidence has come to light in recent years that the American Academy of Pediatrics and the American Dental Association now recommends that infants avoid fluoridated water altogether, and children under 5 years brush with water only.[4]

For these and many other reasons, fluoride has been banned in most of Europe, with 98 percent of Europe being fluoride-free.  And rightly so.

I hope it is becoming clearer that all these healthcare errors make it easier for yeast and fungi to gain a foothold in our bodies.

## Chapter 3

# Back In Time

*"So here is a disease from an organism doctors admit exists chronically in the body, whose presence shows up on laboratory antibody tests, which arguably causes immense physical and psychological problems, the elimination of which can bring dramatic reversals of sickness. Yet, most traditional doctors don't 'believe' in it."*

... Dr. Stuart M. Berger, M.D.

Candida has been called a twentieth century disease, owing to its explosion in the past fifty years. But, in truth, this eminently powerful little microbe has been around since the dawn of time.

Conditions have to be exactly right in order for yeasts to grow–the right temperature, humidity, food supply–all must provide *the proper mix*. In fact, because man lived for thousands of years on a natural diet and lived in harmony with nature, yeast colonies were contained and remained low in the intestines, barely surviving from one generation to the next.

But in the last hundred years, yeast has finally come into its own and hit its stride. With the advent of the so-called "wonder drugs" such as antibiotics, steroids, hormones, and birth control pills, combined with our standard American diet with its heavy emphasis on sugar and carbohydrates, yeast has, indeed, found the proper mix it needs to increase and multiply.

As a matter of fact, if only one yeast cell were given the perfect environment of food and temperature, within twenty-four hours a colony of one hundred cells would be produced. At this rate of reproduction, within eight days one cell would proliferate into a colony weighing one billion tons! The reason this does not happen is that rarely is the environment for its growth that ideal. It is actually *difficult* to grow them. However, this should alert us to its potential.

Just a few years ago, many doctors were calling yeast syndromes "fad" diseases, or "phantom" diseases, or even "yuppie" diseases. They tended to pooh-pooh the anecdotal and even scientific evidence they encountered. Many patients were told their symptoms were "all in their head" and were sent to psychiatrists.

The tide is turning today, and now yeast is the subject of medical seminars, research grants, television ads, books, and articles, and is being called by many the *most important medical issue of our time.*

We know for certain it is neither a fad nor a phantom, but rather a living organism that we had better pay attention to now–or pay the consequences later.

Going back in time, we know from the earliest fossil remains that fungi have been here for millions of years. Paleontologists have some evidence of their existence in the pre-Cambrian period, (1500 million years ago), and also have undisputed evidence that dates from the Devonian period making fungi at least 405 million years old.

Through the ages, this class of micro-organism has been a major player in the ecological balance of the planet, but scientists have had difficulty in classifying it. As we read in a previous chapter, it has features of both plant and animal, and being neither a true vegetable nor a true animal, scientists have relegated it to what is called "The Third Kingdom."

Molds, mildews, yeasts, puffballs and mushrooms are members of this kingdom. So far, over 100,000 different species have been identified, and thousands more are being added to the list every year. They come in different sizes and shapes. Some live in water, others prefer soil. Some thrive in both cool and tropical climates, others like moist shady soil, manure, rotting leaves, dead carcasses, decaying food–*anything that has damaged tissue.*

Yeasts have a mission, which they perform with single-minded zeal. *They are the garbage disposals of the planet.* When airborne yeasts are attracted to and fall upon injured or rotting tissues, they feed on them until they are gone. Their job is to break down tissue further and further in order to digest and eliminate it. This is the process by which the planet keeps a tidy house. Like the Energizer Bunny, they just keep going and going, recycling planetary garbage back into the earth.

Think what it would be like on earth without fungi. How would you like to be sloshing through mountains of plant and animal remains left over from the age of dinosaurs? We should be thankful they are with us.

When man first appeared on the scene, it didn't take him long to learn how to use members of the Third Kingdom to his advantage. Three thousand years before Christ, man was making beer and wine through the process of fermentation.

People observed that when grains were crushed, moistened, and placed in a warm place (the proper mix), yeast landed on them and began decomposing the sugars, causing fermentation. This eventually resulted in the making of beer, wine, bread, vinegar, pickles, cheeses, sauerkraut, etc.

Egyptians were making beer by 2500 B.C. and the Chinese by 2300 B.C., and incredibly an Assyrian tablet dated 2000 B.C. has been found that asserts that Noah attributed his ability to survive the trip on the ark–with all those animals–to his private "stash of mash" on board!

The Chinese knew of and were using antibiotics 2500 years ago. They discovered that when the curd of soybean turned moldy it had a curative effect, and they used it to treat skin infections such as boils and carbuncles.

The history of medicine is full of references to yeast overgrowths in patients. Hippocrates, the father of medicine, knew of and treated yeast back in the golden age of Greece–around 400 B.C., more than 1.500 years before the invention of the microscope. "Thrush" and "vaginitis" have been part of the human condition and well known to the medical profession for thousands of years, but they were rarely reported because they were rarely seen. The *first infectious disease ever diagnosed was a fungal disease called muscardine*, found in silkworms in 1834 in France.[1]

Vaginal yeast infections were first reported in 1849; systemic candidiasis was first described in a debilitated patient in 1861; Candida infections of the nails were first reported in 1907; and Candida cystitis, in 1909. By the 1940s it became evident that candidiasis was the most variable of the fungal infections, commonly appearing on skin, in mucosa, and in the vagina. Even then it was *rarely* reported and *even more rarely* developed into serious, fulminating, systemic disease.

Besides working for the food and beverage industries, pharmaceutical companies have put yeast to work by developing mold-produced chemicals, antibiotics, and chemotherapies following Sir Alexander Fleming's discovery of a blue-green mold growing on top of a colony of *staphylococcal* bacteria in his lab. After investigating further, he observed that the *staph bacteria were being destroyed by mold.* Eventually that simple observation led to the development of penicillin, a drug that has been credited with saving countless lives in life-threatening situations.

Today there are many other positive uses of yeast, fungi, and bacteria. Sewage treatment plants use them to digest and decompose excrement, thereby actively helping to prevent the spread of disease. Citric acid, fermented from sugar, is used in food and blueprinting. Oxalic acid, fermented from yeast, is used by the leather and textile industries to make dyes and condition raw materials. Enzymes from yeast microbes are used to remove stains from clothing. Fungi are even used in the making of stone-washed jeans.

These are a few of the many beneficial uses of The Third Kingdom. But, like most things in life, they have a down side. Any farmer will tell you of the constant battle he has with fungi and mold as they attempt to recycle his crops back into the soil prematurely, causing millions of dollars in crop losses each year. (It has been estimated that 10 percent of crops worldwide succumb to the microscopic monsters.) In the Bible are many accounts of plagues and diseases such as cereal rusts (fungi), which were attributed to sins and offenses against God. Dutch elm disease, chestnut tree blight, and apple scab are only three of many diseases that destroy our trees, all caused by a sac fungus.

Fungi, if eaten, are capable of causing bizarre symptoms. Ergot is a fungal disease that attacks cereal grains, especially rye, and when ingested results in ergotism, characterized by hallucinations. *Ergot is also the source of LSD!*

In recent years there has been a re-examination of the infamous Salem witch trials of 1692. The eating of ergot-infested grains may be what was behind the convulsions and hallucinations of the "bewitched" or "possessed" members of that colony. According to records of the rain and weather patterns for that year, conditions were ripe (the proper mix) for the growth of ergot–a mold. Mold spores in the brain are known to cause hallucinations and bizarre behavior.

The Irish potato famine of 1845-47 has been attributed to the growth of another fungus, *Phytophthora infestans*. Again, favorable warm, moist weather conditions prevailed, and Ireland's potato crop was decimated. As a result, an estimated one million people died, and hundreds of thousands of Irish people immigrated to America. *So yeast even has the power to change the course of history.*

The story of the "curse" of King Tut's tomb is a fascinating mystery that was only recently solved. The fabulous tomb of Tutankhamen was discovered near the ruins of Luxor in Egypt in 1922. Two years later, Hugh Evelyn-White, a British Egyptologist, was among the first to enter. He and eleven other explorers died shortly thereafter, Evelyn-White by hanging himself, immediately after writing in his own blood, "I have succumbed to a curse."

In their zeal to get to the treasures, the excavators didn't notice the pink, grey, and green patches of fungi growing on the walls of the chamber. The fruits and vegetables, which had been placed in the tomb to nourish the pharaoh as he journeyed through eternity, decayed and were decomposed by fungi. Eventually the spores spread to the walls and waited there for centuries for the first unwary intruders.

The first twelve men to enter the tomb of King Tutankhamen apparently died of *severe allergic reactions to mold.*

To bring the subject up to modern times, the Congressional Report of December 2, 2008 contains an article claiming that terrorists were formulating a plan to fly planes over the United States, releasing deadly mold spores which, when inhaled, would contaminate the bloodstream and kill millions of Americans. If this doesn't convince you of the power of this microbe, nothing will.

As you can see, yeasts have played a significant role, both beneficial and harmful, to both planet earth and its occupants. If they weren't held in check, they could consume all life as we know it.

So, why are we not overrun with the little critters?

The answer is that for eons the earth and our bodies have managed to maintain conditions that keep them in check. But today, inside our bodies, the age-old fortifications for keeping them in check have been torn down, and yeast has been unleashed. Because we have finally created and sustained the proper mix *inside us,* many of us are now overrun with the yeast/beast.

*And that is why we are sick.*

**Chapter 4**

---

# The War Within

*"Nature, in order to be commanded, must be obeyed."*

...Sir Francis Bacon

As we have learned, under normal circumstance yeast lives in small quantities both on and in our bodies. (Over three hundred different types of yeasts and fungi have been identified that live on human skin alone.) Inside the body it thrives mainly in our gastrointestinal tract, the surface area of which equals that of a tennis court. It loves the warm, moist, recesses of the mouth, esophagus, linings of the stomach and intestines, vagina and rectum where it lives harmoniously with several pounds of local bacteria and other organisms in a peaceful kind of co-existence.

On closer inspection, we see that sometimes things aren't as peaceful as they seem, and it becomes evident that what we have, instead of a peaceful co-existence, is more of a truce or cease-fire. (The war metaphor works well here to help you grasp what is really going on inside the body when yeast begins its assault.)

A bargain seems to have been struck between the body and yeasts. Yeasts have been permitted to live on surface linings in balance with bacteria, but are forbidden from going into deeper tissue. If they do attempt to breach that truce and colonize in undesignated areas, the immune system will marshal its white blood cells to seek out and destroy them. For ages this seems to have worked well.

Of course, for any immune system to carry out that mission, it must be strong. If the front line of defense is crippled, small bands of yeasts begin to sneak through holes in its fortifications, regroup, and proliferate wildly.

White cells, *the SWAT teams of our immune systems*, are eventually
overwhelmed by yeast and put out of commission.  As a result, the original
bargain is scrapped and the prisoners are now in charge of the prison.  Fungi,
yeasts, bacteria, and other organisms are all rioting for control of newly
taken territory and the establishment of a new pecking order.

Wherever fungi and bacteria live, there is fierce competition for food,
shelter, and space.  It's a jungle in there.  Yeasts even attack and produce
chemicals to suppress the growth of *other* yeasts in an effort to maintain a
balance among species.  Nevertheless, all are vying for their own territories
in a limited space, and things can get pretty testy during the process.  But as
long as the host (you) remains healthy, the normal ecological ratio of
millions of parts bacteria to one part yeast is preserved, and the interaction
between host and parasite continues unnoticed, indicating our bodies learned
long ago to cope with our mysterious boarders.  The body has accepted and
adjusted to them, and a miraculous homeostasis prevails.

Homeostasis is the physiological ability of higher animals to
maintain stability in their organic functions even when threatened with
disruption.  This exquisite function, homeostasis, or ability to remain
balanced and whole, is what all our bodies are constantly striving to achieve.
It is a form of peace.

When homeostasis is compromised by drugs, poor diet, injury or
accident, or any kind of physical or emotional stress, the immune system
falters, and yeast, the ultimate opportunist, over-colonizes and goes on the
attack.  The normal balance of millions of bacteria to one yeast becomes
*reversed*–to an abnormal ratio of *millions of yeast to one bacteria.*

The immune system, already losing steam, valiantly tries to fight
yeast and the poisons they give off, but eventually crumbles under the
overwhelming numbers of proliferating armies of yeast. The medical
profession refers to this as a "depressed immune response."

A vicious cycle is created.  The body begins to pick up viruses and
produce allergies, infections, and illness.  Then to add insult to injury, we

add antibiotics, steroids, and chemical drugs of all types to the mix, which produce even more yeast overgrowths–and as we know now–*more illness.*

Predictably, the immune system continues its downward spiral.

The only way to interrupt this slide into a desperate disease state is to stop the yeast from growing and spreading.  And it can be stopped–*dead in its tracks.*

Any general will tell you that "an army moves on its stomach," and if not well fed, soldiers can neither march nor fight.  The same holds true for an army of yeasts.  *If you don't feed them they curl up and die.*

As they die, and as their numbers are decimated, they keep falling back to former lines of defense.  With each retreat, the immune system builds up its armaments, flexes its muscles, and regains strength.  Slowly but surely, as more and more battles are won, the once-defeated immune system rebuilds itself, and at last claims victory.  The expanded armies of yeasts are vanquished, and a small number of survivors are placed into camps surrounded by armed guards.  The battlefield is cleaned up and the immune system is back in command. Peace once again prevails.

In order to win against overwhelming odds, the victorious general had to take the initiative.  He had to be bold, innovative, and disciplined.  In your case, the general is your mind and will, and the tactics and battle plans that appear in this book will help you chart your strategies for victory.

You will have to be bold, innovative and disciplined, as the war plans are drawn and the battle unfolds.  You will have to take the initiative and strike decisively, again and again.  But it will be worth the effort, because you will recapture, regain, and reclaim that which the yeast/beast has tried to steal from you *as spoils of war:* your immune system, your health, and even your life.

## Chapter 5

---

# The Immune System

*"Today scientists are taking a closer or broader look at the immune system.*
*They are seeing that all parts of the human body participate in its defense."*
                                                            ... Shirley S. Lorenzani, Ph.D.

Our immune system is what keeps us healthy. It is made up of an intricate
and vital network of cells and organs that protect the body from infection and
disease. Except for the nervous system, it is the most complex of our
biological systems. Organs that make up the immune system are called
lymphoid organs, such as adenoids, bone marrow, lymph nodes and
lymphatic vessels, spleen, thymus, and tonsils. This sensitive system is
enhanced by good nutrition, sleep and rest, but impaired by junk food, drugs,
and stress.

All cells, including immune cells, are produced in the bone marrow.
Some cells become lymphocytes, a type of infection-fighting white blood
cell, while others become part of another type of immune cell called
phagocytes, or engulfing cells. Each fights infection differently, but their
mission remains the same–to protect the body from disease *as quickly as*
*possible.*

Lymphocytes, which remain in the bone marrow, become "B" cells
(for bone). They produce antibodies to specific infectious microorganisms
or foreign antigens in order to "ambush" them. Other lymphocytes find their
way to the thymus gland to finish their maturation and become "T" cells (for
thymus). T-cells kill infectious microorganisms by destroying body cells that
are affected. Phagocytes, on the other hand, kill infectious microorganisms
by "devouring" them.

Once mature, some T-cell lymphocytes leave the thymus to reside in the lymphoid organs and wait until called upon. Others travel the lymphatic system and bloodstream, constantly "patrolling" the body for infectious organisms such as viruses, bacteria, parasites and fungi, toxic chemicals, or cancer cells.

The largest immune organ in the body is the gastrointestinal system. It represents almost *eighty percent of our entire immune system.* That is why it is critical for the terrain and flora of the intestines to be balanced with the correct amounts of microorganisms to perform properly. When yeast and bacteria live symbiotically, all is well. If these microorganisms become imbalanced, a state of *"dysbiosis"* exists, meaning digestion is out of sync and something needs to be done to restore it to good health. If probiotics and anti-fungal remedies are not taken to restore balance, yeast multiply rapidly.

We have learned how yeasts in moderate numbers can live harmoniously with their neighbors, not calling attention to themselves as long as normal checks and balances are in place. Not too much harm or damage is done to the host.

However, this amazing little organism actually has the ability to change its own DNA and identity. In medical jargon, it is called *"dimorphic,"* meaning shape-changing. In the twinkling of an eye, it can change both its physiology and anatomy and become a fungus, (*mycosis* or *mycoses*). From then on it can continue to *keep changing* in order to hide or elude our immune system's attempts to kill it. In the end, it can even revert to being a yeast!

As a yeast, it *lives on top of tissue*, consuming and recycling only *dead* tissue. It cannot invade deeper tissues, so contents itself by manifesting as occasional pesky local conditions, such as vaginitis, thrush, nail fungus, "jock itch," dandruff, and ring worm. As long as the immune system remains strong, yeast is unable to penetrate deeper tissue or get into the bloodstream where it can wreak havoc.

Once it mutates into a fungus it is called a mycosis (mycoses are any diseases caused by a fungus). Candida then becomes candidiasis. This is truly a disease because *its fungal stage is an infection.* Infection is disease. The infectious yeast/beast starts consuming and recycling LIVE tissue.

### *That means you!*

In this stage it becomes voraciously hungry and begins to break out of its normal confines in search of food. It grows roots (*rhizoids)*, or tentacles, which enable it to break the barrier that was once impenetrable by yeast. These tentacles begin to break down and penetrate cell walls. When the cell walls are weakened and damaged, fungi easily enter the cells themselves. Some cells are consumed for food, and others either die or survive crippled.

The pact between yeast and the body now has been broken. The yeast/fungus has learned how to attack and enter the body proper. You could say it has developed an "attitude." It sinks its evil tentacles deep into tissue, and when it hits the bloodstream, it goes berserk. It seems that once it has a taste of blood, it wants more and more, like a vampire, and goes on a wild feeding frenzy.

The bloodstream is the 'highway' to every cell in the body. Its 60,000 miles of blood vessels feed our 1,000 trillion cells. Penetration into this once sacrosanct and off-limits area by the fungal, or *mycelial* stage of yeast, is the turning point for the immune system. All organs and glands, all tissue are fair game, and all bets are off.

Now yeast/fungus has access to the entire human organism, and like a kid in a candy store, it wants everything it sees.

The intestinal lining, or lumen, acts as a filtering system, which keeps food particles from improperly digested food, plus chemicals and toxins from entering the bloodstream. It is the bloodstream's first line of defense. With the fungi's new root-like structures, the once peaceful parasite can poke holes through all the mucosal linings of the body, especially the digestive tract, on its way to blood.  The linings become damaged in the process, as the little rhizoids puncture these linings with tiny holes. The walls of fortification are breached by the invading yeast, and the war widens.

Once the fortification has been breached by invading yeast and the lining is punctured and weakened by its fungal tentacles, yeast spores and their poisons slip through the holes into the bloodstream and start spreading to cells and organs.  Immediately they start to disarm and depress the immune system. Some even reach the brain.

The tentacles, or rhizoids, act like pipes as they leak yeast toxins or poisons, called mycotoxins, directly into the bloodstream, where nature never intended them to go. To date over eighty different mycotoxins have been identified. From the bloodstream they circulate wildly throughout the entire body, infecting tissue wherever they go.

And so a new twentieth century disease has been born, called *"leaky gut syndrome."*  (*Note*: Psyllium hulls do a wonderful job in healing the holes.)

The first organ to be invaded usually is the liver–our primary organ of detoxification.  From there yeast cells spread easily throughout the body to heart, lungs, and other organs and glands.

The immune system is stimulated and reacts swiftly.  It sends out an alarm that 'foreign agents' have been spotted, and immediately begins manufacturing antibodies to intercept the upstart antigens and defend its territory.

Anyone who suffers from allergies and allergic reactions knows what happens next in the battle.  Hay fever, eczema, dizziness, fatigue, anxiety, muscle aches are only a few of the miseries commonly experienced.

In the beginning you may react only to the yeast *inside the body*, but as the immune system deteriorates you may begin to react to *outside* yeasts, such as those found in antibiotics, bread, beer or wine, or to fungus foods, such as Stilton, Roquefort, blue cheeses, or mushrooms. Molds and mildews in the bathroom, old buildings, or damp basements are notorious for stimulating allergic responses.

As the infection becomes more widely disseminated, you may experience reactions to a wider variety of food. Now allergies to the environment, such as chemical and gasoline fumes, perfume, out gassing from carpeting, etc., begin to raise their ugly heads. A new illness called MCS (Multiple Chemical Sensitivity) has been added to the lexicon of modern disease.

You feel bad all over.

The battered immune system has to work harder and harder to deal with the ever increasing populations of yeast and their toxic by-products. It literally becomes crippled and is prevented from doing its job. After a while of being stimulated too many times by too large an enemy, the system tires and refuses to recognize any antigens at all. It simply tolerates and accepts them, no longer able to attack and neutralize them.

With the immune system down, the body is vulnerable to any and all disease.

This is exactly what happens with homosexually spread AIDS, or Acquired Immune Deficiency Disease. Sperm is seen as a foreign object, or antigen, by the body, so it automatically manufactures antibodies to combat the sperm. In cases of promiscuously spread AIDS, either heterosexual or homosexual, because of multiple partners, the immune system is constantly stimulated to make antibodies to combat multiple sperm. This over-stimulation tires the immune system, thereby making the host vulnerable to overgrowths of fungi and opportunistic viruses. The immune system simply cannot keep up with the demand. *It becomes deficient.*

AIDS means *Acquired Immune System Deficiency* Syndrome.

The weakened immune system slowly grinds to a halt.  It has fought the good fight.  In defeat, it waves a white flag.  In victory, the invading troops of yeasts, fungi and their toxins joyously break ranks and overrun their newly won territory.

*Tomorrow the world!*

**Chapter 6**

---

# Symptoms of Yeast Overgrowth

*"The war being waged inside your body due to yeast overgrowth boasts its own casualties. You develop a variety of troublesome symptoms that can crop up just about anywhere in your body. That's one of the worst parts of candidiasis. Symptoms can be so varied and scattered that they don't even seem related to the same condition. The result? It's easy to miss candidiasis."*

...Dennis Remington, M.D.

Before we go any further, let's look at some of the most common symptoms of yeast to see if you are a "Candida candidate." After you finish reading the lists you will wonder if there is any disease or condition that *isn't* related to candidiasis! That is what makes it so hard to diagnose. Symptoms are so varied, and many even conflict. (For example, both dry eye syndrome *and* wet eye syndrome can be caused by yeast.)

To add to the normal amounts of yeast found in a healthy body, yeast gains entry into the body through four other avenues.

1. The first is through respiration. We inhale invisible clouds of mold spores in every breath we breathe, even in the Arctic. Concentrations of spores are found in musty old houses and buildings, moldy basements, behind wallpaper and in swampy areas, etc. (Mold only needs seventeen percent humidity to grow. It even grows in sand!)

2. The second way we add to normal yeast loads is through ingestion. We take them in through antibiotics and vaccines,

eating moldy leftovers, blue and Roquefort cheeses, balsamic
vinegars, etc., drinking alcohol (brewer's yeast), eating bread
(baker's yeast) and grains (mold contamination).

3.      The third way fungi can gain entry into the body is through
broken skin or a wound, i.e., a gardener can pick them up while
digging in the garden. The deeper you dig into the soil, the
heavier the concentrations of fungi there are. (Fungi in the soil
stunt, retard and even kill plant life. Any seed hardy enough to
outsmart fungal attacks underground and survive is a potent
antifungal agent. Eat your veggies.)

4.      Couples can transfer yeast organisms back and forth to each
other through intercourse. That's why *both* need to go on the
diet.

Because each human body is unique, yeast will proliferate in various
sites in different bodies. Once in the bloodstream it will tend to gravitate to
individual "shock organs," or those areas of the body that are weaker.

Everyone has these vulnerable areas. In one body the favored site
might be the warm, moist lining of the lungs and bronchial tubes, and the
"host" will exhibit symptoms of asthma, bronchitis, or persistent cough. In
another body, yeast finds a happy home burrowing deep into the lining of
the colon, and the hapless patient will find himself battling recurrent bouts
of colitis, chronic diarrhea or bloating and gas. In some bodies there is a
light overgrowth scattered everywhere in the body, and in others it localizes
into small condensed areas. But wherever it goes, and wherever it grows,
there's trouble. The unwelcome, invasive army continues on its march,
looting, pillaging, killing anything in its path, and taking no prisoners.

In researching this book, I found that most of the books on yeast
infections contain questionnaires or quizzes for readers to take, so they can
rate themselves as to the likelihood of systemic yeast. You can find them
and fill in the questionnaires if you like, but for our purposes here, I feel that
when you finish reading the lists of symptoms, you will know intuitively if
yeast is your problem.

If you see yourself many times in many lists, the answer will be clear–you are growing a bumper crop of yeast. If you see yourself sometimes on some of the lists, chances are you have a moderate overgrowth. If you don't find yourself on *any* list, you are probably from another planet.

In any case, keep in mind yeast grows in cycles which wax and wane. On days when they really get going (after being stimulated by rain, caffeine, or antibiotics, etc.) you may exhibit many symptoms. On other days, when your stress level may be low, and you are more rested, and your diet has contained less of the foods that feed yeast, you may exhibit fewer or no symptoms. That is the elusive nature of this organism.

Another feature you need to be aware of is that yeasts produce poisons called *mycotoxins* (literally fungal poisons). They are the toxic byproducts that fungi excrete. (In other words, *"yeast poop."*) Yeasts produce 80 toxins in their poop, including formaldehyde. Tissues impregnated with mycotoxins become irritated and swell in an attempt to dilute the poisons, leading to inflammation and many of the symptoms and diseases listed below. Fungal poisons are powerful *immune suppressants* and are capable of producing illness and death in animals and humans. (Antibiotics and alcohol are examples of mycotoxins.)

If you still feel the need for medical confirmation of yeast infection, by all means go to your doctor. There are several tests which can be run, using blood and urine, or stool cultures, or smears to confirm the existence of yeast. But since a small amount of yeast is normal to the body, everyone will test positive. On top of that, there is an extremely high incidence of false positives and false negatives in the testing, which makes them unreliable and limited, as well as time consuming and expensive.

But their biggest drawback is that lab tests done on blood don't give any idea of yeast's presence in the gastrointestinal tract–one of its favorite places to grow.

*Candida* often runs rampant in the esophagus, stomach, and intestines, areas from which it is very difficult to obtain samples for cultures. Mouth or vaginal swabs may prove negative and, at the same time and in the same patient, invasive candidiasis can still be raging. Even autopsies performed on cancer patients after their deaths have revealed candidiasis throughout the body, *even though blood cultures taken while they were living were NEGATIVE for yeast.* So, in the end, a doctor probably will learn all he or she needs to know about your yeast condition just by taking a thorough history and carefully going over all your symptoms.

Also, if you choose to have a doctor monitor your progress while on this program, it only makes sense that you choose one who is holistically oriented, or at the very least, open-minded and interested in what you are doing. Nothing will sabotage your efforts faster than a physician who is adversarial or impatient with your efforts at self-help.

Please bear in mind that all the symptoms listed here can be caused by conditions other than yeast, such as nutritional deficiencies, parasites, and side-effects of drugs. The only way to know for certain what is behind your physical problems is to give the diet a "therapeutic trial." Remember, Candida prefers people! You will know shortly if you are on the right track.

### *Common Symptoms of Candida Albicans Overgrowth*

**In the digestive tract or gastrointestinal system:**

>       abdominal pain
>       acid indigestion, gastroesophageal reflux disease (GERD),
>           gastritis
>       belching
>       colic
>       constipation, diarrhea, spastic colon
>       gas and bloating
>       gastric ulcers
>       heartburn

mucus in stools
nausea
rectal itching, hemorrhoids

**In the respiratory system:**

allergies
asthma
bad breath
bronchial infections
canker sores
chronic stuffy nose and post nasal drip
dry mouth and throat
nasal itch
pain or tightness in chest
pneumonia, persistent cough
sinus infections and sinusitis
sinus pressure
sore throat and mouth
thrush
wheezing or shortness of breath

**In the cardiovascular system:**

anemia
atherosclerosis and arteriosclerosis
cold and clammy hands and feet
congestive heart failure
endocarditis
fluid retention
heart attack
high blood pressure
mitral valve prolapse
palpitations
phlebitis
poor circulation

rapid pulse and pounding heart

**In the reproductive and urinary system:**

birth defects
cystitis
endometriosis
erratic menstrual periods
failure to menstruate
fibrocystic breast disease
fibroid tumors
flare-up of yeast infections after intercourse
frequent urination and burning
hormone imbalances
infertility
itchy rashes on genitals
"jock itch"
lack of bladder control and bedwetting
loss of sex drive
menstrual cramps
miscarriages
"PMS" and hot flashes
prostate problems
recurring bladder and kidney infections
scant or extremely heavy menstrual flow
too frequent menstrual periods
urethritis
urgency to urinate
vaginal burning or itching
vaginal discharge
vaginal yeast infection
water retention

**In the musculoskeletal system:**

arthritis and rheumatoid arthritis

easy bruising
fibromyalgia
hiatal hernia
joint aches or pain
leg cramps or night muscle pain
muscle soreness, pain, or swelling
muscle weakness, stiffness, pain, or cramps
numbness and tingling
osteoporosis and osteopenia
pain in neck and shoulder area
paralysis
restless leg syndrome
tension headaches

**In the skin:**

acne
athlete's foot and "jock itch"
body odor
chronic urticaria
dandruff
diaper rash
dry skin
hair loss or excessive hair growth
hives and eczema
nail fungus
psoriasis and eczema
ringworm
seborrhea dermatitis
skin rashes and infections

**In the central nervous system:**

> agitation
> anxiety and panic attacks
> being overly defensive
> brain fog
> confusion or fuzzy thinking
> dementia
> depression
> dizziness or vertigo
> drowsiness
> drunk feeling
> dying sensations
> fatigue
> feelings of being "drained"
> feelings of low self-esteem
> feelings of unreality or "spaciness"
> hallucinations or hearing voices
> headaches–all kinds–tension, migraine, and cluster
> hyperactivity and learning disorders
> irrational fears and phobias
> irritability, restlessness
> jittery behavior
> lethargy
> light-headedness
> memory loss and lack of concentration
> moodiness and mood swings
> numbness and tingling
> outbursts of anger
> poor coordination
> procrastination
> sadness
> short attention span or attention deficit disorder
> sleep disturbances
> suicidal thoughts

**In the eyes, ears, and mouth:**

>blurred vision
>burning or tearing
>chronic inflammation of eyes or eyelids
>coated tongue
>crusty eyelids
>deafness
>dermatitis
>ear pain
>failing vision
>fever blisters or canker sores
>fluid in ears
>itchy ears
>night blindness
>pyorrhea
>recurring ear infections
>sore or bleeding gums
>spots before eyes or floaters
>tinnitus
>tonsillitis
>trouble focusing
>white patches in mouth

**Generalized symptoms or conditions:**

>aching all over
>alcoholism
>cold hands and feet
>constant hunger
>drug addiction
>excessive underarm perspiration
>flu-like symptoms
>food allergies
>food cravings

frequent colds or other recurring infections
hay fever
high cholesterol and high blood pressure
impaired sense of taste or smell
increased sensitivity to chemicals, odors, perfumes, and
   smoke
insomnia
junk food cravings
low blood sugar
lowered immunity
sugar and carbohydrate cravings
weight gain or loss


## *DISEASES CONNECTED TO CANDIDA ALBICANS*

Addison's disease
AIDS
alcoholism
allergies
Alzheimer's
anorexia, bulimia, or any eating disorder
arthritis
asthma
autism
Bell's palsy
blood poisoning or septicemia
cancer
chronic fatigue syndrome (CFS)
chronic mononucleosis
cirrhosis of the liver
Crohn's disease
diabetes, juvenile, adult onset, and gestational
drug addiction
edema
Epstein-Barr syndrome

glaucoma
hepatitis
herpes
Hodgkin's disease
inflammatory bowel disease
leukemia
Lou Gehrig's Disease or Amyotrophic Lateral Sclerosis
    (ALS)
lupus erythematosis
manic depression or bi-polar disease
Multiple Chemical Sensitivity (MCS)
multiple sclerosis
myasthenia gravis
obesity
pernicious anemia
psoriasis and eczema
rheumatoid arthritis (RA)
schizophrenia, including catatonic
scleroderma
"Sick Building Syndrome" or SBS
Sjogren's syndrome
thyroid, parathyroid, and adrenal gland disease (Addison's
    disease)
vitiligo

## *DRUGS, THERAPIES, AND CONDITIONS THAT STIMULATE THE OVERGROWTH OF YEAST*

alcoholism
antacids
antibiotics
AZT, Interferon, and most prescription drugs
chemotherapies
cigarettes
disturbances in the electromagnetic field of the body
fluoride and fluoridated water

food additives, preservatives, and colorings
high blood sugar
high humidity
hormones, including Premarin® and Norplant®
immuno-suppressive drugs
oral contraceptives or birth control pills
other infections, especially ones that disrupt the intestinal
    flora
parasites
pesticides and herbicides
pregnancy, which contributes to hormonal changes
radiation therapy
silver-mercury amalgam fillings in teeth
spermicides
steroids or corticosteroids
stress–both physical and emotional
tobacco smoke, perfumes, dyes, diesel fumes, and chemical
    odors
use of marijuana, cocaine, heroin, and methamphetamines
vitamin and mineral deficiencies

It is impossible to list all the symptoms there are. However, at least you have an idea of the range of havoc the yeast/beast wreaks.

Truly, yeast overgrowth is "the disease behind disease." I will discuss what I mean by that phrase a little later in the book, but for now let's look at how symptoms arise.

**Chapter 7**

---

# What Causes Symptoms?

*"Among the more important and recently recognized connections are those between the immune system, the endocrine system and the brain. And since Candida toxins affect each of these systems and one system affects the other, the yeast connection can cause all sorts of symptoms."*

... Dr. William G. Crook, M.D.

In chapter 6 there are long lists of symptoms that occur when *Candida albicans* is doing its dirty work. Let's look now at what *causes* symptoms to arise and what diseases can result.

We will be examining seven different body systems, plus the general areas of allergies, fatigue, and weight gain.

I'll bet you find yourself somewhere!

### First is the Gastrointestinal System.

The G I tract is the favored site of all for yeast. From the mouth to the rectum, it is full of nooks and crannies where yeast can hide. It has the ideal moisture and warmth which yeasts require, and as long as the host keeps sending down lots of sugar and carbohydrates for them to eat, they are fat, dumb, and happy.

Rampaging fungi invade and damage the mucosa or protective lining of the colon. Afterwards the linings themselves become clogged with growing colonies of yeast, blocking the absorption of essential nutrients. Candida organisms can actually "eat" enough of the ingested nutrients to produce a state of *malnutrition* or semi-starvation in the host. Then allergens slip through the holes in the colon and spill into the bloodstream, along with partially-digested food, dead yeasts, and their poisons causing leaky gut syndrome. The colon no longer is a barrier that keeps allergens and toxins out of the bloodstream. *It becomes a screen door!* Allergies, fatigue, depression, and headaches soon follow.

If food you eat is high in sugar and simple carbohydrates, yeasts eat the sugar and produces a lot of carbon dioxide–*gas*. The host suffers from uncomfortable gas and bloating.

Direct assault on the intestinal lining can result in abdominal pain, gastritis, gastric ulcers (*Candida albicans* has been found in the craters of gastric ulcers), cramping–often called "spastic colon" or "irritable bowel syndrome"–and diarrhea.

Because of increased pressure in the stomach from gas, the valve between the stomach and the esophagus can be forced open. "Reflux" from the corrosive stomach acids and digestive juices flow up the esophagus, burning and irritating its lining, causing heartburn, burping, and indigestion. These acids also can burn the cardiac valve, weakening it and allowing acids to burp up into the mouth when the host is asleep, destroying tooth enamel.

Constipation is common because the friendly lactobacillus bacteria have been decimated by yeast overgrowths in the intestines. Yeast loves to set up housekeeping in old, encrusted fecal matter and the sacs of diverticulosis. Many times there is a pattern of alternating constipation and diarrhea as the yeast and the immune system wax and wane.

### Second is the Respiratory system.

Since yeast is in every breath of air we breathe, it is not surprising that we would find a respiratory involvement with Candida. The mucous membranes from nose to lungs become irritated from constant exposure to yeast and its toxins. If the nose and sinuses are affected, sneezing, runny or stuffy nose, post-nasal drip, and sinus infections may appear. Direct invasion by yeast in the mouth can manifest as sore throat and mouth ulcers. Sometimes white patches appear on the throat and inside the mouth. Oral thrush coats the tongue with a creamy film. Gums may be spongy, sore, and bleed easily.

Studies have proven that yeast organisms are present in almost all lung conditions.[1] Bronchial candidiasis, characterized by coughing with sputum, rales, and thickening of the bronchial tubes, is a form of chronic bronchitis, and in advanced cases yeast patches can be seen with the naked eye growing on the bronchial tree. Asthma and pneumonia have powerful links to Candida.

### *Third is the Cardiovascular system.*

Candida lives on and attempts to digest the lining of blood vessels, causing coronary artery disease. The damage is patched up by the body in the form of scabs called atherosclerosis or arteriosclerosis. Candida can live on heart valves (causing mitral valve prolapse) and both in and on arteries. By interfering with the balance of hormones that regulate the cardiovascular system, especially stress hormones, Candida can cause heart palpitations, pounding heart, rapid pulse, and changes in electrocardiograms.

When the circulatory system is slowed by yeast, all cells are poorly supplied with blood and the nutrients therein, including oxygen. Without oxygen, human cells either suffocate or survive crippled. Unfortunately, the wily yeast cells are so adaptable they can thrive with or without oxygen. Anemia and low energy are examples of slowed circulation, as is slow healing of wounds.

Without oxygen the activity of the defender white cells is severely restricted. Fungal overgrowth appears on and under fingernails and toenails, often accompanied with a thickening of the nail. Poor circulation also contributes to fluid retention, excessive perspiration, and cold and clammy feet.

Biofeedback has clearly shown that anxiety, tension, and the stress of modern day living contribute to restricting blood flow. When thoughts are shifted from anxious to peaceful, skin temperature rises, indicating increased blood flow.

Conversely, the more anxious we become, the slower the blood flows. *And the more blood slows, the more yeast has a chance to grow.*

Congestive heart failure, memory problems, confusion, and slow healing of wounds are indicative of impaired circulation.

### *Fourth is the Genitourinary system.*

What woman in this day and age has never heard of or experienced vaginal yeast infections? All you have to do is turn on a television and count the ads for those over-the-counter remedies to realize the enormity of this epidemic. Our grandmothers and great-grandmothers virtually *never heard of yeast infections or PMS in their day.* Today they are two of the most common complaints a doctor hears.

How are our twenty-first century female bodies different from the bodies of our grandmothers and great-grandmothers? In a nutshell, our intestines are different. Grandma's intestinal flora was balanced with lactobacillus but ours aren't. Their flora was strong enough to resist Candida overgrowth, and ours, having been weakened by drugs, wrong food, and stress, can't stem the tide.

Vaginal yeast infections, characterized by itching, swelling, discharge, pain, and burning are the result of direct invasion of yeast into the vaginal wall, or allergic reactions to the yeast themselves. If a woman can't contain and control the yeast in her vagina, she surely can't contain and control it in the rest of her body!

Yeast can attack the lining of the bladder directly, causing burning upon urination, frequent urination, lack of bladder control, and bedwetting.

Males may develop penile rashes and chronic prostate problems, as well as sexual dysfunction problems such as impotence and premature ejaculation.

In women, yeast can attack the ovaries and fallopian tubes. If ovaries are covered with yeast, they cannot function or make the hormones needed. Menstrual problems and PMS result. If the fallopian tubes are clogged with Candida, conception is thwarted, resulting in infertility.

Candida also makes the body very acid, which makes conception even more difficult.

### Fifth is the Musculoskeletal system.

As Candida damages cells, it is nearly impossible for nutrients to get into muscle tissue and for waste products to get out. This has a wide range of effects all over the body. Weakness, charley horses, deep muscle pain (especially in the neck and shoulders) soreness, stiffness, poor coordination, and tension headaches all fall in this category.

Arthritis has a definite connection to yeast. *Arthritis appears in bodies that are too acid.* An overgrowth of Candida tilts the body from alkaline to acid, and acid is the medium that yeast likes best. Antibodies the body manufactures to attack yeast attack the joint tissue as well! Rheumatoid arthritis is an excellent example of this. As the joint swells, it attracts more yeast that comes to attack and devour the injured tissue. The constant swelling and destruction from yeast eventually deforms the joint, ligaments, and muscles. In the back, muscular stress can actually pull vertebrae out of line and cause pinched nerves. Osteoporosis is due mainly to yeast living inside bone, eating the marrow and nutrients.

### Sixth is the Skin.

Yeast can directly invade the skin, usually breeding in warm, moist areas under the breasts and in the groin. Alkaline and anti-bacterial soaps are implicated in the growth of yeast on the skin since they kill beneficial flora, doing the same thing as antibiotics in the body–creating a favorable environment for yeast.

Almost any skin condition can be traced to yeast activity. Diaper rash, dry itching or scaling skin, psoriasis, hives, and eczema are common. Virulent forms of Candida on the skin can be transmitted sexually, so husbands and wives or sex partners continually exchange yeast with each other during intercourse. (That's why you *both* need to go on the yeast-free diet together.)

The skin of diabetics is especially vulnerable to fungi. Their sweat is high in sugars, which provide a lush medium on which to grow.

Many yeast patients exhibit skin lesions of some type. Acne nodules, when examined under a microscope, reveal skin layers infiltrated by yeast. And what do dermatologists prescribe for most of their acne patients? Antibiotics, of course, which make more yeast, that make more acne. Voila! Acne soon becomes a *chronic* disease.

When the skin of the victim of athlete's foot is examined, the presence of fungal hyphal elements, or spores, is found. Athlete's foot is considered to be allergic reactions to yeast mycotoxins. Inflammation of the nail bed, skin cracking in the corners of the mouth, and seborrheic dermatitis are skin disorders that have definite yeast connections. *Psoriasis is a fungal infection of the skin*, and is very curable with the yeast-free diet and anti-fungals.

### Seventh is the Central Nervous System

Yeast affects the central nervous system through endocrine hormones and muscles. In the brain, the hypothalamus, which serves as a switchboard for the entire body, becomes stressed because hormones have been blocked or destroyed (eaten) by yeast. When the hypothalamus is stressed, or gets out of sync, "messages" get re-routed or lost, and the body's metabolism is affected.

When Candida is present, stress hormones act like irritants to nerves. Headaches, migraines, anxiety, sleep disturbances, low blood sugar, panic attacks, and herpes may manifest.

The brain itself is very sensitive to the yeast/beast, and a proliferation of yeast there is especially cruel. Autopsies often reveal Candida 'caps" on the brain. When colonies set up housekeeping on top of and inside brain tissue and begin excreting their toxic waste, a myriad of symptoms ensue. Short-term memory loss, confusion, short attention span, ADD, ADHD, depression, irritability, mood swings, lethargy, emotional and behavioral problems, hearing voices, hallucinations and convulsions are only a few. People suffering from schizophrenia and bi-polar disease find *immediate relief* from the yeast-free diet and anti-fungals.

When people lose control of their behavior, they first have lost control of their mental processes. Many madmen and their brutal killing sprees can be traced directly back to the dark side of yeast.

Adolph Hitler was termed a "sugar drunkard" by those close to him. "The *Fuhrer*" could never get enough of his favorite whipped cream cakes, and he took a box of candy with him wherever he went. He even put sugar in his wine! Richard Speck, the killer of eight student nurses in Chicago years ago, constantly munched on candy bars. In 1991 George Jo Hennard went on a shooting spree in Luby's cafeteria in Killeen, Texas, killing twenty-three and wounding twenty before he killed himself. He reportedly drank a quart of coffee and ate a dozen sugar donuts before he picked up his weapon. He was a known junk food junkie.

I don't think anyone today would argue that this country has a huge problem with crime. Our prisons and jails are filled to the max. Too often we read and hear about people going on rampages and killing large numbers of people. My bet is that if you looked at the diets of all criminals who have committed aggressive and brutal acts, you will find yeast-stimulating food as the major portion of their diets.

One of the saddest and most visible deteriorations of a human being was that of Howard Hughes, the wealthy industrialist, aviator, film producer and director, and chairman of Hughes Tool. This creative giant with a genius I.Q. bought into the prevailing medical orthodoxy that "sugar provides energy" and ate it hand over fist. He soon began exhibiting symptoms of obsessive-compulsive disorder and bizarre behavior. He became so obsessed with the size of peas that he insisted on using a special fork so he could sort them by size. At one point he holed up in a darkened screening room *for four months*, watching movies over and over in the nude, picking up objects with tissue, stacking and re-stacking the same Kleenex boxes, and *subsisting on nothing but candy bars and milk*. Later he became fixated on Baskin Robbins Banana Nut and French Vanilla ice cream.

Another source of fungus was his business. Several of the warehouses at Hughes Tools were known to be infected with mold. Mr. Hughes personally inspected them, found the mold and had the buildings remediated. Between the sugar-laden diet and the mold spores in his warehouses, it didn't take long for yeast to take hold and lead to his terrible physical and mental decline. Soon drugs were prescribed and shortly, the once stately and handsome man with a brilliant mind, one of the wealthiest men in the world, deteriorated from a strapping 6 foot 4 inch man into a shrunken, 90 pound, delusional hermit. The best medical care couldn't save him. By the time of his death, the yeast/beast had rendered him so unrecognizable the FBI had to use fingerprints to identify the body.

### The first area of general interest is Allergies.

Like the chicken and the egg, we're not sure which came first, the yeast or the allergy, but what we do know is that people who have allergies are susceptible to Candida, and people who have Candida are susceptible to allergies.

In any case, anyone who exhibits an allergy to a substance is exhibiting an intolerance or unusual sensitivity to it. In allergic situations, high levels of yeast keep the immune system on high alert, causing the immune system to *overreact to allergens*. But Candida overgrowths can also cause an *underactive* or depressed immune response. This shifting back and forth creates an imbalanced immune system, which then encourages more yeast to grow. With the proliferation of Candida and their poisons, the immune system is further weakened and more allergies appear. As you follow the yeast-free diet, these swings of hypo- and hyper-immunity flatten out, and allergies slowly disappear.

Allergies in some cases are very easy to identify. You react swiftly after exposure to the offending allergen. You also react every time you are exposed, and the results are predictable: sneezing, headaches, runny nose, burning eyes, dizziness, and wheezing. Asthma and depression also can be allergy related.

In other cases, it's not so easy. You may not react for hours after exposure or you may not react at all. Or you may react only once after repeated exposure. Hives, nasal itching, and contact dermatitis are examples of delayed reactions to allergens.

*The good news is that the longer you stay on the diet, the more of an offending substance is needed to elicit a response.*

The lower the yeast levels in the body, the more your tolerance improves. In just a few months of diet therapy you probably won't be aware of any adverse reactions.

### The second area of general interest is Fatigue.

It has been said that *fatigue and depression are the hallmarks of yeast infection.* With yeast living in both the body and the brain, it makes sense that both are tired and functioning at low levels.

If body cells cannot get enough nutrients and fuel because of impaired metabolism and damaged enzymes, metabolism is slowed and malfunctions. Instant fatigue, drowsiness, lethargy, and lack of interest in mental or physical activities occur. When you don't have the energy to participate fully in life, the enjoyment of life slips away. When life holds little joy or hope and there is no light at the end of the tunnel, depression fills the growing void.

With fatigue and depression, and the withdrawal from life activities, come feelings of inadequacy, low self-esteem, and hopelessness. A psychiatrist may enter the picture, with anti-depression and mood altering drugs to help you "snap out of it," because this is "all in your head." But these prescription drugs are chemicals. Chemicals are only band-aids, which don't cure the problem because they AREN'T the problem.

The problem is most probably the "disease behind disease"–yeast.

### *The third area of general interest is Weight Gain.*

This is a "biggie," no pun intended. Overweight is one of the most universal complaints of people loaded with yeast. By now you are probably able to figure out some of the reasons why. If you have a weight problem, think back carefully and you probably will be able to *trace the beginning of the scale's climb back to your first prescription for antibiotics or birth control pills.*

Fatigue and a slowed metabolism obviously contribute to the burning of fewer calories. When all you want to do is sleep, the body systems need less fuel, and the pounds pile up due to decreased activity. Add to that the constant cravings for food because damaged cells can't take up nutrients, plus the unremitting sugar and carbohydrate cravings from the yeasts themselves who are screaming to be fed. To top it off, malfunctioning insulin hormones keep blood sugar levels high, which add more pounds.

Water retention, or edema, is another common complaint. If the kidneys are sprouting a nice stand of fungus, it is impossible for them to do their jobs of filtering blood, producing urine, getting rid of wastes, and balancing minerals and salts. "Water weight," puffiness, and swellings are inevitable.

Candidiasis disrupts sugar, fat, and protein metabolism in your body. Most people tend to gain weight under these circumstances, but occasionally we see someone who is so severely debilitated from candidiasis, that he or she has gone the other way and has developed eating disorders such as anorexia and bulimia, or has become emaciated from constant diarrhea or vomiting. As soon as the yeast is brought under control and normal metabolism is restored–especially to the thyroid and pancreas–normal weight soon follows.

I hope I have impressed upon you the magnitude and scope of destructive activity that *Candida albicans* can cause. It seems this little organism can go anywhere and do anything it pleases.

That is, *until the yeast-free diet comes on the scene.*

**Chapter 8**

---

# The Damage

*"Untreated systemic candidiasis has a mortality rate approaching 100%. Delay in treatment is dangerous and will almost certainly end in the death of the patient."*

...Dr. Rosalind Hurley, M.D.

Now that we have an overview of what yeast is and how it grows, let's look at actual ways it harms the basic functioning of our body. There are three major areas where yeast's handiwork does the most destruction:

1. It *damages* cell membranes.
2. It *destroys* or blocks enzymes.
3. It *interferes* with normal hormone responses.

How does that happen?

As yeast lives, reproduces, and dies, it releases a number of chemicals during those processes. Two of the most deadly are *acetaldehyde and ethanol*. Both are *poisonous to tissue*. Our bodies can handle small amounts of both toxins as long as yeast levels are normal. But as yeast levels rise, we can literally become intoxicated by them!

Just as yeast is used by the alcoholic beverage industry to convert different sugars into ethanol (a type of alcohol), yeast in our bodies converts sugars in the food we eat to produce ethanol as a by-product. Ethanol is broken down further into acetaldehyde, a close cousin of formaldehyde. (That's embalming fluid, folks!) Unfortunately, acetaldehyde is six times more toxic to brain tissue than the original ethanol, and wreaks great havoc in the body as well.

Years ago in Japan a rare and mysterious disease appeared called *"meitei-sho"* (drunkenness disease). An affected person appeared to walk, talk and smell like he was totally intoxicated. Even his blood alcohol tests indicated high levels of alcohol in the bloodstream. Yet the person had not drunk one drop of alcohol. (In America they were called "drunken liars.")

After years of frantic research the mystery was solved. Researchers found that those patients were *walking distilleries* due to the huge load of yeasts in their gastrointestinal tracts. Overgrowths of *Candida albicans* created their own personal 'stills' by converting refined carbohydrates directly into alcohol. When carbohydrates were greatly reduced and their yeast infections were treated, the patients got well.

Another bizarre phenomenon, which may be yeast related, is that of "spontaneous human combustion." Stories of people bursting into flames (known as human fireballs) have been around for centuries. Could it be that this is also caused by Candida creating so much alcohol in the body that it causes it to ignite spontaneously and burn itself to ashes? Maybe we will see this mystery solved in the years ahead.

So, two chemicals, acetaldehyde and ethanol, both by-products of yeast, are highly suspected in causing much or most cellular damage that results in disease.

Now let's look at the three areas of destruction.

### *Number 1–Damage to Cell Membranes*

Normally the membranes of cells are moist and pliable. However, *the chemicals released by yeast make these membranes hard and rigid*. In the case of red blood cells, this makes it impossible for them to mold and squeeze themselves into tiny capillaries, thereby depriving tissues and organs of life-giving oxygen. Without oxygen, these tissues and organs become impaired and lose their ability to function.

White blood cells are affected the same way. They are a large part of our immune systems, and constantly gobble up bacteria and other foreign invaders in an attempt to keep us infection free. When their cell walls become too brittle to wrap themselves around and devour the enemy, the enemy can break through, and you lose the ability to fight off infections easily.

When cell membranes are damaged, the body's primary fuel, blood sugar or glucose, *has trouble getting inside various cells to feed them,* so it remains in the blood instead of penetrating cells. The body, not getting enough glucose, calls for more insulin. High levels of insulin are known to stimulate the conversion of sugar to fat. Both high and low blood sugar problems and weight gain can result.

Thyroid hormones also have difficulty penetrating rigid cell membranes, resulting in slowed metabolism, low body temperature, fatigue, etc. Unfortunately, lab tests are useless in pinpointing this problem since they only reflect the level of hormone circulating in the bloodstream, not its metabolic ability to function within the cell.

Minerals, such as sodium, calcium, and potassium are deflected by rigid cell walls, causing fluid retention, and electrolyte imbalances.

Yeast toxins also interfere with our cells' ability to communicate with each other. Normally, when one cell wants to send a message to another, it releases a special chemical that contains the message. Then a nerve or muscle cell absorbs the chemical to "take its message." But, because the cell membrane is defective, the message is garbled and soon lost. Muscle and nervous system symptoms and diseases result. Poor coordination and myalgias plus other symptoms of multiple sclerosis and Lou Gehrig's disease (ALS–Amyotrophic Lateral Sclerosis) may appear.

### *Number 2–Enzyme Destruction*

Enzymes are a very large class of protein substances that are produced by living cells. They are essential to life, acting as catalysts in the metabolism and metabolic processes in the body. They are chemical helpers which spark or jump-start everything from digestion to ovulation. They help both to build and break down, start and stop, and also maintain the body's energy and heat.

Yeast poisons cripple or kill some enzymes, and as a result all functions of the body can become sluggish or erratic. Diabetes, weight gain or obesity, and indigestion are only a few examples of enzyme impairment.

### Number 3–Interference with Hormone Response

Hormones are the secretions from various endocrine glands (pituitary, thyroid and parathyroid, pancreas, thymus, adrenals, ovaries, and testes), which travel in the bloodstream to control and adjust certain metabolic processes. Some target a particular organ while others affect the entire body.

Yeast toxins interfere with the functioning of *all endocrine glands* by blocking or impeding their chemical messengers–hormones–from getting to their intended destinations. *Candida actually EATS hormones*, creating hormone imbalances. Here again, blood tests may indicate an adequate level in the bloodstream, but if enough hormone doesn't reach its targeted organ, it can't do its job. Edema and PMS are two conditions that illustrate an abnormal hormone response in the body.

This presents a pretty grim picture, but I hope you are beginning to get the big picture. *When the yeast/beast goes from local to global, the landscape changes.*

Instead of a serene and bucolic painting, we are now looking at a canvas from hell. All systems are disrupted and malfunctioning. Chaos and confusion reign. Yeasts are everywhere, gleefully gorging everything they land on in an incredible feeding frenzy, belching, and excreting their toxic wastes as they go. Dead and dying tissues are strewn around their colonies, along with rotting garbage and filth. The smell is horrible.

The weary, disheartened, and weakened host now comes down with strep throat and goes to the doctor.  He comes home and dutifully swallows another round of antibiotics.

The yeasts let out a resounding cheer.

**Chapter 9**

---

# The No–No's

*"If only a fraction of what is already known about the effects of sugar in relation to any other material used as a food additive, that material would promptly be banned."*

...    Dr. John Yudkin, M.D., Ph.D.

It is now time to look at what really is going to heal us–food, or should I say, the absence of some foods. Food can be your best friend, or your worst enemy.

The food we choose to eat has the power to alter our biochemistries, the chemical processes of the body and mind. By the same token, what we choose NOT to eat has both the power to alter our body chemistries *and to heal us.*

Following this simple eating program allows you to balance your body chemistries; wipe out massive colonies of yeast; and restore your metabolism and immune system to their intended purposes. It is a very simple and straightforward approach.

You are going to *starve* the yeast/beast.

By eliminating yeast-stimulating food and drink from your diet, you will slow down and start reversing the yeast load your body has had to cope with. For too long yeasts have been living high on the hog, eating *you* for breakfast, lunch, and dinner. Now, instead of their absorbing and eliminating *you, you* are going to turn the tables and absorb and eliminate *them.*

Instead of their eating *you* alive, *you are going to eat them…dead.*

The average duration of the diet is three months. Don't forget that Nature is a slow but steady healer. You didn't get sick overnight and you are not going to get well overnight.

If you have a very *serious* illness, stay on the diet for at least *six months*. If you have severe *mental symptoms*, commit for *a year*. After the diet most people feel so good they choose to stay on it and allow for occasional lapses and treats. In any case, look at this program not as a "diet" but a "die-off" because that is in essence what is happening. If you view it *not* as a life sentence, but a *sentence to life*, you will help yourself stay on the straight and narrow.


### Sugar and Carbohydrates

*Yeast's favorite food is sugar.* It is no coincidence that Candida overgrowth is being called "the twentieth century disease" since refined sugar is the "twentieth century food." *Fructose is now the number one source of calories in the United States!* In 1700 the average American consumed **4 pounds** of sugar a year. By 1800 it had risen to **18 pounds** per year. In 1900 the average was **90 pounds** per year. In 2009 it was estimated that we are consuming a whopping **180 pounds** of the stuff per year, or ½ pound per DAY! Our bodies have not been able to adjust to such high levels of sugar and they are *telling* us so.

Most people who have Candida-related health problems have been habitual eaters of sweets. We are a nation obsessed with sugar and carbohydrates, gulping them down from our sugar-coated cereals in the morning until that last bowl of ice cream at night. Much of the sugar we get is neatly hidden in ketchup, salad dressings, soft drinks, canned soups, snacks, and processed foods.

Even health food purists and vegetarians can maintain huge overgrowths of yeast by eating diets loaded with grains and whole grain breads, granola, tofu, mushrooms, brewer's yeast, honey, fruits, dried fruit, and fruit juices. Yeast and fungi LOVE tofu! (It is spongy and moist.)

Sugar (a carbohydrate), contains almost no vitamins and minerals, and has been dubbed by nutritionists as "dead food." Cane sugar is a notoriously moldy food. It provides only empty calories and interferes with the ability of minerals to perform properly. Sugar is the primary source of fuel for yeasts such as *Candida albicans.*

All of us are born with a set of genes, but the *expression* of those genes is not set in stone. Just because you may have a gene for breast or colon cancer does *not* mean it is a foregone conclusion that you will develop those diseases. Genes can be activated or neutralized by many variables, including diet, lifestyle, and even your thoughts and emotions. For instance, cancer genes can be "switched on" with the wrong diet, and conversely, the cruciferous vegetables (broccoli, cauliflower, brussels sprouts, cabbage, kale) greatly modify gene expression. So it is not your genes that dictate your future health, but rather the *expression* of those genes that is critical.

Recent studies have demonstrated that human genes actually remember a "sugar hit" for *two weeks!* In other words, the impact from ingesting sugar lasts fourteen days, during which time cells switch off genetic controls designed to protect the body against both diabetes and heart disease.[1] With controls in the "off" position, disease is given free reign.

Also, sugar neutralizes your body's natural 'happy pill', called endorphins. Depression is rampant among 'sugarholics' (and alcoholics).

The number one item to remove from your kitchen during the diet is sugar. That means white sugar, brown sugar, turbinado sugar, date sugar, agave syrup (a highly processed sap that is eighty percent fructose and spikes blood sugar just like regular sugar), molasses, corn syrup (especially high-fructose corn syrup), and anything that ends with "ose", e.g., fructose (especially crystalline fructose), sucrose, lactose, maltose. "Ose" means sugar.

Most versions of yeast-free diets severely restrict or eliminate honey, maple syrup and all fruit for the first three or four weeks of the diet. Sylvia's diet does not. She feels that by taking away all sugars all at once, you run the risk of shocking the body, especially the pancreas and adrenals, and the body is already in shock enough from the yeasts and all their poisons. Small amounts of sugars actually stimulate the immune system. She recommends one or two pieces of fruit a day, preferably at breakfast, for the first month. This will prime the pancreas for its day's work and kick the metabolism into gear.

Honey, maple syrup, rice syrup, *small* amounts of evaporated cane juice, and barley malt are allowed occasionally since they are metabolized slowly and gently. It seems that they can slip by the yeast without the yeast noticing they were there. These small amounts of sugars are actually *necessary to stimulate the immune system* so it won't become depleted. Even most diabetics (except brittle diabetics) can indulge in a little honey and maple syrup without disturbing blood sugar levels. As long as you use it cautiously you won't be harmed.

Sylvia and I have by now worked with thousands of people who have weathered this diet successfully and become Candida free while eating small or moderate amounts of fruit, honey, and maple syrup. So, since there seems to be no good reason to restrict them, we don't. Besides, being able to eat these sweets makes the whole program more palatable and enjoyable. That goes a long way in keeping us content, satisfied and on course, rather than bored, frustrated, and on the verge of throwing in the towel.

Complex carbohydrates and starchy food, while allowed, have to be kept in *very moderate portions.* If you remove sugars, but double the amounts of rice, pastas, potatoes, grains, etc., you are eating, you won't be helping much. Yeasts are so crafty and adaptable, that when they realize that sugars have been removed, they learn to content themselves with whatever carbohydrates are around. So, keep the carbs to one moderate portion per meal, and you will get well much faster.

### *Breads*

*Of course, all breads and foods that contain yeast or yeast extract must be eliminated.*

If you want to see first hand how yeast works, get a package of baker's yeast and place the contents into a bowl. Add a little warm water and watch as the yeast begin to bubble and ferment. Then, sprinkle on a little sugar. The yeast will *explode* in numbers as they metabolize the sugar, produce ethanol (alcohol), and release carbon dioxide. (Baker's yeast is used to produce glycerol, an ingredient in the manufacture of *explosives*.) In the bowl you are witnessing exactly what goes on inside your body. The proper mix of warmth, moisture, and sugar provide the perfect environment for fermentation. This is a wonderful way to teach your children and grandchildren how yeast grows.

After the population of the United States reached 200 million, we had to store grains in silos–huge metal vats that sweat. The moisture and warmth spur the growth of yeast, mildew, and mold. Consequently *all grains are contaminated to some degree.* Corn now is 100 percent contaminated with mold. Fungi attack grains from planting, through growth and storage to harvest for their carbohydrates–fungi's favorite food. One of the most common grain molds, aflatoxin, is the most carcinogenic substance known to man. So eat minimal amounts of grains and breads, even yeast-free.

I am often asked why the yeast in baked bread isn't killed by the heat of the oven. The answer is that yeast is indeed killed by the baking process. But their mycotoxins in the grains are heat-stable and are NOT killed by the heat. They are still viable and destructive.

Read labels on all processed foods and everything that goes in your mouth. You will be amazed to find yeast or yeast extracts in canned soups, crackers, even Grape-Nuts®. There are some excellent yeast-free sourdough breads on the market that use only wild yeasts from the air for leavening. French Meadow Bakery makes delicious yeast-free breads. You can order from their website and their breads freeze beautifully. Please keep even these breads to one or two thin slices a day for the first month to keep your carbohydrate count within boundaries.

*Alcohol*

All alcoholic beverages contain yeast because all alcohol is the result of fermentation. Alcohol kills the friendly bacteria in the gut, leading to yeast over-growth. *Alcohol itself is pure yeast mycotoxin.* Any fruit juice with a high sugar content can be used to produce an alcoholic beverage. Grape juice is the most common.

Fermentation begins as soon as the grape skin is broken. In Europe wild, natural strains of yeast are used to ferment wine. But in the United States wine makers usually seed their vats with specific strains of yeast. As sugar is consumed by the yeast, vats bubble with carbon dioxide. Soon ethyl alcohol is produced. When the alcohol level reaches 14 percent, the yeast stops growing and the fermentation process comes to an end. All the yeast cells fall to the bottom before the wine is bottled.

Brewer's yeast is the fungus used to ferment grain into alcohol. Beer, (liquid bread) the "yeasty-ist" of brews, is made in much the same manner as wine, only malt (made from barley or oats) is used instead of grape juice. While fermenting, yeast is fully distributed throughout the beer and then flocculates, or clumps together, and then falls to the bottom of the vat when fermentation ends. This clumping action, which gives beer its clean, clear look, gives yeast the ability to hide from view. Unfortunately it is this same clumping ability that allows yeast to hide from attacks by the human immune system.

Liquors are made by yeast fermenting corn mash into bourbon, barley malt into scotch, sugar cane into rum, rye grains into rye whiskeys, fruit juices into brandy, and potatoes into vodka. Fermentation is the key.

Inside the human body, yeast *can ferment you into mush* as it creates disease. Even a moderate intake of alcohol increases a woman's chance of developing breast cancer. For women who consume one-to-two drinks per day, the risk of developing breast cancer is approximately 10 percent and rises to 30–40 percent in women who consume four or more drinks a day.[2]

Alcoholics have huge crops of yeast screaming to be fed. *Alcoholism is basically a yeast/sugar addiction.* The yeast-free diet has helped many alcoholics to overcome this terrible disease by quieting and eventually silencing the continuous cravings set up by the yeast/beast.

### Milk and Milk Products

These are difficult for many people to give up. Cows, cow's milk, and country settings of bucolic beauty have become part of the American idiom. We have been reared on the marketing of the "four food groups" driven mainly by a powerful dairy lobby in Washington, D.C. But we should get wiser as we get older. Now the prevailing wisdom is pointing out irrefutable evidence that *all milk and milk products (except organic raw milk) are just plain bad for the human body!*

Cow's milk was designed for baby cows. Period. Man is the only mammal that continues to drink milk after infancy, *and* is the only mammal that drinks the milk of another species! It is very hard for the human body to break down and digest the milk of cows because cows' milk cells are much bigger than the cells of human breast milk. Milk requires rennin, a digestive enzyme, for complete digestion. *Rennin is found only in infants.*

The homogenization process forces milk under high pressure through tiny openings. This makes all the cream or fat particles smaller so that they can become equally distributed and united with milk particles. That enables fat to enter *directly* into the blood or lymph stream and attack the heart and arteries, as many people in their fifties and sixties are made so painfully aware by their doctors. The new *ultra* pasteurized milks and creams are even worse. Pasteurization sterilizes milk through heat. Unfortunately high heat (ultra pasteurization in particular) destroys enzymes found naturally in milk, making milk a dead food.

Cow's milk provides very little calcium that can be assimilated; has a poor balance of protein; an even worse balance of fats; and the lactose, or milk sugar, it contains feeds yeast like crazy. There are twelve grams of lactose in every eight ounces of milk! (Even yogurt, so don't eat it while healing.)

Cow's milk, unless organic, also contains concentrated levels of *cow growth hormones!* Hormones regulate the rate of growth, and all animals have hormones that are unique to their species. The natural rate of growth for cows is much faster than the natural growth rate for humans. Many researchers now believe that the ingestion of cow hormones causes children to grow too fast and physically mature sooner than normal, and contributes to the crowding of teeth, gum problems and the need for braces. Also, antibiotics added to the cows' feed appear in their milk, adding more fuel to the fire for the yeast/beasts. All play major roles in our current epidemic of obesity.

Looking even further, when you add acid rain, herbicides, and pesticides to the antibiotics, steroids, and hormones in milk (all of which are further concentrated into cheeses), the result is a very harmful food product.

### *Margarine*

Margarine, like cow's milk, eats up your arteries. In 1994 Harvard researchers reported that people who ate partially hydrogenated oils had twice the risk of heart attacks as those who did not.[3] It is high in trans fatty acids; increases LDL (the bad guys) and total cholesterol; lowers HDL (the good guys); lowers the quality of breast milk; decreases immune and insulin response; and increases the risk of cancer up to five-fold. The hydrogenation process, which is used to turn a liquid oil into a solid, makes margarine every bit as saturated as butter. In actuality, hydrogenation makes the molecular structure of oil *one molecule away from PLASTIC*. Our digestive enzymes do not assimilate plastic. If you want to see this for yourself, purchase a tub of margarine. Put it in a garage or shady place. Take off the lid. Come back in a couple of days and you will notice two things. No insects, no flies, or even pesky fruit flies, will go near it. (Sometimes insects are smarter than humans.) It does not rot or smell any different. Nothing will grow on it–not even mold! Why? *Because it's mainly plastic!* Would you melt a plastic bag and pour it on your popcorn? Yum.

Margarine also contains a lot of preservatives, emulsifiers, artificial colors and flavors, plus synthetic vitamins. Yeast laps them up.

### *Fruit to Avoid*

Bananas must not be eaten because they are practically pure sugar, even though the sugar is natural. Grapes and plums contain too much natural yeast, which you can see as a white film usually around the stem. Dried fruit, since it is dehydrated, is a concentrate of sugars and harbors mold.

### *Caffeine*

Caffeine is an addictive drug and a powerful poison. A single drop of this alkaloid in its pure form injected into the skin of a small animal will produce death within minutes. When injected into the brain, tiny amounts will bring on convulsions. Caffeine is habit-forming and when taken away from the addict, "withdrawal symptoms" are suffered. It also removes oxygen from the bloodstream. We need oxygen in our bloodstreams because cancer and Candida cannot survive in an oxygenated environment. Read labels carefully.

Coffee, all teas except herbal teas, and all food and beverages that contain caffeine must be removed from your diet. Caffeine is a powerful stimulant, and anything that stimulates the body will provoke it to ferment more yeast. That is why steroids are so dangerous. Steroids are powerful stimulants of yeast and should be saved for life-threatening situations only. Coffee is also extremely acidic, which is the medium *all diseases like to grow in, and is like fertilizer for yeast.*

Caffeine is known to produce gastrointestinal ulcers in animals, which later turned into cancers, and contributes to hardening of the arteries and decalcification of the bones.

Decaffeinated coffee may be even more dangerous than regular coffee. Solvents–usually toxic–must be used to remove caffeine. The most commonly used solvent is methylene chloride, which the FDA has banned in hair sprays and cosmetics because it is a carcinogen!

### *Chocolate*

No one likes this no-no. Chocolate contains caffeine. A lot, too. One ounce of dark chocolate contains 20 milligrams of caffeine, and one ounce of milk chocolate contains 6 milligrams of caffeine. Cocoa or chocolate drinks contain from one to two percent theobromine (which is closely related to caffeine) *plus* caffeine. Children (and adults) who consume large amounts of chocolate, hot cocoa, cola drinks, and candy bars usually are addicted to the caffeine in them, plus the sugar. Chocolate also contains *oxalic acid,* a yeast mycotoxin, which has the unfortunate ability to bind with calcium and render it useless for assimilation in the body. So adding chocolate to milk neutralizes whatever small amount of calcium is present. But it makes the yeast ecstatic.

Cocoa and chocolate are implicated clearly in calcium deficiencies such as female disorders, decayed teeth, osteoporosis, nervous problems, and arteriosclerosis. Chocolate cravings, most of the time, are indications of yeast overgrowths and mineral deficiencies, especially magnesium.

### *Artificial Sweeteners*

The bad news about artificial sweeteners is finally coming to the fore. Aspartame (NutraSweet® and Equal®), Splenda® and Sweet'N Low®, etc., have to be eliminated. And not just for the duration of this diet, but for the rest of your life, PLEASE.

The manufacturing of artificial sweeteners is now a multi-billion dollar industry. Note that Aspartame and Splenda® are not manufactured by food companies. They are manufactured by *drug companies!* There are over 6,000 foods and products now that contain them, including OTC medications, chewing gum, and children's vitamins. In Europe they are banned in children's products.

The brand names for aspartame, a synthetic sweetener made by the *drug company* G.D.Searle and Co., are NutraSweet®, and Equal®, Spoonful®, Canderel®, and Equal Measure®. Aspartame's sweetness is two hundred times more intense than white sugar. The constellation of symptoms associated with its use is called Aspartame Poisoning or Aspartame Disease. Worldwide consumer action has exposed this artificial sweetener for the deadly poison it is, and, with any luck, it will be banned in the next few years.

The FDA denied aspartame approval for over eight years because it was continuously shown to cause brain tumors and seizures in lab animals. As food additives, artificial sweeteners are not subject to the same scrutiny of FDA safety trials as pharmaceutical drugs. Additionally, most of the funding of trials was done by the food industry itself, which has an obvious vested interest in the outcome. So, after bowing to enormous political and financial pressure, the FDA gave its final approval in 1981, making it one of the most contested approvals in FDA history.

The FDA lists ninety-two official symptoms and side effects linked to aspartame–including *death*! (Since when is death a *side effect*? I would call it a *direct effect*!) There have been more reports to the FDA about aspartame reactions than for *all other food additives combined.* As of 2010, over 10,000 complaints have been filed. However, by the FDA's own admission, less than one percent of those who have a reaction to a product ever report it. That means that 10,000 translates into nearly a million adverse reactions. Evidence is mounting that it causes or aggravates headaches, seizures, memory loss, neurological disorders (especially multiple sclerosis or MS), visual problems, birth defects, tinnitus, diabetic complications, hypoglycemia, female hair loss, Alzheimer's disease,

Parkinson's disease, chronic fatigue syndrome, cancer, and many other diseases.

Aspartame is made from two amino acids, *aspartic acid and phenylalanine*, which occur naturally with other amino acids in protein. Aspartame uses aspartic acid and phenylalanine *alone,* making an unnatural product *that becomes neurotoxic without the missing amino acids.* It is 40 percent aspartatic acid. When ingested, it passes the blood-brain barrier and significantly raises your level of aspartate, which slowly affects the central nervous system and destroys neurons in the brain. Aspartame and other artificial sweeteners are classified as "excitotoxins," and can literally *stimulate the neurons of the brain to death,* causing changes to the chemistry of the brain and brain damage of varying degrees.

Phenylalanine breaks down into DKP, a brain tumor agent. It is known to lower the seizure threshold and deplete serotonin–*your calming neurotransmitter (*no wonder people who ingest artificial sweeteners complain of insomnia), causing seizures, manic depression, panic attacks, rage, and violence. Suppressed serotonin levels also create cravings for carbohydrates–exactly what you don't want on the yeast-free diet–or any diet!

Aspartame is the main ingredient in NutraSweet® and Equal®. It is 10 percent methanol (wood alcohol), the same poison that causes blindness and death in "skid row" alcoholics. Methanol is highly toxic–the adult minimum dose for toxicity is two teaspoonfuls. If heated above 86 °F, methanol converts to formaldehyde (embalming fluid!), and then into formic acid–the same poison found in the sting of fire ants! Yikes! Our Desert Storm troops drank huge amounts of aspartame-sweetened beverages that had been heated to well over 86 °F in the hot Saudi Arabia sun.

Could the mysterious neurological symptoms many of our service men and women exhibited after they returned from the Middle East have been caused by methanol/formaldehyde poisoning? Formaldehyde is grouped in the same class of drugs as cyanide and arsenic–lethal poisons–

and during research was recently found in the retina of the eye. It doesn't kill as quickly as cyanide and arsenic, but quietly takes its time.

Recent experiments show conclusively that artificial sweeteners interfere directly with the balance of brain chemicals. Just five years after its introduction, the March, 1986, issue of the *Journal of Clinical Nutrition* warned that aspartame (NutraSweet®) in diet colas was linked to depression, mood swings, insomnia and fatigue, due to the creation of an imbalance of neurohormones in various parts of the brain. Powerful lobbying has kept it on the market.

There is excellent evidence that artificial sweeteners actually make you fatter. They can be from 50 to as much as 1,000 times sweeter than sugar, which can cause an abnormal rise in insulin. *When insulin levels are raised, fat is stored.* This is one of the reasons we see weight gain instead of weight loss in those who use them. They can also cause rashes, headaches, mental confusion, and water retention. (More pounds,)

Don't get excited about the new kid on the block, Splenda®, either. It also is manufactured by a drug company–Johnson&Johnson.

Splenda® is made by adding chlorine molecules to sugar molecules. *It is chlorinated sugar.* Chlorine is a powerful carcinogen. It is a chlorocarbon in the same family as chlordane, lindane, and DDT–pesticides! In lab experiments on animals it reduced the amount of good bacteria in the intestines by a whopping 50 percent. Animal studies have shown many problems, such as severely shrunken thymus glands (the keys to the immune system), enlarged livers and kidneys, and decreased red blood count. It also contributed to increased body weight. Oops! Chemically, Splenda® may be more similar to DDT than sugar.

The long-term safety of Splenda® has never been established, as no human research has ever been done. Unbelievably, there is no established system for monitoring and tracking adverse reactions and side effects. It's no wonder European countries have not approved it use, awaiting further review.

Like caffeine, aspartame and most artificial sweeteners are addictive, which makes their manufacturers happy. The more people are hooked, the more money they make. The high-intensity sweetener market is huge–bringing in $1.5 billion a year, providing drug and chemical lobbies with very deep pockets. It seems like greed and profits come before people's lives and health.

Doctors and health professionals everywhere who are informed about this subject are referring to the use of artificial sweeteners as a "plague," causing a "major health disaster," and a "world epidemic." There are many sites on the web that you can visit and study, such as: doorway.com, sweetpoison.com, aspartamekills.com, mercola.com, and many others.

One of the primary benefits of becoming yeast-free is that you lose your cravings for sugar, so why continue to try to thrill your taste buds with artificial sweeteners that will enhance and fuel your desire for sweets?

Artificial sweeteners have no useful function at all, and can only create problems for you. *Banish these menaces from your diet.*

## *Vinegar*

Vinegar is usually a ferment of wine, grain, or cider. It has an alcohol base, and except for distilled vinegar, contains live mold spores. It acidifies blood and tissues, promoting the growth of bacteria, yeast, fungus, and mold. Distilled vinegar is a synthetic made from a petroleum product called glacial acetic acid. Most prepared food products contain vinegar, and unless the label specifies a natural vinegar, in all probability the product contains the cheap distilled kind. Do not use it, or eat anything pickled in it.

## *Artificial Colorings and Preservatives*

More than 2,000 preservatives are allowed in food and drink products in the USA, but only eight in France, five in Belgium and Sweden, and none of those is allowed in food in those countries. The United States government permits *679 artificial ingredients to be used in the mass production of soft drinks alone.* Artificial colors have been linked to cancers. Additives and preservatives decompose food and remove oxygen from whatever they decompose. *This helps yeast to grow.* Also, the liver and pancreas are severely stressed by having to deal with additives, colorings, and preservatives. *Any stressed organ invites yeast to "eat" its damaged tissues.* Monosodium glutamate (MSG) is a flavor enhancer used in processed foods, fast foods, TV dinners, canned foods, seafood, crackers, poultry, and Chinese food. It has been found to cause brain damage in lab animals and has been *banned* from baby food. Ban it from your "grown-up" food also.

### Beef, Pork, and Veal

Almost all commercially raised beef, pork, and veal in the USA are laced with antibiotics, steroids, hormones, herbicides, and pesticides. Pork is forbidden in the Bible, and is the *only meat broth medium on which cancer cells can be encouraged to grow.* Pigs eat anything and everything, *including their own feces!* The cells of pork meat are hard to digest and are so huge they can clog up your kidneys. Pork is also notorious for harboring parasites. Nearly seventy percent of all the antibiotics produced in the United States now go into animal feed. *You eat what they ate!*

Avoid smoked and aged meats as they are often contaminated with yeast mycotoxins.

### Mushrooms

Most people think mushrooms are vegetables. They are not! Mushrooms are *big molds*, or fungi, or more correctly they are the fruit of the fungus which remains underground. They grow on rotting compost in dark, dank bins away from sunlight. Or to put it less politely, they grow in doo-doo in the dark. Yuck. Why would anyone want to eat that! They contain no healthful chlorophyll and contribute to yeast overpopulation in the gut. In the body, mushrooms disperse fungal spores throughout blood and tissue. Mushrooms are known to cause bladder cancer. Don't ingest them ever, if you can help it, including mushroom preparations and extracts sold in health food stores. Mushrooms are polysaccharides, meaning *many carbs.*

We are doing everything we can to *rid* the body of fungi. Why ingest them. Enough said.

### *Condiments*

Condiments, like mustard, mayonnaise, ketchup, soy sauce, and barbecue sauce contain vinegar, sugar, milk products, and loads of preservatives. Read labels carefully.

### *Soft Drinks, Fast Foods, and Frozen Dinners*

In 2005 soft drinks dethroned white bread as the *number one source of calories in the American diet.* In 1946 the average consumption of carbonated soft drinks was 11 gallons per year. In 2000 it had risen to 49 gallons per year. In 2010 it is estimated Americans drink nearly *60 gallons per year*, contributing directly to the rising rates of obesity and diabetes. The American Heart Association recently sounded the alarm about the fact that Americans are now swallowing on average *22 teaspoons of sugar a day* (355 calories), mostly from candy and soft drinks.

As stated above, United States government agencies permits 679 artificial ingredients to be used in the mass production of soft drinks. *Yeast feeds on all 679 of them.* There are 2 teaspoons of sugar per ounce in soft drinks or 10 teaspoons on average in one can. The only reason you don't vomit as a result of the overwhelming sweetness is that the phosphoric acid in soft drinks cuts the flavor. (It also sweeps minerals out of the blood stream. *Soft drinks mean soft bones!*) Soft drinks sweetened with artificial sweeteners are even worse because they are neurotoxic to the brain. Yeast is in heaven when you swig them down.

Fast foods in general are loaded with trans fatty acids, so harmful to the heart and circulatory system, and MSG. Chicken nuggets are the worst. Most chicken made into "nuggets" in fast food franchises are fed a continual diet of antibiotics along with their pesticide-laden feed. Chickens from factory farms are notoriously ridden with many bacteria and viruses. The meat to make nuggets is finely ground with as much skin as possible. (Skin holds all the toxic pesticide, antibiotic residues, and other environmental toxins.) Then partially hydrogenated soybean oil is added (trans fatty acids) to the meat/skin mixture, which are fried in even more hydrogenated soybean or vegetable oil (more trans fatty acids). After that they are served up with another pile of trans fatty acids called french fries! Trans fatty acids go straight to the cell membranes, damaging them and contributing to metabolic syndrome, heightened sugar cravings, obesity, and the inability to lose weight. But their most dangerous characteristic is that they are carcinogens. Lobbying from the huge food manufacturing industry has kept them in our food supply. For your health's sake, keep them out of yours.

As for eating frozen dinners, aside from the cheap ingredients, high sodium content, and artificial colors and flavors that feed yeast, remember that *nobody who made them loves you.*

### Canned Fruits and Vegetables

All canned fruits and vegetables are virtually dead food with very little nutritional value. The canning process destroys valuable enzymes, and vitamins and minerals. Please eat fresh, living food to assist the body in healing itself. Canned tomatoes, tomato sauce, tomato paste, water chestnuts, beans, and tuna can be used on occasion. In addition, make certain cans are not lined with plastic that contains Bisphenol–A (BPA), a powerful toxin.

### DRUG USE

Antibiotics, birth control pills, prescription drugs and hormones should be avoided at all times unless your physician finds them absolutely necessary. They are largely responsible for getting us into this yeast epidemic in the first place.

In the end remember that *diet is the key to the padlock* on the yeast/beast's cage.

## Chapter 10

---

# Eating Yeast–free

*"The wise man should consider that health is the greatest of human blessings. Let your food be your medicine."*

...Hippocrates

Now we are coming to the good part–looking at what you *can* eat. There's hope! As you will readily see, there is a lot to choose from and no one is going to starve to death. Shopping in the grocery store will be very simple, quick, and easy. You won't be buying half the stuff you bought in the past.

Begin by cleaning out the refrigerator and cupboards of everything on the "no-no" list. No reason to keep temptation around. Then head for the health food store or your grocery store and stock the pantry and kitchen with healing foods.

Normally, my family sticks very closely to the diet most of the time, and every three or four months we do it strictly for three weeks to make sure our yeast levels remain low. That way, when we eat out or travel, we feel free to eat whatever we want, but get right back into our usual yeast-free way of living when we get home.

At home you will be modifying your favorite recipes, and most recipes make the transition very well. Have fun and get creative. In recipes that call for mushrooms, eliminate them or substitute water chestnuts. If a recipe calls for bread crumbs, use rolled oats or crushed yeast-free crackers. In recipes calling for milk, use soy, rice, coconut, or almond milk straight or diluted by half with water. You can hardly tell the difference.

It may seem expensive at first as you look at the prices of alternative milks in comparison to cow's milk, or organic meats and vegetables, or yeast-free breads and butter.  But if you look again at the prices of soft drinks, beer, alcohol, beef, pork, bacon, veal, sugars and sugar-filled cereals, cookies, ice creams, etc., things you *won't* be buying very often (or hopefully ever again), you may be spending less.  On top of that, think of the antibiotics and other drugs you won't have to buy (hopefully ever again).  In every way you will come out ahead.

In our house, food is of prime importance. The quality of the food you eat determines the quality of the life you live.

### *Chicken, Fish, Turkey, and Lamb*

Please try to get these organically grown and fresh if possible–*not smoked*. Smoked food is irritating to our digestive systems and can lead to cancer of the stomach and intestine. They also contain polycyclic aromatic hydrocarbons (PAHs ) and mycotoxins.  Seventy percent of conventionally grown broiler chickens in the United States are fed ARSENIC[1], a class-A carcinogen! Lambs are slaughtered early so there is no need to fatten them up or use steroids, antibiotics or hormones.  It is a very clean meat.  Eat wild-caught fish only–not farm-raised.  (In view of the 2010 Gulf of Mexico oil disaster, always check where the fish you purchase comes from.) Canned tuna, salmon, and sardines are okay.

### *Fresh Vegetables*

Organic if possible. The more vegetables you eat, the better. Because veggies contain natural fungal inhibitors which keep them from being consumed by the fungi in the soil, they are naturally anti-fungal and anti-cancer. They protect the body from cancer *by countering the effects of mycotoxins.* They contain vitamins and minerals for healing, and chlorophyll for cleansing. When we eat them, they help inhibit yeast overgrowth in the intestines.  Carrot juice is particularly anti-fungal.

### Beans, Pastas, Potatoes, Rices, and Grains

Remember to eat small to moderate amounts, because of the high carbohydrate counts and the tendency to mold. Rice–actually a seed–not a grain, is very easy to digest. Brown and wild rice are high in protein and very nourishing.

*Eat corn in limited amounts.* We eat high quantities of corn since it is ubiquitous in our food supply. Cattle, poultry, pigs, sheep, and farm-raised fish are fattened on corn. We eat eggs from corn fed chickens. It is in corn starch, corn oil, corn syrups, and many processed foods. It is in juices, soft drinks, and even toothpastes. You'll find it in yogurt, ketchup, mayonnaise, mustard, deli meats, salad dressings, and vitamin pills. If we are what we eat, guess what. *We're corn!* Considering the fact that most of our corn is genetically modified (GM) and is contaminated with mold, please eat sparingly.. Sorry popcorn lovers.

### Fruits

Eat only one or two a day from the acceptable list the first month, preferably for breakfast. One small glass (4–6oz.) of juice counts as one serving.

### Butter

Enjoy! It is made from pure fat and contains only traces of lactose or milk sugar to feed yeast. It is a good natural source of gamma linoleic acid known for its anti-inflammatory properties, and is full of vitamin A. It is rich in short and medium chain fatty acids and has strong anti-tumor and anti-cancer properties. It also increases the absorption of many other nutrients found in other foods. Be sure to buy hormone-free, organic butter if you can.

### Eggs

Purchase organic eggs when possible. They are much more nutritious than factory-farmed eggs. They come from chickens that are raised naturally and are allowed to scratch on real ground for their food. Also, they benefit from natural sunlight and from being around roosters, which keeps their hormones balanced. Commercial chickens are raised in unnatural environments, where they live in crowded cages, never see sunlight, and are artificially stimulated by artificial light to make them lay more eggs. Their feed is mixed with antibiotics, dyes, hormones, tranquilizers, plus their own *recycled waste*. To add insult to injury, they are fed growth steroids which cause bacteria to proliferate, and *then* they must be fed antibiotics to control the bacteria!

### Soymilk, Rice Milk, Almond Milk, Hemp Milk, and Coconut Milk

There are many wonderful and delicious soymilks and other alternative milk products on the market now. Vitasoy®, EdenSoy®, and Westbrae® are three favorites. Better Than Milk® really does taste better than milk. Some make Lite lines if you want to cut calories. The new hemp milks and coconut milks are excellent. Much of our soymilk in the USA is now genetically modified, so be sure to buy only organic soymilk or soy products. Do not be concerned with small amounts of evaporated cane juice in these milks. Actually, it is good to introduce small amounts of sugar (in the form of honey, maple syrup and cane juice) into the body to stimulate the immune system–especially the pancreas–in a homeopathic manner. If there are no stimuli, the immune system will become lazy and depleted!

### Yeast–Free Breads

They are out there, and most are delicious. I always toast and butter them and add a sprinkle of sea salt. French Meadow makes a superb line of yeast-free breads. Most tortillas are yeast-free, but read the labels. Rice cakes can be used for bread in a pinch. Toast lightly to crispen them.

### Nuts and Nut Butters

Some of the other versions of the yeast-free diet restrict peanuts and peanut butter, if not all nuts, because of their tendency to mold. Most of our patients eat nuts and nut butters in moderation and get well anyway, so we don't see any reason to eliminate them. Please, *always stir one-half teaspoon of powdered vitamin C into your nut butters* before you refrigerate them. This will neutralize any molds that may have started growing there. Try cashew butter and almond butter, or sunflower butter for a change. My husband is hooked on almond butter.

### Honey, Maple Syrup, Rice Syrup, Unsweetened Apple Butter

Honey is the only food on the planet that will not spoil or rot. (Never boil or microwave it.) Moderate, occasional amounts won't hurt, such as a couple of cookies made with honey, or 2–3 tablespoons of honey or maple syrup on pancakes once a week. Refrigerate maple syrup and any unsweetened jams or fruit butters.

### Baking Powder Breads, Pancakes, and Waffles

Muffins, biscuits, cornbread, pancakes, and waffles can all be made using half water and half alternative milks for the milk. Most recipes are easy to convert, and taste very good. Use aluminum-free baking powder. Rumford baking powder, found in health food stores, is excellent.

### Beverages

Pero®, Roma®, and Dandy Blend® are delicious coffee substitutes, as is Take-A-Break® herb tea by Bigelow. Herb teas are fine, plus occasional fruit juices diluted by half with water are acceptable. Drink filtered or spring water only, to keep chlorine and other additives out of your body. Perrier and other natural mineral waters with fresh lemon or lime are delicious.

If you do buy juices, please read labels like a hawk. The front label may say "100% natural, no sugar added," but when you read the list of ingredients you may find the sweetener is concentrated grape juice–a big no-no, since grapes are forbidden. *Always dilute fruit juices with water or Perrier to cut the sugar content.*

One of our favorite beverages, especially during the summer, is tea made by brewing 2 teabags of Lemon Zinger, 2 teabags of Red Zinger to

make 4 cups, and add 4 cups unsweetened apple juice.  Refrigerate.  It is
delicious.  Experiment with other herb teas for variety.

### Condiments

Mayonnaise, mustard, and ketchup must be homemade.  Check my recipes
in *The Yeast-Free Kitchen.*

### Snacks

Popcorn – occasionally only. Corn is a grain, not a vegetable, and our corn
crops are now genetically modified and very contaminated with mold.
Roasted and salted pumpkin seeds, rice chips with homemade salsa, hummus
or guacamole make delicious snacks. Yeast-free crackers and nut butters are
my favorites. Also, almonds, walnuts, and pecans are good high protein,
anti-inflammatory foods.

### Cheeses

These have to be soy or rice cheeses, of course. They bake especially well.
Check labels carefully as some alternative cheeses have started adding yeast
extract for flavor! In the third month you may have small amounts of sheep
or goat feta. (Goat and sheep cheeses and fetas are alkaline producing,
whereas cow's milk cheeses are acid producing.)

### Oils

Be careful of corn, safflower and canola oils as their omega 3 and omega 6
ratios are not the healthiest. Your best oils are *cold-pressed olive oil, coconut
oil, nut oils, and flax oil.*

### Salt

Be sure to use *unrefined sea salt only.*  The stuff from the grocery store is
over-processed and most of the natural minerals have been removed.
Unrefined sea salt contains over eighty minerals essential to human health.

Salt is as important to life as oxygen and water. (Animals walk miles to find natural salt licks.) Salt and water work together to carry out important functions in our bodies, including stimulating metabolism, assisting in detoxification, and making sure our nerve, hormone, and immune systems are working properly. Many people who have been put on salt-restricted diets have found they can eat sea salt with no elevations in blood pressure.

So as you can see there is *plenty* to eat. There is no reason for someone who doesn't need to lose weight to lose weight, and there is every reason for someone who needs to lose weight, to do so.

If you are already underweight, try to eat five or six times a day. Drink almond milk, eat nuts, potatoes, oils, etc., and you shouldn't lose weight. In an overweight person, as the body balances and the metabolism wakes up, the pounds drop off naturally.

Following is a partial list of foods by brand names you can find in health food stores. It will help you get started. Some may be found in grocery stores. If they don't carry them, ask the manager to order them for you. Most are very obliging. Also, please continue to check ingredients as manufacturers change recipes frequently. Most of these items can be found in Whole Foods.

# In Health Food Stores

*Frozen Foods*

>Amy's Tamale with Roasted Vegetables
>Amy's Thai Stir Fry
>
>Rice Dream Ice Creams:
>Strawberry, Wildberry, Vanilla, Carob Bars–Vanilla dipped in Carob Coating

*Cheese Substitutes*

**Rice Vegan:**
Cheddar
Mozarella

**Lisanatti:**
Almond Jalapeno Jack
Almond Mozarella
Almond Cheddar Style

*Seasonings*

Bernard Jenson's Natural Vegetable Seasoning and Instant Gravy
Bragg Liquid Aminos
De Souza's Solar Sea Salt
Herbamare
Morga Instant Extract of Vegetables
Santay Garlic Seasoning
Trocomare
Vege-Sal–does contain a small amount of soy sauce, but okay

*Instant Soups*

**Nile Spice:**
Black Bean
Chicken Noodle
Italian Tomato
Lentil
Lentil Curry
Sweet Corn
Tomato Minestrone
Vegetable Chicken

*Dried Soups*

**Montebello Kitchens:**
Peanut Soup

**Frontier Soups:**
Corn Chowder
White Bean
Wild Rice

**Bob's Red Mill:**
13 Bean Soup Mix
Vegi Soup Mix

*Canned Soups*

**Health Valley:**
Black Bean
Minestrone
**Amy's:**
Curried Lentil
Minestrone
Split Pea
Tuscan Bean
**Lucini:**
Italian Minestrone
Umbrian Lentil

*Spaghetti Sauces*

**Lucini:**
Rustic Tomato Basil Sauce

Spicy Tuscan Tomato Sauce
Tuscan Marinara
**Amy's:**
Family Marinara

**Mario Batali:**
Marinara
Tomato Basil
**Rao's:**
Marinara
Tomato Basil
**Paesano:**
Roasted Garlic

## *Soydrinks or Acceptable Milk Substitutes*

Almond Breeze
Better Than Milk
EdenSoy
Hemp Dream
Rice Dream
Silk
So Delicious Coconut Milk
Soy Moo
Vanilla Almond Milk
Vitasoy Creamy Original or Carob (chocolate substitute)
WestSoy

## *Cereals, Dry*

Rusketts from La Loma

**Arrowhead Mills:**
Puffed Wheat
Shredded Wheat Bite Size

**Udi's:**
>Vanilla Granola
>Au Naturelle

*Cereals, Hot*

>**Arrowhead Mills:**
>>Instant Oatmeal
>>Rice and Shine
>>Steel Cut Oats

>**Bob's Red Mill:**
>>Creamy Wheat
>>5 Grain
>>Oat Bran
>>Steel Cut Oats

*Mixes*

>Organic Buckwheat Pancake and Waffle Mix
>Organic Gluten Free Pancake and Baking Mix
>Montebello Kitchens Virginia Spoonbread Mix

**\* Whey is allowed after 21 days.**

*Chips*

>**Lundberg** Rice Chips
>**365** Veggie Chips
>**Kettle** Potato Chips

>**Garden of Eatin':**
>>Black Bean Chips
>>Mini Yellow Rounds
>>Pico de Gallo
>>Red Hot Blues
>>Sesame Blues

Sunflower Blues

**Terra:**
Stripes and Blues
Sweet Potato Carrot Chips
Sweet Potato Chips
Taro Chips

## *Crackers*

**Bible Bread** crackers:
Oregano and Sesame
Five Whole Grains

**Blue Diamond:**
Almond Nut Thins
Hazelnut Nut Thins
Pecan Nut Thins

**Brown Rice Snaps**
Onion Garlic

**Carr's** Table Water Crackers

**Lundberg's** Brown Rice and Wild Rice Cakes

**Margaret's Artisan Bakery**
Rosemary & Sea Salt
and others

**Susie's:**
Rosemary and Sesame Crackers
Kamut Puffed Cakes
Puffed Rice Thin Cakes

**365** Baked Woven Wheat

**Wasa** Light Rye Crispbread

*Cookies*
> Jennies Macaroons–plain, carob, carob chip

*Yeast–Free Breads:*

> Rudolph's Rye

> **French Meadow:**
>> Hemp Bread
>> Sourdough Rye
>> Spelt Bread
>> Spelt Muffins
>> Summer Bread

> **Essene Breads:**
>> Five Seed
>> Multigrain
>> Rye

*Spreads*:

> **Bionaturae:**
>> Apricot Fruit Spread
>> Organic Bilberry
>> Strawberry
>> Wild Berry

> **FiordiFrutta:**
>> The entire line

> **Kime's** Apple Butter Spread

> *365* Organic Almond Butter

**365** Organic Creamy Peanut Butter
**MaraNatha** Creamy Peanut Butter
**Redmond's** Creamy Almond Butter

*Boxed Grain Dishes:*

**Casbah:**
   Couscous
   Couscous Pilaf

**Near East:**
   Couscous Moroccan Pasta
   Falafel Vegetable Burger Mix
   Spanish Rice Mix
   Tabouli Wheat Salad Mix

**Fantastic Food's** Tabouli Mix

*Miscellaneous*

Roma, Pero, and Dandy Blend are excellent coffee substitutes.
Asman's Baba Ghannoug, Hommus, and Tabouleh are highly
   recommended
Bubbies Kosher Dill Pickles have no vinegar and are delicious.
Jane's Crazy Mixed-Up Salt
Chebe Focaccia Flatbread Mix
Chebe Pizza Crust Mix

# In the Grocery Store:

*Spreads:*

Tap'n Apple apple butter spread
Laura Scudder's Peanut Butter

Smucker's Natural Peanut Butter
Camp's 100% Pure Maple Syrup

*Crackers:*

Carr's Table Water Crackers
Hol-Grain's Brown Rice and Whole Wheat Crackers
Lawry's Taco Shells
Manischewitz Matzos
Quaker Rice Cakes and Butter Pop Corn Cakes
Sesmark Sesame Thins
Triscuits Original

*Dried Soup Mixes:*

Bean Cuisine soup mixes and many others

*Canned Soups:*

Imagine Organic Creamy Butternut Squash
Imagine Organic Free Range Chicken Broth
Imagine Organic Harvest Corn
Imagine Organic Vegetable Broth

*Spaghetti Sauces:*

Alessi Homemade Marinara Sauce
Classico Sun Dried Tomato
Classico Tomato and Basil
Hunt's Italian Garlic and Herb
Tasty Tomato Basil and Garlic
Lucini Spicy Tuscan Tomato Sauce
Rao's Homemade Marinara Sauce

*Fruits and Juices:*

Del Monte Pineapple in its own juices
Martinelli Apple Juice
Mott's Natural Applesauce with Vitamin C
Mott's Natural Fresh Pressed Apple Juice
Ocean Spray 100% Grapefruit Juice
Old Orchard Premium 100 % Tart Cherry Juice
Tree Top Apple Juice
Treetop Unsweetened Applesauce
V-8 Juice

*Cereals:*

Aunt Jemima Grits, old fashioned or quick cooking
Cream of Rice
Cream of Wheat
Hodgson Mill Oat Bran
Nabisco Shredded Wheat and Spoon Size Shredded Wheat
Old Fashioned Quaker Oats and Multi-Grain
Post Original Shredded Wheat
Uncle Sam

*Chips:*

El Galindo tortilla chips
Fritos corn chips
Lay's Classic Potato Chips
Tostitos tortilla chips
Utz Kettle Classic Crunchy Potato Chips

**Remember–it is always cheaper to stay healthy than it is to get sick!**

**Chapter 11**

---

# The Healing Diet in a Nutshell

*"Those who think they have no time for healthy eating will sooner or later have to find time for illness."*

*...Edward Stanley*

As you know, this book is about a tiny one-celled microorganism–*Candida albicans*, which normally resides in our gastrointestinal tract in a contained fashion. Because of extraordinary circumstances, which I explore throughout the book, this normally benign "germ" escapes from its cage, the intestines–where it was designed to live–and goes on a rampage. The little yeast transforms itself into a ravenous beast–dangerous, destructive, and deadly.

The only way order can be re-established in our bodies is for the yeast/beast to be subdued, cornered, and backed into its original cage (the intestinal tract). The lion is my metaphor for the menacing, ferocious yeast/beast searching for his supper. This metaphor is a simple and effective way of helping you picture in your mind what has happened inside your body. It will also help you visualize the victory you will achieve as you learn how to establish control over the voracious monster. YOU become the "lion tamer," cracking your whip over the beast, showing it who is boss. YOU become the healer. YOU become the Victor. Once the yeast/beast realizes it has no power over you, it will settle down and behave, living peacefully inside its cage.

My aim is to teach you how to become that lion tamer. With practice and commitment it isn't hard, and can even be fun. But most important of all, as you gain mastery over the beast, you will regain mastery over your health and your life.

The first step is to pick up your whip, and:

# *For an average duration of three months do not eat or drink:*

*Sugar or artificial sweeteners of any kind,* including fructose, maltose, lactose, sucrose, galactose, molasses, date sugar, maple sugar, turbinado sugar, glycogen, mannitol, monosaccharides, polysaccharides, Agave, NutraSweet®, Equal®, Sweet'NLow®, Splenda®, and saccharine.

*Alcohol* in any form, including anything fermented such as cider or root beer.

*Breads* containing yeast, including pita bread and most crackers.

*Milk products* of all kinds, including yogurt, cheese, cottage cheese, ice cream or dry milk solids. Whey allowed after three weeks.

*Red Meats*, such as beef, veal, pork, or any smoked meats.

**Caffeine**, including coffee, de-caf, tea, and chocolate.

*Bananas, Grapes, Plums, Raisins, and All Dried Fruit*, including prunes.

*Mushrooms*

*Brewer's Yeast and Yeast Extracts*

*Vinegar* of all kinds or anything pickled, such as sauerkraut.

*Condiments*, such as ketchup, commercial mayonnaise, mustard, pickles, Worcestershire, soy sauce, miso, tamari, barbecue sauces, relishes, steak and chili sauces, green olives, and horseradish.

*Preservatives, artificial colors and dyes*

*Margarine*

*Soft Drinks and any drinks in aluminum cans*

*Canned fruits and vegetables,* except for tomatoes, tomato sauce and paste.

*Chocolate*

*Antibiotics*, birth control pills, prescription drugs, steroids, and hormones should be avoided unless your physician finds them absolutely necessary.

*NOTE:* Artificial sweeteners, brewers yeast, bakers yeast, soft drinks, margarine, and mushrooms should be banned from your diet forever.

# *You may eat and drink:*

Chicken, fish, turkey or lamb, preferably organic, not smoked

Venison, rabbit, and all wild game

Fresh vegetables, preferably organic

Potatoes, yams, pastas, corn, beans, and rice in moderation

Grains, such as wheat, barley, rye, oats, millet, quinoa, amaranth, buckwheat, grits, and couscous in moderation

Oranges, lemons, limes, strawberries, kiwi, apples, pears, peaches, raspberries, blueberries, watermelon, cantaloupe, papaya

Butter

Eggs (preferably organic or non-GMO)

Oils, such as safflower, soy, corn, flax, coconut and extra-virgin olive, non-GMO

Soymilk and soy cheeses without yeast extracts, rice, almond hemp and coconut milks (preferably organic or non–GMO)

Yeast-free breads, including yeast-free natural sourdough

Tortillas, wheat or corn, and rice cakes

Tortilla chips and homemade guacamole

Nuts and nut butters, such as almond butter, cashew butter

Honey, maple syrup, rice syrup, barley malt, evaporated cane juice (very small amounts), and unsweetened apple butter in small amounts

Muffins, cornbread, biscuits, pancakes made with soymilk, almond milk, etc.

Tofu in small amounts

Herb teas and unsweetened juices

Filtered water, spring water, mineral waters

Popcorn, (in small amounts) pumpkin seeds, sunflower seeds

Carob powder and unsweetened carob chips

Roma®, Pero®, "Dandy Blend®" or Take-A-Break® herb tea instead of coffee

Rice Dream® and Purely Decadent® Coconut ice cream (small amounts)

You have just read the best "prescription" there is for your health. It is called simply, "the yeast-free diet." This miracle of a diet is transforming lives everywhere, every day, as news of its healing power spreads from friend to friend, family to family, and slowly but surely from doctor to patient.

Tell everyone you love.

**Chapter 12**

---

# Supplements

*"He causeth the grass to grow for the cattle, and herbs for the service of Man."*

...Psalms 104:4

To assist the body as it detoxifies and heals, there are a number of supplements that Sylvia recommends to most of her patients. All of these can be found in health food stores or large grocery stores.

Physicians who treat Candida have been using a drug called Nystatin® for years. It is effective, especially when a patient is close to dying from being eaten alive by Candida, but it does have some drawbacks:

Number one, it is a drug.
Number two, it is an antibiotic!
Number three, Candida has a tendency to return with a vengeance when Nystatin® is stopped.

It is important to remember that drugs do not cure, and Nystatin® is a drug. It only kills Candida in the gastrointestinal tract–and in the vagina if used topically. It does not affect Candida in the blood or tissue. It is not effective for all types of fungus, since many strains are resistant to it. Also, Nystatin® itself is a mold by-product (a derivative of *Streptomyces noursei*), and people who are sensitive to molds may react adversely to it.

The good news is Nystatin® is not a broad-spectrum antibiotic that wipes out yeasts *and* bacteria, creating the perfect scenario for the proliferation of yeast. It is a *single* target antibiotic that kills only yeast. The intestinal flora is not disturbed very much.

The bad news is we are beginning to see new and more resistant strains of yeast that are not responding to Nystatin® and drugs like it, e.g., ketoconazole, fluconazole, itraconazole, and miconazole.

Many people have found Nystatin® to be only a temporary cure, and as soon as they stop taking it, the yeast flares up again, known as a "rebound reaction." It seems drugs only drive the pathogens deeper into tissue, and stronger and stronger drugs have to be developed to cope with them. We have witnessed this many times in medical history. Now it is taking stronger and stronger drugs and antibiotics to knock out diseases.

Are we really helping ourselves when the treatment of disease with drugs only encourages new, more resistant strains of viruses, bacteria, and yeast? The very use of these drugs has harmful and, in some cases, fatal side effects. The liver and kidneys are hit especially hard by drugs. Even before drugs are prescribed, vital organs are valiantly struggling to perform, while coping with large colonies of fungi that are sapping the very life force from them.

*Doesn't it seem strange to treat a condition CAUSED by drugs and antibiotics, WITH drugs and antibiotics?*

As I said before, drugs do not cure the body, only the body can cure itself–and only if it is given the proper tools. Drugs just mask symptoms and reroute enzyme systems. They do nothing to correct the basic imbalance that paved the way for disease to take hold. They don't get to the *cause* of disease, they just drive it deeper into tissue where it waits until another stress–mental, physical, or spiritual–comes along to activate it and *cause the original disease to erupt again, many times disguised as a more serious disease.*

So, for that reason, Sylvia only works *with* nature and the natural laws of cure. Using only diet, herbs, vitamins and minerals, homeopathics, and other natural remedies, she skillfully guides the body back to its memory of wholeness.

If you are very ill or severely debilitated with cancer or any other major illness, or you are obese, or have symptoms of yeast in the brain, such as hallucinations or hearing voices, please commit to three to six months or longer of supplementation. Use your own discretion here.

### *Natural Anti-Fungals*

In the health food store, look for grapefruit seed extract, olive leaf extract, oregano oil, caprylic acid, Kyolic® garlic, or Candida Cleanse® by Rainbow Light. All are excellent yeast fighters. Use one product at a time. It is best to rotate them.

All will start killing yeast immediately, and as long as you don't feed existing yeast with the food they like, no new colonies will form. Yeast grows in cycles, some hours long, some days long, and some weeks long. If you keep ingesting antifungals and watching your diet, all the cycles will be interrupted and their forward progress will be stopped.

- *NOTE*: Do not take yeast control supplements if you are pregnant. Instead drink Pau D'Arco (also called Taheebo) tea every day. It is a tea made from the bark of the Pau D'Arco tree in the Brazilian rainforests. Rainforests are notorious for moisture, warmth, and the subsequent growths of mold, but the bark of the Pau D'Arco trees miraculously remain mold-free and doesn't decay. Two cups made with one tea bag daily will do it.

### *Kidney Cleansers*

It is a good idea to cleanse the kidneys of Candida while on the diet. Use KB-11 herbs in capsules (KB stands for kidney–bladder), Cran-Aid capsules®, or K-Help®, by Hannah Kroeger. I have seen people with as little as 14 percent kidney function (from yeast clogging and damaging the delicate tubules of the kidneys) go up to 90 percent renal function in a matter of weeks, just using the yeast-free diet and kidney herbs. Both clean and rebuild kidneys as well as speed up detoxification. Both are wonderful in eliminating unwanted water weight.

## *Vitamins, Minerals, and Fatty Acids*

A moderate amount of vitamins and minerals may be taken–all natural, yeast and dairy free, of course. Sylvia usually recommends 1,000 to 3,000 milligrams extra vitamin C and 400 IU of vitamin E daily, along with 50-100 milligrams B complex (be sure B complex vitamins are extracted from veggies and contain no yeast!), and 1 gram of calcium with 500 milligrams of magnesium. Take the B complex with lunch and the calcium/magnesium with the dinner meal or a bedtime. If you are anemic, take some organic iron or a homeopathic for iron as directed. Anemia invites yeast to grow.

Sylvia directs many patients to supplement their diets with fatty acids of some kind to combat inflammation. Omega-3 fatty acids, primrose oil, or flaxseed oil are acceptable. When cooking, use only cold-pressed oils from the health food store, such as olive oil or coconut oil. They will help the formation of healthy prostaglandins, which are hormone-like substances vital to your immune system.

## *Probiotics*

Be sure to supplement daily with a high-quality probiotic to rebuild healthy intestinal flora. They are live beneficial microorganisms that aid in digestion and help restore the immune system. There are many excellent brands to choose from. Check with the folks at your health food store and ask which one they recommend. Probiotics help replace the beneficial bacteria the yeast/beast devoured and help you to absorb more of the nutrients from your food.

## *The Bath*

Another facet of Sylvia's healing program is her soaking bath. The purpose of this bath is to open the pores of the skin so toxins can come out more quickly. At least once a week, and no more than three times a week, at the end of the day, put two tea bags of chamomile tea in a pot with eight cups of water. Bring to a boil, and boil for fifteen minutes. Then dump the chamomile water plus the tea bags into a bath tub full of comfortably warm-hot water, along with one-third cup sea salt and one-third cup hydrogen peroxide. Get under the water up to your chin, and relax and soak for twenty minutes. Use a wash cloth and trace circular motions on the skin to help open the pores further. *Use no soap!* Towel dry, and go straight to bed. You will be relaxed by the chamomile tea, and ready for sleep. After you are well, these baths can be used anytime you feel you are coming down with something, or just as a part of your general program of prevention.

Basically, this will keep you busy, and we don't want to overwhelm you or your body with too much to do. The diet and simple supplementation will knock the yeast for a loop, and the body will slowly but surely adjust to its new levels of health.

Always remember healing is gradual, and several months will be needed to normalize body functions. You didn't get sick overnight, and you won't get well overnight. Healing is similar to peeling the layers of an onion. You have to peel one layer at a time. Yeast that has burrowed deep into tissue will remain there until the layer of yeast on top of it is starved.

Be patient and trust in the healing forces of nature to do their jobs.

They know what to do.

**Chapter 13**

# The Healing Begins

*"Wherefore fear not ye that have suffered, for healing shall be your portion."*

...Enoch 96:3

After a few days on the program you may feel worse. As hard as it is to believe, *that's good. It means the yeast overgrowths have started dying.*

When alive, yeast can evade the immune system by changing its shape and identity, but when killed, yeast cell-wall proteins are absorbed through damaged and weakened mucous membranes and start causing allergic reactions. There are antibodies in the body at various sites wherever *Candida albicans* has lived. They react and start triggering the immune system to seek out and destroy those foreign antigens.

As large numbers of yeast die, the membranes absorb their toxic products so your symptoms may worsen temporarily.

This is called a "healing crisis," "die-off," or the "Herxheimer reaction." The most important thing to remember is it is normal, will not hurt you, and is not terminal. It is simply the body healing so quickly that it is producing symptoms as a result of toxic or allergy-like reactions to the dead and dying yeast being dumped into the bloodstream. The body is actually being sickened by dead fungus. *But not to worry,* they eventually will be eliminated through the bowels, kidneys, or skin.

Symptoms can arise in the body wherever yeast toxins have acted most strongly, and any symptom of yeast overgrowth which you had before can become worse. Headaches, body aches and soreness, extreme fatigue, bloating, stuffiness, sore throats, diarrhea, flu-like symptoms, and general misery are all common. As yeast die, they need to come out of wherever they have been living and, unfortunately for us, that process can become uncomfortable. But fortunately for us, it usually doesn't last very long. Two to seven days is the average.

At times the body will *crave the very food it is cleansing from the body.* Sometimes these cravings can be excruciatingly strong. Just keep remembering it is only the yeast screaming like spoiled, demanding children, to be fed again. Don't fall for their whining.

Because each body is unique, and each body has its favored avenues of detoxification, each will reflect "die off" individually. In some people, the healing crisis may be so mild as to be unnoticeable. In others, they close the curtains and crawl into bed to wait it out. In some, the route of detoxification may be the colon in the form of diarrhea, while in others it may be the skin in the form of acne. I have received phone calls from a number of patients in their forties, moaning that they looked like they had teenage acne, and felt like walking around with a paper sack on their heads! Occasionally–two or three weeks into the diet–some clients break out in rashes, which is indicative of the liver throwing off more toxins. But, never fear, this too shall pass.

When Sylvia gets phone calls from patients complaining they feel worse after seeing her, she always says "Congratulations!" In this case, worse means better, and is a wonderful sign the body is swinging into action and the yeast/beast is on the run.

One of the best things you can do to help yourself through this uncomfortable time is to drink plenty of fluids and remember to take your detox baths. Cran-Aid tea is a godsend here as it cleans the kidneys and bladder clogged with yeast. Get plenty of rest because your body is going through a lot of changes quickly while working hard to clean itself. A lot of energy is required in this process, so it is no wonder you may feel fatigued, if not exhausted.

Also, don't be surprised if you have a few days when you feel great and then, WHAM, you feel like you have run into a brick wall, as old symptoms return. That is normal, too, because yeasts live in cycles. Your bad days, or hours, are just corresponding to the start of another cycle of growth spewing out more mycotoxins. As long as you stay on the program and don't feed them what they want, they, too, will die.

The entire healing process, using Sylvia's diet, usually requires three months. It takes that long to catch all the cycles of yeast that try to get footholds. And, as I have said earlier, if you have a serious disease (especially cancer), are obese, or have mental manifestations of yeast overgrowths, it can take up to six months to a year.

As you come to the end of the three months and are ready to try some of the restricted foods, please do so very slowly. You can't run out the first day and celebrate with pizza and beer. You may have severe reactions, so we advise you to go slowly and gently.

The first day you may want to try half of a banana, but stay on the diet for the rest of the day. The next day, add another item and stay on the diet for the rest of the day. That way you can watch for allergic reactions such as headaches, muscle aches, nausea, etc. If they do occur, hop back on the diet for a little longer and try other no-no's very gingerly.

To me, the real beauty of this diet is that you will be changed. You will be changed both mentally and physically. Slowly but surely, cravings and addictions, which originated from the yeast themselves, no longer exist. Mood swings, fatigue, aches and pains–all are gone. Pounds have melted away, the skin glows, eyes are bright, and energy has returned.

Mental processes are clear, memory returns, and attitudes become positive. A beautiful serenity comes over you and the world seems like a nicer place.

People will start noticing these positive changes and comment on them. Some may even ask you what you have been doing. I hope you tell them! You may even be asked if you had a facelift!

I have seen people literally become transformed while following the yeast-free program. One sweet lady in particular comes to mind. She appeared to be in her late fifties.

She arrived at our office for her first appointment with Sylvia within a few days of checking out of a mental hospital where she had been treated for severe depression. While in the hospital, she was put on six different powerful mood-altering drugs, none of which helped, and had experienced severe side effects. She was dirty, her clothes were rumpled and torn, she was thirty pounds overweight, and she smelled bad. She was hunched over, wouldn't look anyone in the eye, seemed confused, and mumbled when she spoke.

When she returned for a check-up just four weeks later, she came in standing erect, was neat and clean from head to toe, had lost ten pounds, and exuded self-confidence. She also looked ten years younger. It took her several more months to complete the transformation, but she did it.

Several times we have witnessed people who arrived for their first appointment actually hallucinating from yeast in the brain. It must have been terrifying experiences for them. One client had lost twenty pounds in one month prior to her appointment due to anxiety alone. In 48 hours on the diet, the hallucinations vanished and she came back into her own consciousness.

In metaphysical terms, *yeast infection is a form of possession.* And the yeast-free diet can be considered a form of exorcism. If you are a slave to whatever you are addicted to, you are not in control of your consciousness or behavior. That constitutes the classic definition of possession. Conversely, if you are free of addictions and are in control of your thought processes, you are free from any outside control and truly are liberated.

The yeast-free diet has the power to raise you into a higher consciousness and liberate you from the junkyards of your past. As the body becomes clean and the mind becomes clear, you truly will look, think, and act differently. You truly will be transformed. You will have recreated and reinvented yourself.

Just as you are happier living in a house that is clean, harmonious and peaceful, your soul requires a body to live in that is clean, harmonious, and peaceful as well.

Both benefit and prosper as a result.

**Chapter 14**

---

# The Body–Mind Connection

*"Mind is ever the builder. That which the body-mind feeds upon, that it gradually becomes."*

...Edgar Cayce(3102–1)

In working with her patients, Sylvia, in most instances, assigns "homework." She is a firm believer that "emotions always make the nest for disease," and has preached this philosophy for many years. Negative and unmanaged emotions set the stage before disease makes its debut. They will feed the disease unless they are resolved, removed, and forgiven. After the negative memories and emotions are addressed, she works carefully to re-program the subconscious mind in order to "seal the healings."

Our conscious minds are only able to process approximately 50 bits of information per second, *while our subconscious minds process approximately 11 million bits* per second. In other words, our unconscious minds process information 220,000 times faster than our conscious minds![1] This powerful part of our brains has extremely important ramifications in our lives and must be attended to if we want to be successful in changing our beliefs about ourselves, the world, and others, or want to make changes in our habits, preferences or behaviors. Accessing the subconscious and re-programming it is critical for healing to be complete and lasting. A simple exercise helps facilitate this process.

Patients are sent home with an assignment. Before they return for their next appointment, they are instructed to write about any and all of the painful issues, events, and memories of their lives. They are to look carefully at their relationships with their parents, spouses, or ex-spouses, children, friends, etc., living or dead, current or going back to childhood, and write about any part of those relationships that resulted in anger, guilt feelings, or painful memories.

Some patients return with short, simple letters while others return with reams of paper. In those letters and papers is healing. The simple act of writing about their feelings, no matter how old or deeply buried, enables them to get in touch again with their original emotions.

These emotions are buried within the cells of our bodies, not just the cells in our brains. Edgar Cayce said many times that each cell has its own consciousness. In releasing our emotions through pen and paper, we can stop running the "old tapes" of remembering or reliving old hurtful memories. That process allows us to heal properly and completely.

Sylvia provides her patients with a form to use that helps them write their letters. I included a copy at the end of the chapter. Place a sheet of paper next to the form and write at the top of the page the name of the person you had issues with, such as "mother". Then go down the list and write about whatever seems appropriate. Every lead-in sentence on the template form does not need to be completed, only the ones that spring to mind. Then place another sheet of paper next to the form and write another person's name. Write until you can't write anymore. Most especially, write until the tears come. *Then cry until you can cry no more.* With tears comes the releasing of emotions that are connected to the memories. And when the original emotions are released and healed, the body will follow. ***The body always follows the mind.***

Over the years I have witnessed time and again this profoundly simple–but not always easy–approach. These healing letters carefully guide you from feelings of anger, resentment, fear, pain, and guilt, to feelings of understanding, forgiveness, and love. They are powerful. And they work.

The next step after the letter is written is to *read it out loud.* The best person to hear it is a family member, a good friend, or a therapist. (The Bible affirms this practice by telling us to "bear ye one another's burdens," and "therefore confess your sins to each other and pray for each other so that you may be healed.") They are to listen and make no comments or judgments on what you have written. They are there to encourage and assist you in healing yourself. It might not be easy, but it will be worth it. When you are finished, rip the letters into pieces, and either burn them or flush them down the toilet. The Bible affirms this practice in James. "Therefore confess your sins to one another and pray for each other so that you may be healed."[2]

The subconscious is not stupid, but takes its clues *literally*–from what it sees and hears. The subconscious "sees" the toxic thoughts coming out of the brain, down the arm, into the hand, and out through the pen and onto paper. Then it "hears" the paper being ripped into pieces and flushed away. It sees, hears, and even smells–if the paper is being burned–the damaging memories being destroyed. This act literally "re-programs" the subconscious.

By going through this process you are teaching the subconscious mind, that the *original thoughts and memories which were responsible for initiating the disease process are being released and healed–both at cellular and soul levels.* The subconscious gets the message that those old "tapes" are now "disconnected" from the body and can no longer manifest as disease.

In Proverbs we are told, "As a man thinketh in his heart, so is he." This is one of the most powerful statements in the Bible. Notice the implication that we think *not only* in our brains *but also* in our hearts! In actuality, our "brains" are located in all cells throughout our bodies. Each cell has a consciousness that is connected to the whole.

The ancient Hebrews were trying to tell us of the intimate connection that exists between our minds and our bodies, and that our bodies truly are manifestations of the workings of our minds. That may be hinted at in the Lord's Prayer when Jesus said, "Thy will be done on earth as it is in heaven." In a metaphysical interpretation, earth is our body and heaven is our mind. He may have been alluding to that body-mind connection.

Just a few years ago, it was impossible to find a textbook on immunology that even mentioned the brain. As a matter of fact, not only was there *no* chapter on the brain, *"brain" wasn't even listed in the index!* Yet for centuries medicine has known of and employed the placebo effect, one of the most powerful "mind medicines" there is. Go figure.

There is overwhelming evidence that our nervous systems, endocrine systems, and immune systems are in constant dialogue, communicating with the brain through messenger molecules called neuropeptides. These same peptides are the biochemicals of emotion and are found in the parts of our brain that control emotion. Because they control opening and closing of the blood vessels in the face, when the emotion of embarrassment comes along, you blush. Throughout the body they carry messages inside the brain, then from the brain to the body and from the body back to the brain, alerting each as to its status and needs.

*Quantum Healing*, by Deepak Chopra, M.D., is one of the best books ever written on this subject. It clearly underscores the mind-body link. Chopra even refers to it as *bodymind,* and at one point says that *the immune system and the mind are one and the same!* Both operate within the same chemical framework, and it is not possible to separate them. The astounding placebo effect demonstrates this. Albert Einstein was alluding to this fact with his quantum theory formula $E=MC^2$ which means that energy and matter are inseparable and are, in reality, one and the same.

With the advent of quantum physics we have learned that the invisible, immaterial realm is far more important and has a more profound influence in our lives than the material realm we see. Our thoughts actually shape and create our environment in a way physical matter cannot. Albert Einstein was quoted as saying, "The field is the sole governing agency of the particle." Translation: *Invisible energy is the sole governing agency of matter, or the physical world.* This echoes the Biblical passage that states, "the unseen is more real than the seen."

Recently, neuroscientists have found and traced the nerve threads that run like wires between the human nervous system and the immune system that enable the mind and the immune system to communicate with each other in a continuous loop. For years western medicine assumed they worked independently of each other. Now it is being proven that they never were separate, but actually are two sides of the same coin. Mind and body are parts of an integrated, interdependent whole.

Actually, the root of the word "heal" means to "make whole," or "to bring together." Holy and health come from the same root also. The word "religion" means "to link together." *Religion brings together that which has become separate,* that is self and God, linking again what was fragmented. We are beginning to see that healing and spirituality are at last being reunited after centuries of being perceived as separate. They are and always have been *one.*

*We can actually change our GENES with the power of our minds and changes in diet and lifestyle.* Dr. Dean Ornish, M.D., head of the Preventive Medicine Research Institute in Sausalito, California, and well-known author, recently published a study in the *Proceedings of the National Academy of Sciences* that followed thirty men diagnosed with prostate cancer.

For three months they made major lifestyle changes–eating a diet rich in vegetables, fruits, whole grains, soy products (sounds very close to the yeast-free diet), getting moderate daily exercise, and practicing an hour a day of stress management methods, such as prayer and meditation. They had no surgery, chemo or radiation. Biopsies were taken before and after the study. The results were startling.

After three months, the men had changes in activity in about 500 genes–including 48 that were turned on and 453 genes that were turned off! The activity of disease-preventing genes *increased,* while a number of disease promoting genes had *shut down!* The biopsies taken after the study showed the men in much better health and their cancers in retreat.[3]

We also have learned that a mother's diet during pregnancy can turn DNA off or on–another good reason to stay close to the yeast-free diet!

Astoundingly, one of the few triggers that has ever been proven to BREAK a strand of DNA is a *fungus!* More on that subject later.

In the last few years an emerging field of study called "epigenetics", which may be the most important discovery since DNA, is turning our understanding of genes and how they function on its head. Epigenetics (epi means above) is the study of the chemical reactions that switch parts of the genome off or on at strategic times and locations. The "old" biology taught that we are all beholden to the genes we inherited. Epigenetics is proving otherwise.

We are learning that the true secret to life doesn't rest within our DNA, but rather the mechanisms within the *cell membrane.* In actuality, it is the cell membrane that controls the "reading" of the genes inside! Epigenetic studies are proving that cell membranes operate in response to environmental signals picked up by the receptors on the membranes of cells. This response controls the reading of the genes. How the membrane reacts to your diet, thoughts, and lifestyle is what influences your tendency to express disease. Our DNA is simply a blueprint we have the ability to modify.

In other words, our minds control genetic expression and our thoughts are the creative impetuses in our lives. Cells respond to the energetic messages emanating from our positive and negative thoughts. This epigenetic "malleability" helps to explain why identical twins, with identical DNA, can develop different diseases, and why genetically identical cells placed in different Petri dishes exhibit different gene expressions depending on information received from various environments. The best book on this fascinating subject is *The Biology of Belief* by Bruce H. Lipton, PhD. I highly recommend it.

All this proves we are not victims of our own heredity. Genes and DNA do not control our biology. It is our thoughts, attitudes, perceptions, and diet that have mastery over our genes and dictate which genes are turned on and which genes are turned off. Our emotions can literally trigger our genes to express either health or disease So we can no longer wail, "Oh, it's all in my genes so what can I do?" This proves there is a LOT we can do. Indeed we can change our genetic codes by what we eat and how we live and think. *Indeed, changes in diet and lifestyle can TRUMP genes!* When that occurs we become masters of our lives instead of victims of our lives.

Recap: We know there is an intelligence in every cell in the body. Emotions (and their memories) are stored in the cells of our bodies, not just our brains. The mind cannot be relegated to the three pounds of grey matter found within our skulls. The "mind" exists throughout the brain and body, and this "mind" communicates through the same chemicals that are involved in emotion. We are beginning to understand that those chemicals of emotion *may be the current that provides the link, on an unseen level, between mind and body.*

The suppression of anger or emotions has been shown to be associated with a higher statistical probability of cancer. Could cancer be literally suppressed emotion stored in the cells of the body? (What's eating you?) A great part of the healing of this vicious disease is the art of gently leading the patient to paper and pen.

That is what modern medicine has forgotten: The sick body being treated is attached to a mind that is sick with worry, stress, old wounds, and negative thought patterns. In order for it to heal completely, physicians must address the mind and help their patients rid themselves of their old baggage. Otherwise the disease will be driven deeper and deeper into body tissue through prescription drugs and erupt later in a more virulent and deadly form when the immune system is low.

Prayer, meditation, and visualization also are recommended to help patients "repent" (which means to *rethink*) faulty or negative thought patterns. In Matthew, Jesus told the centurion, "Go thou way, and as thou hast believed, so be it done unto thee." Jesus knew the value of thinking right thoughts, the power of positive thinking, and creative visualization. He knew and taught the power of faith.

Jesus also implored us in John, "Let not your heart be troubled, neither let it be afraid." He knew that worry and fear can make a "nest" and eat up the mind, and at some point would manifest as disease. By the same token, laughter, gaiety, and fun are very important components in any healing program. Again we are told in Proverbs, "A merry heart doeth good like a medicine: but a broken spirit drieth the bones." (Candida eats bone causing osteoporosis!)

Sylvia never attempts to heal the body without addressing the mind. To me it is the most awe-inspiring part of her work.

She skillfully and lovingly points out the errors in our living *and* thinking, and attempts to bring all of us to the end of the healing letter. It is there where we abandon judging others–and ourselves–release guilt and pain, and find ourselves in a place of peace and understanding called *forgiveness.* When we forgive others of mistakes, faults, and sins, we forgive ourselves of our own mistakes, faults, and sins. Soon, emotional and physical healing will follow as the heavy burden of lugging around anger, resentment, fear, hatred is removed and discarded.

Jesus reminded us many times of the importance of reconciliation and forgiveness. Just as God lovingly forgave mankind for the many sins that were committed against Him, so must the followers of Christ forgive their friends, families, neighbors, enemies, and themselves for their faults and sins. They must love each other unconditionally and without reservations, having regard for nothing but the soul.

This is made especially clear in Matthew when Jesus instructed his followers to never approach the altar for worship if they had unresolved issues, telling them,

"Therefore, if you bring your gift to the altar,
and there remember that your brother has something against you,
leave your gift there before the altar, and go your way.
First be reconciled with your brother, and then offer your gift."

No one can honor God by bringing festering issues to His table. Reconciliation and forgiveness, a pure heart and a clear conscience are required before we can open a dialogue with Him. Only then can we approach the altar and offer Him our gift.

Through forgiveness and reconciliation, the "sins" and mistakes of others, and ourselves are relegated to the past, *which doesn't exist anymore*. They no longer have a grip or hold on us, and we find ourselves living in the "eternal now", in a space of love.

Only true healing can take place in this space of love, for a person cannot be healed—mentally, physically, and spiritually— if he is riddled with hate, envy, resentment, and emotional pain. Only when they are lifted can love fill all the empty spaces. That love will enable you to *think only the thoughts that serve you.*

# Writing a Healing Love Letter

*"Be ye transformed by the renewing of your mind."*

Romans 12:2

Begin your letter by expressing your anger, resentment, and pain. Then move on through other levels until you work and write your way to love and forgiveness. You will feel relief...and peace.

I don't (or didn't) like it when...
>> I resent...
>> I hate it when...
>> I am fed up with...
>> I am tired of...
>> I want...

I feel (or felt) sad when...
>> I feel hurt because...
>> I feel awful because...
>> I feel disappointed because...
>> I want...

I feel (or felt) afraid...
>> I am afraid that...
>> I feel scared because...
>> I don't understand...
>> I want...

I am sorry that...
>> I am sorry for...
>> Please forgive me for...
>> I didn't mean to...
>> I want…

I love you because...
I love when...
I thank you for...
I understand that...
I forgive you for...
I want...
I am willing to…

**Chapter 15**

---

# Tips

*"There is nothing so complex that it cannot be explained simply."*

...Albert Einstein

Through the years I have kept a running list of helpful hints or tips. The list has grown to fill a entire chapter! I hope these tips help you on your journey to health.

1.  Throw out your microwave oven (or at least use it as little as possible). Microwave cooking is not natural or healthy, and actually is dangerous. Microwaves work by creating friction in water molecules thereby creating heat. Artificially produced microwaves are created from alternating current that forces a billion or more polarity reversals per second in every food molecule they land on. This violent agitation causes substantial damage to food molecules, often tearing them apart or deforming them. Impaired cells then become sitting ducks for waiting viruses, fungi, and other microorganisms. Microwaves are especially destructive of B-complex vitamins, C and E, and essential minerals. Disturbing changes in blood samples have been shown in volunteers who ate microwaved food. (In 1991 a woman in Oklahoma died after receiving a transfusion of blood that had been warmed in a microwave oven. The microwaves damaged the blood components.[1]) Carcinogens have been found in virtually *all food tested*. Microwaves render all food acid-forming, the environment most favorable for the growth of yeast. Every microwave oven leaks microwave radiation, and patients with implanted defibrillators are told not to use them or stand near them.

Microwaves also negatively affect hormones, especially male hormones. *In 1976, Russia banned the use of microwave ovens* after years of research proved their dangers, even showing that a human did not even need to eat microwave prepared food to be adversely affected–just standing near the energy field itself was enough to cause harm.[2] (Unfortunately, Gorbachev lifted the ban in the 1980s.) If a microwave is installed at eye level, eyes can be damaged. Every time you use one, the yeast/beast is waiting for all the cells damaged by microwaves to feast on. I don't even own one.

2. Get rid of all your non-stick cookware. Teflon is far more dangerous than people realize. The Environmental Protection Agency (EPA) is calling for a nasty chemical found in Teflon (C–8) called perfluorooctanic acid to be removed because it is a proven carcinogen. As soon as you heat the pan Teflon starts to vaporize, is inhaled, and goes straight to the bloodstream. It targets the liver and kidneys; has been found in breast milk; and has been linked to birth defects and infertility. Teflon is found in the lining of some paper bags, especially microwave popcorn. The safest cookware to use is porcelain enamel, or enamel-coated cast iron or steel, such as Chantal, or glass such as Pyrex or Corning Ware. OrGreeniC™ kitchenware is a superb, non-toxic, non-stick line of cookware.

3. Fill a small spray bottle with Bragg Liquid Aminos, and spray a small amount on popcorn, instead of using butter. Add garlic powder if desired. Less calories, different and delicious.

4. Don't buy juices in boxes that are lined with aluminum foil. They tend to be contaminated with yeast. Buy juices in glass jars and dilute with water (half) during the first month.

5. Squeeze fresh lemon juice into your drinking water. Lemon is healing to the liver and will help speed up detoxification. It is also

alkalizing in the body, which is so important to outwitting the acid-loving yeast. *Alkaline blood is anti-fungal blood.*

6. Get out the crock pot! It is so wonderful for cooking chicken, turkey, lamb, stews, soups, beans, etc. It is one of the best ways to prepare food from a nutrition standpoint. I use mine several times a week.

7. Check all your supplements to make sure they don't contain yeast. Buy only natural, yeast-free products. And never buy mushroom extracts or products that contain them. More about this later.

8. Never drink distilled water–it leaches valuable minerals from the body. It also is acidic, which yeast loves. It is dead water, containing no oxygen. Fish can't live in it. Drink filtered, mineral, or spring water only. Try to drink 1 to 2 quarts of water daily. Water hydrates internal organs–especially the brain–enabling them to function properly, removes waste and toxins, and keeps elasticity in the skin to help you look younger.

9. Wash cantaloupe and strawberry skins carefully before cutting into them. Their skins are porous and they may harbor mold.

10. Eat leftovers in the refrigerator within two days.

11. Use oatmeal instead of bread crumbs when called for. Or use crushed yeast-free crackers. Arrowroot can be used in dredging chicken pieces.

12. Substitute water chestnuts for mushrooms.

13. Pour apple juice on cereal instead of soy or rice milk for a change.

14. *Always eat breakfast* to set your metabolism for the day. This is the best time to eat your one or two pieces of fruit.

**15.** Do not use yogurt or vinegar douches or coffee enemas under any circumstances.

**16.** Substitute coconut milk (in a carton) for milk and canned coconut milk for cream. Delicious!

**17.** Fasting is not allowed. Fasting causes minerals to disappear from the bloodstream.

**18.** For patients who are highly allergic to chemicals, mix one tablespoon lemon juice and one tablespoon sea salt into one gallon cold water. Soak vegetables and fruits in the bath for 5–10 minutes and rinse thoroughly. This will remove insecticides, preservatives, colorings, metal salts, fungi, and bacteria.

**19.** If you can't find organic chicken, remove skin and sprinkle sea salt over the meat. Let stand thirty minutes and rinse carefully. This will remove toxic substances from the meat and the taste is delicious. You may want to cut down on salt in your chicken recipes since a small amount will remain in the tissue.

**20.** Use only sea salt. It contains more than eighty sea minerals in perfect balance. The trace minerals and macro-nutrients present in naturally harvested sea salt are in a precise dosage identical in composition to that of our body fluids. It is both a food and a medicine. (As a preservative, salt maintains flesh! It is the nature of flesh to spoil, but salt-cured meats remain unspoiled.) Chemically produced table salt has been stripped of its nutrients and is unbalanced and harmful. It can legally contain up to two percent chemical additives, such as bleaches, anti-caking agents, and conditioners. Salt to which iodine has been added contains about twenty times the naturally occurring amount of iodine in sea salt. This imbalance can be dangerous.

**21.** Never skip a meal. Low blood sugar makes yeast hungry too.

**22.** Eat carbohydrates moderately. One medium-small portion per meal, please. Yeast learns to eat other carbs after the sugar is taken away. (Remember how adaptive they are.) Do *not* go on a no-carbohydrate diet, however. It will shock your systems, especially the pancreas and adrenals, and throw them off balance.

**23.** Avoid irradiated foods at all costs. They produce huge amounts of free radicals and will stress the immune system further by adding more toxic chemicals to the total body load. Radiation is used to kill bacteria, such as E. coli, to mask the filthy slaughtering and unsanitary food processing practices so prevalent in factory farms and agribusiness today. It also renders most nutrients worthless. (Note the growing number of recalls on contaminated meats, fruits, and vegetables we've seen in the last few years.)

Food is bombarded with ionizing radiation, using gamma rays (generated from radioactive cobalt), x-rays, or high speed electrons from electronic guns to kill bacteria and extend shelf life. In the process cell walls are broken up, chromosomes are shredded, enzymes are killed, nutrients are destroyed (especially vitamin A– one of the most radiation sensitive of the fat soluble vitamins) and dangerous free radicals are formed which could become cancers down the road. *And the FDA claims irradiated food is safe!*

In the last twenty years it has become legal to irradiate beef, chicken, pork, fruit, vegetables, eggs, juice, spices, almonds, spinach, iceberg lettuce, sprouting seeds, oysters, clams, scallops and mussels.

Buy local and organic as much as possible, and avoid any food labeled "treated with radiation" or "treated by irradiation" or has the radura–the symbol for irradiation (which, oddly enough, is a flower in a circle)–on the label. Sadly, the FDA is considering a proposal to ease off labeling guidelines because too many people are being scared away by the "irradiated" label! *The only way to make sure you are not buying nuked food is to buy organic.*

**24.** Don't cook with aluminum pots and pans or use aluminum foil. Aluminum dissolves when it touches organic acids and alkalis that are found in fruit and vegetables. Salt and baking soda speed up the corrosion. Once "aluminumized" food is eaten and is dissolved by the hydrochloric acid in the stomach, it enters the bloodstream and is deposited in organs, muscles, and other tissue. Aluminum has been found in the brains of Alzheimer's patients.

**25.** Use only aluminum-free baking powder. Rumford is excellent.

**26.** Check ingredients in underarm antiperspirants and deodorants. Most have aluminum and other harmful ingredients. Try Aubrey's E Plus High C all natural roll-on deodorant. Burt's Bees also makes good products.

**27.** Don't panic if a no-no slips into your diet on occasion. You won't undo everything. Even though you stimulated a few yeast, if you get right back on the diet and don't feed them, they will die also.

**28.** If you can't find a good yeast-free bread, go online and search for yeast-free breads and bakeries. My favorite is French Meadow at www.FrenchMeadow.com.

**29.** If you have arthritis, eliminate members of the nightshade family from your diet. Many arthritics are allergic to them. They include white potatoes, peppers, eggplant, tomatoes, and tobacco. Be sure to alkalize with a green drink daily since arthritis is an acid condition. See tip 31.

**30.** Have a live blood cell analysis done. You can actually see how your blood is teeming with bacteria, yeast, fungi, mold, and other unsavory characters. Very motivating! Then have a re-check when the diet is over. You'll be astounded.

**31.** Add a "green drink" to your regimen to help alkalize your body. Look for one containing a wide variety of grasses, including wheat grass, barley grass, lemon grass, shave grass, kamut grass, oat grass, or organic liquid chlorophyll from alfalfa. (If you can't find them, just barley grass will do.) Green drinks help regenerate new cells to replace the ones the yeast/beast ate. *Alkaline blood is antifungal blood.* Don't buy green drinks that contain algae or *mushrooms.*

**32.** Try stevia powder to sweeten drinks, fruit sauces, etc. It is an herb that is thirty times sweeter than sugar, does not alter blood sugar levels or feed yeast. It has no calories and a little goes a long way.

**33.** If you smoke, now is the time to *quit!* Get that monkey off your back. Smokers are literally poisoning themselves. Smokers live an average of 9–13 years less than non-smokers. Tobacco is very, very high in fungus (a causal factor in the development of lung cancer) as it is a sugar- and a fungally- "cured" product. There are 599 approved additives in cigarettes and over 4,000 chemical compounds are created when cigarettes are burned, many of them toxic and carcinogenic, including carbon monoxide, nitrogen oxides, hydrogen cyanide, and ammonia.

The largest purchaser of refined sugar in the United States is, of course, the baking industry. The second largest purchaser of refined sugar is the tobacco industry! Flue-cured tobacco contains as much as 20 percent sugar by weight, and even air-cured tobacco has sugar added in the blending process. Every time you inhale you are getting a sugar fix, your blood sugar rises and yeast is ecstatic! *Tobacco addiction is basically a yeast-driven sugar addiction.*

More than 700 chemicals are found in cigarettes, some classified as so toxic they aren't allowed in food! Additionally, they contain over 50 carcinogenic materials. The temperature of a lit cigarette reaches nearly 2,000 degrees. This high heat spurs the release of thousands of chemical compounds, including poisons like carbon monoxide, cyanide, methanol, formaldehyde, acetylene, and ammonia, all of which are inhaled into the body. Yeast and fungi welcome them with open arms.

Nicotine is another driver in this equation. *All stimulants taken into the body stimulate the growth of more yeast and fungi.* Nicotine is one of the most powerful stimulants known. Between the sugar and nicotine, yeast levels can reach astronomical proportions. No wonder they want to be fed every few minutes or hours. No wonder cigarettes are so "addictive." No wonder it is so hard to quit. And no wonder the yeast-free diet, as yeast levels fall and the cravings are diminished, makes it easier to help you become "un-hooked."

**34.** If affordable, find a good massage therapist and treat yourself to a massage once a week while you are healing. This will help break down the accumulations of toxins in muscles and tissues and will speed the healing.

**35.** Once a week take a soaking bath that will open the pores of your skin and allow toxins to escape. Before bedtime, bring 8 cups of water to a boil, add 2 chamomile tea bags and boil for 15 minutes. Pour tea, with bags, into a tub full of comfortably hot water; add 1/3 cup sea salt, and 1/3 cup food grade (3%) hydrogen peroxide. Soak, using no soap, for 20 minutes. Rub a washcloth in a circular motion all over your body several times during the soak. Towel off and go to bed. This bath *really* speeds up the healing.

**36.** Do not use antibacterial soaps, sprays, or wipes. They are another fear-driven fraud foisted on the gullible public. We have become so germaphobic that now we have antibacterial soaps, laundry detergents, shampoos, toothpastes, body washes, dish soaps, even cutting boards! The active ingredient in most of these products is Triclosan, a dangerous and toxic bacterial agent that kills bacteria and inhibits its growth. Unfortunately, *it also kills human cells!*

The overuse of these products causes bacteria to mutate into resistant strains. Such products are, after all, antibiotics. When absorbed into the bloodstream, they adversely affect immune, lymphatic, endocrine, reproductive, and neurological systems. Sound familiar? You are inviting yeast to proliferate wherever they are used. (It is good for the immune system to be challenged with a little bacteria or dirt on occasion to keep it humming.) Use essential oils such as Thieves, a wonderful line of all-natural, non-toxic, immune boosting antimicrobial products for the home, and good old soap and water. Remember, you want clean, *not sterile!*

37. Do not use air fresheners unless they are all natural. Commercial air fresheners are loaded with toxic chemicals that add to the load of the already over-burdened immune system. Instead order a natural air purifier called Aclare from Healthy Perceptions. It is a fabulous product which removes bacteria, yeast, and mold from the air. It is a plug-in model the size of a flashlight that makes it easy to travel with. Call 800–340–0247 or go to www.HealthyPerceptions.com. It can make a huge difference in your health.

38. Check your urine and pH levels at home with pH strips found in pharmacies. Your body should be slightly alkaline at a pH of 7.365. Anything lower than that indicates an over–acid body. Yeast loves acidity, and over-acidity causes many of the symptoms of Candida. Find an acid and alkaline list of foods to follow. If you are too acidic, eat foods mostly from the alkaline list until you normalize.

39. Go to Home Depot or a health food store and buy inexpensive "mold detectors". If you have mold or mildew growing anywhere in your home–behind wallpaper, in the bathroom, in the basement, in the air-conditioning, in the humidifier–have it remediated at once. There are companies that help you find it and remove it. If you continue to live in a moldy environment, you constantly will be reinfecting yourself and you will never get well.

**40.** Do not drink fluoridated water or use products that contain fluoride. Never have fluoride treatments in the dentist's office. Fluoride is a corrosive poison and is the *active toxin found in rat poisons and roach powders.* Its toxicity rating is slightly higher than lead and slightly lower than arsenic. Most of the fluoride added to municipal drinking water is a chemical pollutant and by-products of aluminum, steel, copper, iron, cement, phosphate, and *nuclear weapons manufacturing.* Ingestion of as little as one percent of a tube of children's fluoridated toothpaste can produce acute fluoride toxicity in a young child.[3] Since 1997, all fluoridated toothpastes are required by the FDA to carry warning labels that read: *"Warning: Keep out of reach of children under 6 years of age. If more than is used for brushing is accidentally swallowed, get medical help or contact a Poison Control Center."* Some tubes even carry the poison symbol of skull and crossbones! Fluoride is known to cause dental fluorosis, osteoporosis, arthritis, hip fractures, brain damage, thyroid disorders, and infertility. It increases the uptake of aluminum in the brain by 600 percent, making a nest for Alzheimer's.[3] It is a known carcinogen and neurotoxin, and is banned in Scandinavia and most of Europe. It is found in Teflon and Tefal cookware. Drink pure spring water, artesian well water, or reverse osmosis water from *glass* containers only.

**41.** If possible, have all the silver/mercury amalgam fillings removed from your teeth. Replace them with composites. Chewing, grinding, and drinking hot beverages release toxic mercury vapors which are absorbed into the body with devastating effects on the kidneys, blood vessels, and central nervous system. Mercury also kills the beneficial bacteria in the gut, leading to the creation of more yeast. Healing from Candida will be much slower, or even thwarted, if your immune system is constantly dealing with mercury poisoning. Find a dentist who is well qualified to do this procedure, as extra training is needed to extract and dispose of the hazardous waste.

**42.** Try to avoid farm-raised or "pen-reared" fish. Most are raised in overcrowded, feces-infested pens with little swimming room that makes them prone to diseases. Farm raised fish are fed more antibiotics by weight than any other form of livestock. Even so, many are infested with sea lice. Most farm-raised fish are fed ground-up fish to which genetically modified *corn* has been added (fish don't eat corn), contain mercury, cancer-causing PCBs, and dioxin. The omega-3:6 ratio is very unfavorable, as farm-raised fish contain up to 400 percent more omega 6 fatty acids than wild-caught fish, an unhealthy imbalance that *contributes to inflammation* in the body. The flesh of salmon raised in pens is actually grey, so artificial color has to be added to make them look normal and pink. In the grocery store and when eating out, always ask for wild-caught fish only.

**43.** Eliminate plastic containers for storage and leftovers. They contain cancer-causing chemicals which can leach into your food and slow down your healing. The connection was discovered in 1987 at Tufts Medical School when researchers were culturing breast cancer cells in test tubes made of plastic. The chemicals in the plastic leached into the test tubes causing the cancer cells to proliferate wildly. Some plastics are safer than others. The way to tell which ones are safe and which ones are dangerous is to look at the bottom of the container. You will see a little triangle with a number inside it. Containers with a 3, 6, or 7 are the most dangerous, containing a volatile chemical called BPA. Avoid at all costs. Containers with a 4 or 5 on the bottom are generally regarded as safe, but use sparingly, and *never* use in a microwave. Containers with a 1 or 2 on the bottom are the safest, and again, *never* use in a microwave. Use glass. Also, never use Styrofoam cups or plates. Styrene is a poison.

**44.** Try to remain cheerful while healing yourself. Leave your martyr complex at the back door. Nobody enjoys being around a whiney person.

**45.** Get plenty of sleep and rest while you heal.  Remember, the body will be using much energy to detoxify and rebuild itself.  You may feel real fatigue the first few days or weeks, so keep exercise to a minimum.  This is not the time for a marathon or heavy exercise as they will strain the immune system.  Use this time to nourish, balance, and heal the whole person, body, mind, and soul.

**46.** Never refer to the disease or condition you are dealing with as "my cancer," "my asthma," "my colitis," "my candidiasis," etc. *You do not own it,* and when you say "my" you are, in effect, claiming it.  Your subconscious is always listening to what you are thinking and the words that you are saying and will program them for the future.   Just say "the cancer" or "this condition" or "this temporary disease."

**47.** Pray daily for healing to be complete.  Learn to meditate and reconnect with our Creator.  All healing is simply activating our God within.   In Exodus we read: "I am the Lord God which healeth thee."

**Special Note**: While Doctor Buttram was reading my manuscript in order to write the Foreword, he realized that I had not addressed an important family of chemicals that can affect body chemistry, e.g., pH balance, free-radical formation, DNA, and Candida *albicans* (yeast) flare-ups.  So, I asked him if he would write something about Volatile Organic Compounds, which he did, and I include below.

## Volatile Organic Compounds (VOCs): A Neurotoxic Class of Chemicals

Many who have some familiarity with the field of environmental medicine are becoming aware that toxic chemical pollution of air, food, and water in the United States, largely of commercial origin, has reached such an extent that it has become a significant source of mental and physical illness today. As far as current awareness of the VOCs and their dangers is concerned, it appears to be very nebulous, similar to the times when Pasteur and Lister were first bringing to light the role of microbes as sources of deadly diseases and the role of sanitation in controlling these diseases.

VOCs are a very large class of commercial chemicals that tend to evaporate into and contaminate indoor air of buildings. They enter the human system not only by inhalation but also through skin contact. VOCs all share one important characteristic. Being largely derived from petrochemicals, they are fat or lipid soluble and therefore have an affinity for the fatty or lipid tissues of the body. Conversely, VOCs are water insoluble. Once in the blood stream, which is predominantly aqueous, they are rapidly sponged off by fatty tissues of the body. The brain is a prime target because of its high lipid content (approximately 60 percent of solid weight) and rich blood supply.

Of the many thousands of chemicals used in commerce, several hundred are known to be neurotoxic. However, except for pharmaceuticals, only a small percentage of VOCs have had any testing at all for neurotoxicity, and only a few of these have been tested thoroughly. (1)

The pervasiveness of these chemicals was reflected in a study that showed that 10 volatile chemicals were commonly found in indoor air, drinking water, and exhaled breathes of residents of New Jersey, North Carolina, and North Dakota. (2)

Because the brain is the primary target of VOCs, symptoms are primarily cerebral in nature. Acute symptoms include dizziness, forgetfulness, headaches, mental fogginess, difficulty concentrating, and poor coordination. One of the centers investigating chronic effects of organic solvent exposures is the University of Pittsburgh where Lisa Morrow, Ph.D. and coworkers have published a series of studies on the effects of solvents on occupationally exposed subjects. (3-7) These findings include social alienation, poor concentration, anxiety, and impairments in learning and memory.

VOCs are taking a heavy toll among American adults in the U.S. with high levels of VOCs commonly found in homes and workplaces today, but the effects may be even greater in infants and children. In the book, Pesticides in Diets of Infants and Children, sponsored by the National Research Council, official advisory body to the national government, it was estimated that children may be ten times more vulnerable to toxic chemical exposures than adults because of their rapidly growing tissues and relatively immature organ systems. (8)

It is more than coincidental that the present epidemic of hyperactivity and behavioral problems among school children has coincided with steadily increasing levels of VOCs found in modern buildings.(1) Standard neurotoxicology texts point out that behavioral problems may be the earliest sign of chemical toxicity. (9,10)

In an investigation of three Sick Building Syndrome (SBS) outbreaks, which included two high schools, it was concluded that the Chronic Fatigue immune Deficiency Syndrome (CFIDS) is often associated with the SBS. By way of explanation, CFIDS is a condition characterized by overwhelming fatigue, muscle aches, inability to concentrate, and other symptoms predominantly affecting young adults. (11)

The Sick Building Syndrome, in turn, refers to buildings in which a significant portion of persons in the building is made ill by combinations of airborne chemicals that have reached toxic levels. In the study, respiratory and neurologic symptoms often overlapped with CFIDS. Symptoms included headaches, fatigue, low-grade fevers, eye irritation, tearing, and light sensitivity. The authors suggested that the cause may be low levels of contaminants acting "in concert" or synergistically to produce overlapping syndromes. (12) This principle has been substantiated by three studies showing that combinations of toxic chemicals may bring exponential increases in toxicity. That is, two toxic chemicals in combination may bring a 10-fold increase in toxicity. (13-15)

Categories of VOCs include pesticides, organic solvents, glues, formaldehyde, fumes from auto exhaust, fumes from oil or coal-based furnaces, household sprays, passive smoking, moth balls (naphthalene), foam rubber, Teflon®, and Freon® leaks from refrigerators.

Recommended Reference Books:

- Gorman, CP, Less Toxic Living, Environmental Health Center, 8345 Walnut Hill Lane, Suite 205, Dallas, Texas 75231, 214-368-4132.
- Dadd, DL, The Nontoxic Home & Office, New York, GP Putman's Sons.
- Bower, J. The Healthy House, How to Buy One, How to Cure a "Sick" One, How to Build One. Secaucus, New Jersey, Lyle Stuart.

....Dr. Harold Buttram, M. D.

**Chapter 16**

---

# Recap and Overview

*"In vain shalt thou use many medicines, for thou shalt not be cured."*
...Jeremiah 46:11

Before we continue, let's simplify the basic essentials of what is important to understand and remember about how yeast behaves in the body.

There are *five basic steps* or levels of yeast growth that take it from local and unobtrusive to fully disseminating and lethal.

**Step 1.** Yeast lives topically, in confined areas, more or less unnoticed. Dandruff and ring-worm are two examples. Small colonies live normally in intestines and vagina. Immune system remains strong.

**Step 2.** Yeast still lives topically, but is on the march. Increasing numbers begin creating infections in the gastrointestinal and genito-urinary tracts. Diarrhea, bloating, heartburn, vaginal yeast infections, weight gain, and cystitis can appear. Immune system is being stressed and starts losing ground.

**Step 3.** Yeast becomes fungus. It burrows into the bloodstream. Yeast is now invasive, meaning it has gained access to the "inner sanctum", or the body proper, and becomes systemic. Yeasts and their toxins circulate throughout the body. Headaches, hives, rashes, asthma, ear infections, acne, fatigue can occur. Embattled immune system breaks down further.

**Step 4.** Central nervous system becomes affected. Dysfunction and deterioration occur from huge loads of yeast toxins circulating in the bloodstream. Memory loss, depression, PMS, behavioral problems, intense fatigue, hallucinations can occur. Immune system barely functioning, approaching gridlock.

**Step 5.** Endocrine systems and organ breakdowns occur. Some parts of the body are literally eaten alive, as the fungus penetrates deeper and deeper into tissue. Low thyroid, adrenal exhaustion, diabetes, overwhelming fatigue, severe abdominal pain, diseases of digestion, cancer, menstrual problems such as endometriosis, infertility, low liver function are indicative of severe infestation of fungus. *Immune system meltdown.*

We must never forget that *Candida albicans* is a potential killer. Because it can disseminate widely to cause infection in almost every tissue of the body, it can become very fulminating and cause rapid death through the destruction of tissue and the production of toxins. The death certificate may read "heart attack," "kidney failure," "pneumonia," "liver disease," "cancer," etc., but you can be sure *Candida albicans* was there first and created the environment needed for the disease to develop. Again, it is the "disease behind disease."

I watched a television program years ago where the mother of a young woman who had just died of AIDS told the painful story of her daughter's courageous battle against that deadly disease. The young woman had spent her last weeks at home where she died. The mother told of her daughter's final hours and described the feeding tube that had been inserted down her throat and the breathing tubes that had been put into her nose.

After her daughter died, all the tubes were removed from her body; all were found to be *completely clogged with yeast.*

AIDS (Acquired Immune System Deficiency Syndrome) is a disease of low immune system function. (The disease name was changed from HIV, or Human-Immunodeficiency-Virus, to Acquired Immune System Deficiency Syndrome when scientists suspected it was a fungal disease, not a viral one.) As the disease progressed and the young woman picked up more and more infections, compassionate and caring doctors prescribed antibiotic after antibiotic to treat each new setback. *Each prescription ignited more yeast*. With each new batch of yeast came lowered immunity, which invited more infections and more antibiotics. It was a lose, lose situation. Eventually her body was both too debilitated to resist and too weak to fight and she died.

Here a sad argument can be made that this young woman didn't actually die of AIDS, but that fulminating *Candida albicans* killed her. Her body was "eaten up" and overwhelmed by fungi to the point that her feeding and breathing tubes were so filled with Candida organisms that she could neither breathe nor swallow. Yet her death certificate cited AIDS as the cause of death. Almost all AIDS patients succumb to fungal diseases.

True, the interventions of antibiotics and other drugs have prolonged and saved many lives in the short run, but now we are finding it's not without a price. It is a tradeoff that needs to be closely scrutinized and evaluated more scientifically.

Instead of dying from infectious diseases early in life, we are now living longer but enjoying it less. We are developing chronic degenerative diseases, such as cancer, diabetes, arthritis, and multiple sclerosis at earlier ages and at alarming rates as trade–offs for the use of synthetic drugs and immunizations. (More about that in later chapters.) We need to decide if that is a fair trade or whether we have been deceived and swindled. The promises of drugs to heal us in too many cases have turned into the ashes of sick and broken lives.

The medical mainstream unfortunately has become fascinated with disease instead of health and mesmerized by pathology instead of wellness. Consequently, American medicine–instead of delivering a "health care system"–is instead mass-producing a "money-making symptom-management system."

As a result of dissecting and compartmentalizing the human body into innumerable specialties, or what is called "body parts medicine," (I call it Humpty Dumpty medicine) the focus of modern allopathic medicine has become specialized and narrow. We have reached the point where the whole person is so out of focus that he cannot be perceived as a total entity. He is only a blur of fragments. Now all the king's horses and all the king's men are frantically trying to put the pieces of old Humpty back together again–to no avail. Consequently, the whole person is rarely healed. The excellent book, *The Four Pillars of Healing*, by Dr. Leo Galland, M.D., illustrates this point beautifully.

Right now as much as two-thirds of the medical research funding in most major academic institutions comes either directly or indirectly from drug companies. Of the 127 medical schools in the United States, *only 24 require courses in nutrition.* Of the top 15 medical schools, only 4 offer such courses. Our modern doctors are basically taught two principles: Number one: diagnose disease and Number two: prescribe drugs. In my opinion, many physicians have become little more than modern-day, legal, third-party payer acceptable drug "pushers."

Is it any wonder we are spending hundreds of billions of dollars on medical care each year? Our health care system is crumbling under the weight of enormous costs of surgeries, drugs, and expensive treatments and equipment. How much of this colossal bill was caused by diseases that could have been prevented in the first place? How much human suffering could have been prevented if doctors had been trained in preventive medicine and natural healing?

It is time for doctors to re-read the Hippocratic Oath, a seminal treatise on medical ethics. Many believe that *"Primum non nocere"* ("First thou shall do no harm") was part of that oath. Actually the phrase originally appeared in one of his private letters. Hippocrates, the Father of Medicine, formulated the beautiful oath 2,500 years ago. In it doctors vowed:

1. "I will first apply dietetic measures for the benefit of the sick according to my ability and judgment: I will keep them from harm and injustice."
2. "I will neither give a deadly drug to anyone if asked for it, nor will I make a suggestion to this effect."

3. "I will not give a woman an abortive remedy. In purity and holiness I will guard my life and my art."

Many medical schools no longer mandate the recitation of the Hippocratic Oath. A modern version was instituted in the 1980s that bears little resemblance to the original. Gone are the references to dietary measures for the healing of the sick. No reference is made regarding deadly drugs. The vow not to give a woman an abortive remedy has been re-written to read: "I will not give a woman a pessary to produce abortion." (A pessary is a plug or cylinder that was used to induce labor.) With the new deceitful wording it is implied that "other" more modern methods of abortion might be employed.

This original oath is violated blatantly by doctors many times every day as most of their prescriptions for chemical "miracles" are, in actuality, harming us and speeding up our deaths by creating a more favorable environment for the great decomposers and recyclers–yeast and fungi.

We have come to a crossroads in medicine and healthcare where some hard decisions about the road we want to follow in our search for health will have to be made. For over one hundred years we have been fascinated with pharmaceutical drugs and synthetic "quick fixes." Some of these "miracles drugs" have indeed eased pain and saved lives and should be made available to those who need them. But, in our pursuit of the quick and easy, we may have become our own worst enemy.

Even though candidiasis or yeast infection is often an "iatrogenic" or doctor-caused and doctor-driven disease, we cannot place all the blame for this epidemic on modern day allopathic (chemical drug) medicine. In fact, we ourselves must bear part of the responsibility.

For too many years we have demanded of our doctors quick and simple solutions to complex problems and put our faith in "better living through chemistry." They have done their best to oblige us, and now our drugged bodies are breeding stronger, more resistant, more *virulent* strains of viruses, bacteria, fungi, and parasites. Now new, stronger, more toxic drugs must be developed to kill them. Our embattled immune systems never have a chance to get ahead.

And what have these drugs been *teaching* our bodies?

They have been teaching our bodies that *they cannot get well by themselves.* Big Pharma's mantra seems to be, "You cannot be well or get well without our drugs!"

By constantly nipping every little infection in the bud with antibiotics and other drugs, our immune systems are deprived of the valuable knowledge that they can rise to the occasion and knock out any invaders *on their own.* The body is denied the experience of winning a battle and then *remembering* how to do it again if needed. That is why having childhood diseases builds up immunity. Once a child has measles, the body "remembers" how to fight it if ever exposed again to the measles virus.

Through practice, the immune system "learns" to become strong and "learns" that it can be victorious. Drugs deny the immune system the chance to practice or exercise. "If you don't use it, you'll lose it" truly applies here because what we are seeing now is an entire generation of younger and younger people coming down *with immune system disorders,* i.e., AIDS and *auto-immune system disorders* such as rheumatoid arthritis, lupus, multiple sclerosis, cancer, and diabetes–diseases historically seen in much older people.

These young people's immune systems were all compromised by pharmaceutical drugs as they grew up. By the time they entered young adulthood they had poorly-functioning immune systems. True, their sore throats, bacterial infections, etc., were knocked out by antibiotics or other drugs. But their bodies *learned nothing from the experience.* The much-needed learning and natural cleansing processes that the body goes through, such as vomiting, diarrhea, coughing up sputum, fevers, etc. were interrupted or halted altogether. The virus or bacteria then went deeper into tissue– into hiding–and a kind of artificial health, or the *appearance* of health, was left to masquerade as well being.

*Instead of learning to become strong, our immune systems actually have been taught to become weak.*

This, in turn, has put a basic law of Nature on "hold." It is called "the survival of the fittest," and has been the way of Nature since the beginning of time. It applies to all living things. Simply stated, it means that when an organism is weak or out of balance with Nature, *dis-harmony* and *dis-ease* develop. Micro-organisms are then stimulated to proliferate and cause illness. If an organism's constitution is strong enough, it will overcome the illness and survive. If not, it will die. This fundamental law of Nature up until now has created increasingly hardy species on earth.

With the advent of antibiotics, the natural order has been interrupted. Since the body and its immune system have been denied their learning experiences, we are allowing weakened, inferior genetic material to be added to the global gene pool. Our potential for creating healthy new generations is disintegrating with that pool. Only time will tell to what extent we have deteriorated.

According to a recent United Nations survey, nearly three-fourths of the population of the world does not use drugs, but uses herbs for healing, and nearly all of those countries are far healthier than the United States! (*We are now fiftieth in life expectancy, lower than some developing countries.*) It is true that we seem to be living longer, but that is due mainly to decreased numbers of deaths from infectious diseases and infant mortality, organ transplants, plus extended critical care and life support–especially toward the end of life–which is not a reflection of overall health.

One of the most persuasive reflections of the deterioration of our overall health, even as we live longer, is the crushing costs of delivering health care during the last years of our "longer" lives. We have substituted quantity for quality and are paying dearly for it.

Today, as enlightenment grows, more and more people are turning to more natural means to heal themselves and their families. People are tired of going from one specialist to another; getting one prescription after another;

and *not getting well.* In their frustration, they are finding health food stores, surfing the web, reading and learning about nutrition and natural healing, growing their own organic vegetables, juicing, and *healing themselves*!

We are waking up to the fact that none of us is a victim of disease. We create ill-health through making wrong choices, thinking wrong thoughts, and living wrong lifestyles. Most disease is our own fault, and we have no one to blame but ourselves.

And, if we are responsible for our ill health, then we can be just as responsible for healing ourselves. By empowering ourselves with knowledge, making the right choices, and changing what needs to be changed, we eventually can assume responsibility back to ourselves *where it belongs.*

*The only thing that has ever cured an illness or disease is the human body itself,* but only if provided with the right healing tools and building materials it was designed to use.

Our biggest error was to think that modern science and modern medicine could, more often than not, "do it better" than Mother Earth and Mother Nature.

We are learning you can't fool either.

**Chapter 17**

---

# The Rise of Big P(harm)a

*"A medicine is always directly hurtful; it may sometimes be indirectly beneficial. I firmly believe that if most of the pharmacopoeia were sunk to the bottom of the sea, it would be all the better for Mankind and all the worse for the fishes."*

...Oliver Wendell Holmes, M.D. (1809–1894)

As we now know, there are many direct and indirect causes of the current epidemic of fungal diseases. Heading the list of direct causes is our *profligate use of man-made, synthetic chemicals called drugs*. They are some of yeasts' favorite foods. They just rub their little tummies every time you swallow them.

Let me state clearly that if ever I were in an accident, badly burned, had a stroke, heart attack or some other medical crisis, the first place I would want to be would be in the emergency room of a good hospital or trauma center, seeking the most competent medical help possible. Drugs for pain and anesthesia, clot-busting drugs, IV hydration, X-rays, etc., are godsends in these cases. An herbalist and other holistic approaches can come later.

The United States has the best in the world when it comes to emergency and trauma care. We are fortunate to have so many state-of-the-art diagnostic and pain-relieving tools in physicians' hands. There are, and always will be, times when prescription drugs are appropriate, necessary, and useful.

That's the good news.

The bad news is that of all the drugs produced in the world, Americans take *half* of them, even though we constitute only three percent of the world population. Today and every day in the United States, seventy–five million people take one or more drugs. Every year in the United States, three *billion* prescriptions are filled, costing patients, the government, and insurance companies $70.3 billion. Add to that the incalculable number of over-the-counter drugs and illegal drugs being sold and we truly are looking at a "mass-medicated society."

It wasn't always so. All healing was natural until the mid-nineteenth century. For centuries the healing art in Europe was not called medicine; it was called *physic* – from the Greek word, *physis*, meaning nature. Our word *physician* actually comes from a root word that *means nature!* Physicians were trained to treat disease with herbs, homeopathics, poultices, tonics, stimulants, and other natural methods. The word *medicine,* which comes from the Latin verb, *medico,* and literally means "I drug", gradually gained acceptance. Soon the old natural ways (some deservedly) were replaced, setting the stage for the growth of modern medicine as we know it today.

In order to further the interests of the modern "physician," a group of doctors established the American Medical Association (AMA) in the United States in 1847. Its stated goals were and are to protect the interests of American physicians, advance public health, and support the growth of medical science. It is essentially a union for doctors and others in the medical field, and is privately run by its dues-paying members.

Shortly after it was established, the AMA quickly banned all homeopathic physicians from their "club" and proceeded to label all homeopathic remedies "quackery." Homeopathy became a "forbidden medicine." Anyone who didn't conform to AMA's rigid codes was roundly criticized or thrown out of the association. It quickly closed half the medical schools and half the hospitals and began a fifty-plus-year-attack upon chiropractic and osteopathy. It wasn't long before the AMA turned into a medical monopoly, eventually exerting incredible influence on medical schools and medical students alike. Once the AMA was in control of medical schools, it arranged that only those who graduated from schools it sanctioned could officially practice medicine. And since it controlled the schools, it controlled what largely was taught–how to use prescription drugs.

In the past, if the AMA didn't approve of certain health care approaches, it worked diligently to banish them from hospitals and suspend the licenses of any doctor who employed them. In its efforts to eliminate competition, it has often coerced state licensing boards and the U.S. Congress into passing laws outlawing natural healing methods. Any non-MD practitioners using them, such as chiropractic physicians, homeopaths, osteopaths, midwives, herbalists, and acupuncturists were sanctioned. It has failed in these attempts due to the overwhelming evidence of their efficacy–plus a huge public backlash. As a result, many of these natural healing methods are now mainstream.

Even though the AMA failed in its attempts to control medicine in general, it has regrouped and recently joined forces with allies in the Federal Trade Commission (FTC), Food and Drug Administration (FDA), and the drug industry to target aggressively those who advocate natural healing methods. It is illegal for anyone to accurately describe the health benefits of the nutritional products he sells. *Illegal!* Now clinics, nutrition-oriented websites, and even churches are coming under their fire.[1]

A case in point is the alarming number of raids carried out by the FDA on health food stores and co-ops, clinics, and nutritional supplement companies in the last twenty years. All over the country armed police marshals and FDA officials have conducted surprise raids on legitimate businesses and medical clinics, terrorizing employees, burning literature, seizing files, mailing lists, lab equipment, personal property of employees and, of course, the supplements in question.[2] In many cases charges were never filed and confiscated property never was returned. In all of these incidents, the constitution of the United States and the right of free speech were also confiscated and trampled into the dirt.

It is the official position of the FDA that there is no such thing as an herb, vitamin or superfood that has any ability to prevent, treat or cure any disease or health condition. Anyone who claims benefits from them is immediately branded a criminal by the FDA and is subject to arrest. The Federal Trade Commission (FTC) in 2009 sent threatening letters to 130 companies selling dietary supplements, telling them if they *made any health claims* for their products they would be subject to confiscation of customer records, banking and financial records, and all their inventories! Non-compliance meant arrest, imprisonment, and eventual trials in the FTC's own court, *which is subject to no law*. There is no right to trial by jury as the FTC's own judges are appointed by the FTC itself. Most of the defendants plead guilty rather than face enormous fines and legal expenses or go to jail.

The wanton persecution by these powerful government agencies (together with the AMA and drug companies) with deep pockets against an almost defenseless health food industry with shallow pockets should make us fearful of what they might do next. Power corrupts absolutely. These FDA and FTC regulations amount to the *gagging of legitimate information the public needs to know about herbs and natural supplements,* and is a suppression of our rights to free speech. No one is allowed to offer alternatives to synthetic drugs without rigorous hoops to jump through and severe penalties to pay. Government medical bureaucrats have become the sole source of *official* information and they get their marching orders from Big Pharma–while you and I are picking up the bill! These and other so called "experts" are the people on government and/or pharmaceutical payrolls who are silencing the debate. Let your congressmen know you want these gag regulations lifted so we can make informed choices in the future.

There may be reason for optimism. In early June, 2010 the United States District Court for the District of Columbia ruled (in the court case, Alliance for Natural Health, et al. vs. Kathleen Sebelius, et al.) that the FDA violated the First Amendment Rights of a nutritional company by censoring truthful, scientifically-backed claims the company made about how the mineral selenium reduces the risk of cancer. Let's hope this is the first of many victories for our right to free speech.

In the last fifty years the membership of the AMA has been dwindling slowly. Out of 900,000 practicing physicians in the U.S. today, less than twenty percent belong to the AMA.[3] It has recently been making efforts to improve its image and boost its sagging membership with well-directed advertising campaigns. Even so, it remains a powerful lobby on Capitol Hill in Washington D.C.

The AMA has literally become the pharmaceutical industry's and Big Pharma's silent partner over the years. The intertwining of the drug industry, AMA, and medical schools was inevitable. The medical model they have used for the last century and a half relies heavily on drugs, surgery, and hospitalizations instead of natural and true healing practices. Together they created the drug-based paradigm for physicians we see in place today, fueling the meteoric rise in the use of synthetic chemicals and the creation of the burgeoning behemoth we call Big Pharma.

First of all, who or what exactly is Big Pharma?

The phrase Big Pharma is used to refer to thirty or more pharmaceutical companies, each with revenues in excess of $3 *billion* dollars annually. They include American companies, multi-national companies, and other companies scattered across the globe.

Most are publicly-traded businesses that compete fiercely among themselves for market share, and are beholden to their investors and their bottom lines. All are profit-based businesses, and they are profitable only as long as we are sick or chronically ill. They are not in business to heal us out of the goodness of their hearts. They are in business to make a profit for their shareholders and have little vested interest in curing disease. If cures were found, there would be little reason for them to exist. With no profit for shareholders, they would have to go out of business.

No one is more of a defender of capitalism and free market systems than I. They have created the highest standard of living for the largest number of people in world history. But I do feel that Big Pharma has lost its moral compass along the way. It has forged a fast track to riches by delivering symptom relief instead of turning its enormous energies and resources to discovering the *cause* of diseases. *Only when causes are established can true cures be found.*

Instead, Big Pharma has become a multi-billion dollar business whose purpose is having everyone take pharmaceuticals–from birth to death. It ensures their survival. Big Pharma actually is in the "business of disease." It is orchestrating the perpetuation and the *expansion* of disease with their synthetic chemicals. The symptoms and side effects from these chemical drugs, most of which are toxic and cause damage to internal organs, *create a whole new set of "diseases"* for which Big Pharma must create even MORE drugs as treatments. What a racket!

Recently, the American Academy of Pediatrics (AAP)–supposed advocates for our children–even announced they will be making the insane recommendation of giving cholesterol-lowering drugs to children as young as eight! (Even though *no* long term studies as to the safety and efficacy of statins on adults *or children* have *ever* been conducted.)

The arms of this powerful lobby stretch far and wide. In 2009, ABC TV network was scheduled to premiere a new comedy/drama, "Eli Stone." The first episode depicted a single mom who sues a drug company for producing a vaccine she feels was the cause of her son's autism.

Several days before the show's first airing, AAP's reps sent an open letter to ABC's executives pressuring them to cancel "Eli Stone" claiming, "If parents watch this program and choose to deny their children immunizations, ABC will share in the responsibility for the suffering and deaths that occur as a result." ABC bowed to the pressure and the show was promptly cancelled.

Fear and intimidation trumped free speech, and Big Pharma breathed a huge sigh of relief.

The AAP is hardly a disinterested party here. If you look at its website you will learn why. Look for the page that lists annual corporate donations to their *"Friends of Children Fund."* Surprise, surprise! You'll find huge donations from Merck, Abbott Laboratories, AstraZeneca, Sanofi-Aventis, Squibb and many others–all pharmaceutical companies.

Surely our children deserve better *"friends"* than these.

Today we are barraged with ads for patented, synthetic drugs that treat every disease or condition imaginable, touting dangerous antibiotics, statins, anti-depressants, meds for high blood pressure, gout, diabetes, heart disease, migraines–the list is endless. No cures, mind you, just relief from symptoms. Big Pharma's mantra continues: *"No one can be well or get well without our chemicals."*

Unfortunately, we continue to fall for their hype and spin.

In 1929 the average American received less than two prescriptions a year. In 2006, the average prescription rate had ballooned into over *4 prescriptions per child, almost 11 prescriptions per adult, and an unbelievable 28 prescriptions per senior.*[4] Even though there are many good physicians who write prescriptions conservatively, today so many people are taking so many drugs that it has lead to the creation of a new word: "polypharmacy." Polypharmacy refers to the poisonous chemical cocktail of multiple drugs which can cause dangerous interactions, especially in the elderly, and is directly responsible for up to 28 percent of hospital admissions![5] So, you can see that Big Pharma, instead of researching disease in search of cures, has chosen instead to *treat symptoms*. That way they cannot only create the drugs to treat the symptoms, but they can create more drugs to treat the new "diseases" caused by drugs!

A case in point is Strattera®, a new drug that treats ADD and ADHD. Here is a disease–ADD or ADHD–which may be caused by drugs–vaccines–being treated by another drug–Strattera®. Drug companies get to make money both ways–by both "causing" a disease and then "curing" it, *all with government assistance and approval.* Big Pharma's investors and bottom lines are well served and disease is perpetuated as we willingly empty our wallets for their wares.

In 2007 the global market for pharmaceuticals topped $693 billion, and by 2013 it is expected to reach $1 trillion. This includes branded prescription drugs, generic prescription drugs, and over-the-counter drugs.

Speaking of over-the-counter drugs, in the U.S. 46 people die every *day* from taking aspirin, and nearly 500 people die every year from taking acetamenophen. Just because they aren't prescription drugs doesn't mean they are without risk. Liver and kidney damage is inevitable with their use.

Disease is big business. That makes prescription drugs big business. Next to software, drugs have the highest profit margin of any industry in the United States. Drug companies have long been known to put astronomical markups on their drugs. Big Pharma claims it needs these obscene markups for research and development *for more drugs.*

Is it any wonder Medicare and everyone else is going broke?

Pharmaceutical companies are the biggest lobbyists on Capitol Hill. In pursuing profits, last year drug companies employed 625 lobbyists in Washington, D.C., and spent $15 billion on "physician marketing"–a euphemistic way of describing the practice of wooing, wining and dining, and indoctrinating doctors into prescribing their medications. $15 billion on lunches for the office, gifts, sponsored medical seminars, visits to pharmaceutical headquarters, and 315,000 parties and events.[7] Many MDs routinely receive huge bonus checks from drug companies for prescribing their drugs. This is not only big business, but "monkey business" to boot.

As I write this, Pfizer Inc, the largest drug maker in the world, is being hit with a record-breaking $2.3 *billion* fine by U.S. federal prosecutors for "illegal drug promotions and marketing" for plying doctors with free golf, massages, and resort junkets. Pfizer was labeled "a repeating corporate cheat" and "repeat offender." (This is the fourth such settlement of government charges against Pfizer in the last decade.) The allegations surround the marketing of 13 different drugs, including the blockbusters Viagra®, Zoloft®, and Lipitor®. Justice Department officials said the overall settlement is the *largest ever paid by a drug company for alleged violations of federal drug rules*: $1.2 billion of the $2.3 billion is a *criminal* fine, the largest ever in any criminal case.[8] Of course this probably will not deter them as the price of fines and lawsuits is apparently built into the price of their drugs (see 1–8 above.) Consumers are really paying for this fine, and Pfizer continues to make buckets of money regardless.

Pharmaceutical companies donate millions of dollars annually to medical schools. If you think that comes with no strings attached, think again. More than $11.5 million was "donated" to Harvard Medical School alone in 2008, earmarked for "research and continuing education classes." Astoundingly, 1,600 professors and lecturers at Harvard (out of 8,900) admit that they or a family member had business ties to drug companies that could influence their teaching or research.[9] No medical professor can teach unbiased and truthful information if he or she is being paid off by drug companies.

But there is a glimmer of hope. In 2009 a group of 200 Harvard Medical School students concerned that pharmaceutical industry scandals, billions of dollars in fines, lawsuits, proof of faulty, sloppy and biased research, and hyped marketing claims have tarnished the medical profession, confronted the school's administration demanding that pharmaceutical industry influence in the classroom and faculty be stopped. Kudos to those moral and ethical young men and women for making efforts to clean up their medical education.

In the January 7th, 2008 issue of *Science Daily*, a new study reported that the U.S. pharmaceutical industry spent almost *twice as much on promotion and advertising as it does on research and development.* That shows where their true interests lie.

One of the recent promotional goldmines for Big Pharma is called "off-labeling." It is a form of marketing to doctors that encourages them to prescribe drugs legally for diseases *not* approved by the FDA *in order to increase profits.* For example, Neurontin®, *an epilepsy drug,* was marketed to doctors for pain management, bi-polar disorders, shingles, fibromyalgia and migraines as well, even though it was *not approved by the FDA for those conditions.* The result? U.S. annual sales of Neurontin® zoomed from $98 million in 1995 to nearly $3 billion in 2004. A whistle-blower and employee of Parke-Davis filed a lawsuit suit against the company charging that "off-labeling of Neurontin® constituted false claims." In 2004, Warner-Lambert agreed to plead guilty and paid $430 million in fines–*less than fifteen percent of the $3 billion the drug company had grossed in 2004.*[10] The cost of fines is built into the product, and is regarded by the industry as "just the cost of doing business."

In 2005 Pfizer's painkiller, Bextra®, was yanked off the market when research proved the drug was associated with marked increases in heart attacks and strokes. *One half* of its $1.7 billion in profit that year was attributed to unapproved, off-label uses. Pfizer's fine amounted to three months worth of profits. Big deal.

Another pharmaceutical company coming under the gun is AstraZeneca. In May, 2010 AstraZeneca agreed to pay $520 million to settle federal investigations into its marketing practices for its blockbuster schizophrenia drug, Seroquel®. The company was charged with using illegal marketing tactics (pushing doctors to prescribe it for off-label conditions such as anger management, ADHD, Alzheimer's disease, and insomnia). It was also charged with misleading doctors and patients by spotlighting only favorable research while failing to reveal research that showed Seroquel® increased the risk of diabetes. Twenty-five thousand civil suits are now waiting in the wings. But, no matter. For every dollar

AstraZeneca is fined–*it makes ten!* According to the *New York Times*, April 26, 2010, Seroquel® raked in $4.9 billion in sales in 2009. What's a measly $520 million fine. Unfortunately, illegal, off-labeling of many drugs is still being practiced throughout the industry.

In an effort to expand it market, Eli Lilly is even repackaging its anti-depressant, Prozac®, for DOGS! In Japan, GlaxoSmithKline is doing the same, by actively recruiting children between the ages of seven and seventeen to test the efficacy of Paxil®, an anti-depressant, against a placebo in children with depression–*despite the elevated suicide risks associated with the drug.*

Just follow the money. You will find that the financial health of pharmaceutical companies has taken precedence over the health of the people they seemingly serve. It seems the medical profession has become an indentured servant to pharmaceutical companies.

Another illustration of this is one of the most popular medical websites today, WebMD. It boasts over fifty million visitors a month. Originally owned by Eli Lilly, a pharmaceutical giant, it is now publicly owned. But guess who primarily funds WebMD. Ta da...*the pharmaceutical companies, of course.* When you go to their website and type in a medical condition, you immediately are taken to drugs. WebMD is simply an advertising arm of the pharmaceutical industry.

Medical research is another area of medicine fraught with deception and medical bias. Dr. William Campbell Douglass III, M.D., one of the top alternative MDs in the country, wrote recently on his website: *"Corruption has become so endemic and intellectual integrity so compromised in pharmaceutical research that drug companies and collaborators in government and universities can now get away with open fraud."*

Even the prestigious *Journal of the American Medical Association* (JAMA) has analyzed the connecting links between clinical research and resultant guidelines and the pharmaceutical industry. They found *over half* the research labs received financial support from the pharmaceutical industry to conduct research, and 38 percent were hired as employees or consultants for pharmaceutical companies.[11] Hmmm. Let's see. How do you suppose they rated the drugs they conducted clinical trials on?

In recent years, industry insiders and whistle-blowers have written books that clearly document the pharmaceutical companies' obscene profits, conflicts of interests, payoffs to research labs, manipulation of results of clinical studies, and the payments to speakers (usually doctors) who promote their drugs. They are eye-opening books to say the least.

One of the most unethical and immoral changes in the industry in the last few years is the advent of what is called "Direct to Consumer" or DTC advertising. We are so used to this form of TV, radio, and magazine advertising now in the United States that it may come as a surprise to learn that *only one other country in the world allows it– New Zealand, a country of only four million.* Visitors to the U.S. are shocked and appalled at the amount of pharmaceutical advertising they see on TV and in electronic and print media. It is overwhelming now.

For years the pharmaceutical industry was allowed to market their wares only to doctors–mainly through sales calls, medical journals, continuing medical education classes, mailers, medical conventions, etc. Under pressure from the industry, the FDA finally agreed to allow the first DTC advertising in 1985, *but with strict guidelines.* Drugs could be called by name, but if they were used to treat specific conditions, the ads were required to list most of the side effects and contraindications.

Under more pressure from the industry, in 1997 those guidelines were loosened further so that only the *major side effects and contraindications* had to be listed, and consequently between 1994 and 2000 the number of TV ads increased forty-fold! The percentage is even higher today.

Gone are the days when we trusted doctors to do their homework and tell us what *they* thought was best for us. Thanks to DTC advertising, now we go to them and demand the drugs *we* want! The pharmaceutical companies love it. Still, there are many doctors of good conscience who refuse to prescribe a drug just because a patient demands it.

In 1991 spending on DTC advertising in the United States was only $55 million. Between 1991 and 2003, spending jumped five-fold, reaching $3.2 billion per year. Today drug companies spend $4 billion each year on direct-to-consumer ads in the United States, but four times that–*a massive $16 billion in influencing your doctor.* That amounts to $10,000 for every doctor in this country[12] and has provided the pharmaceutical industry with a *huge* increase in profits–a whopping 18 to 20 percent of revenues of just a few years ago. The more they advertise, the more money they make. This is made evident by the endless number of pharmaceutical ads in magazines and on our TV screens all day. The best book I have found on this subject is *Overdo$ed America* by John Abramson, M.D. Read it and weep.

Unconscionably, pharmaceutical companies have lobbied for and gotten the government to guarantee that they be shielded from any liability from the use of many of their toxic products. They have already asked for and gotten a bill that would bar any lawsuit or litigation or liability incurred by them for harm done to children by vaccines–arguing that such suits could run them out of business! They want to bear no responsibility for any harm, damage or deaths caused by their drugs.

In 2002 a rider called the Eli Lilly Protection Act, added at the last minute to the Homeland Security Bill, gave the pharmaceutical companies the assurance they needed to continue to manufacture their noxious remedies with impunity. In the future, watch for Gestapo-like tactics and behind the scenes dirty work to coerce and mandate vaccines for everyone. It is a billion dollar gamble they can't afford to lose.

All of this has led to the creation of the powerful behemoth we know today as Big Pharma. Or dare I say, Big P[*harm*]A? To make matters worse, we have few options on how to change it. Big Pharma, FDA, FTC, CDC, medical schools, research labs–all enjoy a cozy relationship among themselves designed to protect their agendas, their jobs, and their awesome power. Add all this to the fact that Big Pharma is the largest contributor to politicians in Washington, D.C. and you can see the enormity of the problem. We all have become tangled in a spider's web and bound so tightly we cannot move or escape. Unfortunately the big fat spider is saving us for a rainy day. Unfortunately also, he is spinning new and bigger webs.

Case in point is the recent story in the news of 13-year old Daniel Hauser who suffers from Hodgkin's lymphoma. He and his mother fled their farm in Sleepy Eye, Minnesota, to travel to Mexico for natural treatments and to avoid a court-ordered round of chemotherapy which doctors said "could" cure him. The judge also issued a contempt order for the mother and custody of the boy was transferred to Brown County Family Services. Alerts were issued to police departments around the country in a massive effort to hunt them down. *Even the FBI and Interpol* were pushed into action to "apprehend and detain" both, citing "his best interests require it". Daniel and his mother's only crime was to say no to Big Pharma and the AMA.

Both came home voluntarily after a week on the run, and the arrest warrant was dismissed. Daniel received the court-ordered chemotherapy against his will, but was allowed to take natural and alternative treatments as well. This is one of many cases where parental rights are being abrogated in favor of the state and its powerful allies. No doctor has the right to unequivocally say his or her treatment is the only cure available. Statistics prove otherwise. As we know, chemotherapy and radiation can create other and worse cancers down the road. This is a thorny issue to say the least, and one that needs to be debated all the way to the highest courts of the land.

One of the few recourses people have at the moment is to sue. Class action suits against a legion of drugs are beginning to appear everywhere. *The number of ads on TV by law firms recruiting victims of drug side effects is beginning to rival the number of ads for the drugs themselves!* People are getting angry and organized. They realize that the real and most powerful option they have is to become educated! We consumers are still the ultimate marketplace.

Even against terrible odds of ever getting justice, more than 4,900 families in the United States have continued to file lawsuits after their formerly healthy children became autistic within days of receiving their MMR shots. Since the system legally is "rigged" against them, the only recourse for many parents has been to seek compensation from the Vaccine Injury Compensation Act, a notoriously difficult achievement. Even so, to date nearly *$2 BILLION dollars* has been awarded to families of injured or killed children *(that were paid for by the U.S. tax payer, not the pharmaceutical companies)*. More about this later.

The FDA, which is supposed to protect us from harm or harmful substances in our food and drugs, truly has not lived up to its responsibilities, and to add insult to injury, *it spends taxpayer dollars to scare people away from alternative medicine.* Campaigns of intimidation, threats, and invasions of doctors' offices by the FDA with guns drawn should not be tolerated in a free society.

Don't forget, natural medicine is now under siege. Big Pharma is desperate to control the "sickness industry." Its next main goal is to close down and destroy the thorn in its side known as the "wellness industries"– the holistic and alternative clinics, practitioners, and practices around the world–in order to eliminate the competition and consolidate their enormous power.

They are taking steps to achieve this goal every day.

In the meantime, let's look at one of Big Pharma's "blockbusters," (a drug is considered a blockbuster when it reaches sales of $1 billion per year)… the money machine known as *statins.*

## Chapter 18

# Statins…Cure or Curse?

*"Saturated fat and cholesterol in the diet are not the cause of coronary heart disease. That myth is the greatest deception of this century, perhaps of any century."*

George V. Mann, M.D.
Professor of Medicine and Biochemistry at Vanderbilt University

Did you know that people with high cholesterol live longer than people with low cholesterol? Not only do they live longer, they feel better, are more fit, more energetic, healthier, and happier than their friends with low cholesterol. Feeling good is actually a symptom of higher cholesterol!

After you stop hyperventilating, take a deep breath. Exhale. I know that sounds like an outrageous statement that flies in the face of conventional medical wisdom, but, nonetheless, it is true. It is a well-kept secret that pharmaceutical companies don't want you to know. *High cholesterol actually may be good for you.*

First, let's take a cholesterol 101 class to learn the basics of this substance that is so critical to the functioning of every cell in our bodies.

Cholesterol is a fat that circulates in your bloodstream. It is essential because it is a building material for *all body cells*. It is a soft, fatty, waxy substance that constitutes the membrane of all cells, and actually makes them *waterproof.* When our bodies don't make enough, cell membranes become porous and literally *leak.* It is estimated that without cholesterol we would lose four to five gallons of fluid a day.

Around 85 percent of the cholesterol in our blood is made naturally in the liver while the rest is created from the food we eat. If our bodies don't get enough from food, the liver will create more to make up the deficit. Our livers churn out between 2,000 and 3,000 mgs. daily–that's more than a dozen times what you would normally get from food in a day. It seems our bodies know intuitively that we need this critically important substance, and plenty of it.

According to prevailing medical dogma, high-density lipoproteins, or HDL, are the "good guys," which help carry the low-density lipoproteins, or LDL, the "bad guys," away from the artery walls and return them to the bloodstream, thereby preventing buildup on artery walls. In this scenario, an elevated LDL (bad) is associated with a greater risk of heart disease, and an elevated HDL (good) is associated with lower heart disease risks. As you will see, both these designations are misleading.

In order to keep the combined LDL and HDL numbers low, doctors and cardiologists recommend low-fat, low cholesterol diets, and cholesterol lowering drugs called *statins* in order to keep in lockstep with the current low-fat, low cholesterol marching band.

What could possibly be good about cholesterol when we've been taught to regard it as our enemy–as something to fear–or as something we want in extremely low amounts?

**Cholesterol facts:**

1. Cholesterol is the body's repair substance, and can be likened to a natural "sticky glue." High levels are found in all scar tissue, including scar tissue in the arteries. Its natural stickiness is what helps cells hang together; without cholesterol we literally would fall apart.

2. Cholesterol is critical to proper neurological functioning, especially in the brain and in the formation and retention of

memory. *The brain actually is the most cholesterol-rich organ in the body*, and there is a direct correlation between the amount of cholesterol in the brain and how well it functions.[1] Cholesterol even constitutes over half the dry weight of the cerebral cortex! It is an essential element of myelin–the protective sheath that insulates nerves and keeps our brains and nervous systems sharp and healthy. Our spinal cord and all nerves are richly supplied with cholesterol.

3. Cholesterol is the precursor to vitamin D, the trigger for so many biochemical processes, including mineral metabolism and immune function.

4. Bile salts, so important to fat metabolism, are made of cholesterol. Many people whose cholesterol levels are too low from heredity, diet or drugs, have trouble digesting fat.

5. Cholesterol is a building block for making sex and adrenal hormones– hormones so important for maintaining energy, vitality, and libido.

6. Cholesterol is absolutely vital for the proper functioning of the liver.

7. Cholesterol is important in building bones and muscles.

8. Cholesterol helps regulate blood sugar and repair damaged tissue.

9. Cholesterol (LDL) protects against infection, especially bacterial infection.

As you can see, it seems this valuable substance has beneficial effects from our heads to our toes. So why is it wearing such a huge black hat these days?

*Because it has been demonized by both the medical profession and the pharmaceutical industry for so many years.*

This process began in the 1950s when studies "linked" high consumption of animal and saturated fats with high rates of heart disease, and voila!, a newfangled disease called "hypercholesterolemia"–high cholesterol–was invented.  Soon doctors figured out a way to measure cholesterol levels in blood, clinical trials were run, and the formulation of a new paradigm was born, called... *drum roll, please:*

### "The Cholesterol *Theory* of Heart Disease"

This intrinsically flawed "*theory*" (known as "the lipid hypothesis") had extensive consequences because it radically changed our eating habits.  We were told to eat trans fat margarine, fake eggs, polyunsaturated and hydrogenated oils, imitation bacon, etc.  It made all fats bad and all carbohydrates good, contributing mightily to our skyrocketing cases of diabetes and obesity.  It weaseled its way into "clinical practice guidelines" and "standards of care" protocols which doctors are expected to follow.  Subsequently it generated the invasive heart surgery industry, based on the notion that cholesterol-laden blockages must be bypassed or propped open with wire cages called stents.  That new theory led to the creation of a new class of medications– statins, which became *the biggest moneymakers in pharmaceutical history*, generating more than $15 billion in sales worldwide every year.  In order to sell the drugs, pharmaceutical companies launched a massive marketing juggernaut to "fat bash" and sell the public on the "dangers" of cholesterol and saturated fat in general. Unfortunately, we fell for it.

Now we are reaping what they have sown, by witnessing the "side effects" of low fat, low cholesterol diets, and statin drugs– and they are not good. *The so-called "heart-healthy" diet that has been foisted on Americans for over four decades has fueled both our epidemics of heart disease and cancer.* On these regimens the body deteriorates and disease becomes inevitable. Here's why.

If, through diet or drugs, you do not have enough cholesterol in your body to perform the above 1 through 9 duties, you could experience at some point: soreness and destruction of muscle (last time I checked, *the heart is a muscle*), liver and kidney damage, increased rate of cancer, suppression of the immune system, depression of mental acuity, violent behavior, anemia, pancreatitis, acidosis, cataracts, fevers, fatigue, and even death. Incredibly, the statin, Zocor®, comes with a *19-page warning disclosure brochure!*

**Here are some of the more common side-effects of all statins:**

1. congestion and persistent coughs

2. muscle pain and weakness

3. allergic reactions, such as wheezing, itching, skin rashes

4. upper respiratory infections

5. decreased libido

6. difficulty sleeping

7. constipation

8. dizziness or light-headedness

9. headache

10. heartburn or indigestion

11. excessive gas or belching

12. abdominal pain

13. nausea and vomiting

14. You further are saddled with the high cost of statins (between $900 and $1,700 or more a year), plus all the other drugs you will need to treat the above symptoms *for the rest of your life!*

Statins contain a major design flaw. They lower cholesterol levels by reducing an enzyme in your liver that cuts down on the production of cholesterol. Unfortunately, statins not only reduce the production of cholesterol, but ironically also reduce another enzyme called coenzymeQ10, (CoQ10), an enzyme so critical it is used by every cell in the body, *and is vital to heart health! Statins attack and destroy your heart's single most important nutrient!* One of the most dangerous side effects of statins is this ability to cripple and create deficiencies of CoQ10. The heart requires huge amounts in order to work well, especially concerning the heart's pumping strength. Without it your heartbeat would come to a screeching halt. Statin-induced CoQ10 depletion can lead to a decline in left ventricular heart function. A CoQ10 deficiency also accelerates DNA damage and premature aging.

With this 'workhorse' locked in the barn, muscles become sore and weak, leading to muscle wasting, severe back pain, neuropathy, inflammation of tendons and ligaments, *which actually can rupture,* and eventually *heart failure.*

Low cholesterol, in general, *hikes* the risk of congestive heart failure. A recent study involving over a thousand patients with severe heart failure showed that people with the lowest cholesterol *died twice as often* from heart failure as patients with cholesterol over 223![2]

Imagine! The pharmaceutical wizards have created statins that purport to cut down on the incidence of coronary artery disease, which can actually create a *more* critical disease called heart failure! Now you get to take *two kinds* of drugs instead of one: One for prevention of heart disease and the other for a heart disease caused by the drug. Stop the insanity! Unfortunately, most doctors and cardiologists today are unaware of the problem and, consequently, do not recommended CoQ10 supplementation to their patients to correct this life-threatening deficiency.

Unless they are self-taught, few doctors have any real knowledge of nutrition, nutritional healing or alternative medicines. Their first loyalty is to the pharmaceutical industry drugs they have been taught to use. Many receive monetary gifts from pharmaceutical companies for prescribing their drugs! Although I personally believe most doctors do have their patients' best interests at heart and truly care about them, the fact remains that most are so overwhelmed in their practices and the constant flood of drug information they must keep current with, they have neither the time nor the inclination to learn about herbs, nutrition, or natural healing.

Another major concern and stumbling block today is medical liability. Doctors are reticent to do anything that does not meet with FDA approval, and are pressured to conform to "standards of care" or to the requirements of their insurance carriers. (87 percent of doctors who decide "standards of care"–the protocols doctors must follow when treating disease–have their wallets filled by pharmaceutical companies.)[3] Doctors also tend to follow "studies and statistics" in treating patients. In addition, they are trained in medical school *to react rather than think outside the box.*

Physicians *react* by reaching for their prescription pads, and those maverick doctors who dare to *think* for themselves are more likely to be hauled before medical boards for non-conformity and risk losing their medical licenses. Consequently, do not expect answers to questions you ask concerning prescription drugs to be unbiased. Their experience mainly lies with synthetic chemicals, and if you ask about side effects or NNT numbers (numbers need to treat–see below), defensive postures are to be expected.

One of the most dangerous side effects of statins is the terrible toll it takes on muscles. Muscle pain and weakness are very common in statin users, and patients are warned to stop taking them immediately if they experience any pain. Remembering that the heart is a muscle, it's not hard to understand why. Already, statins have killed 50 people with rhabdomyolysis, a severe and potentially fatal muscle wasting disease. It occurs when muscles weaken and literally fall apart, oozing a protein, *myoglobin,* into the bloodstream.[4] Once in the bloodstream, these harmful proteins travel to the kidneys, clog the tiny tubules or filters of the kidney and inflict massive damage. Sometimes the kidneys are rendered useless and the patient must go on dialysis to live. (Drug companies hope you don't remember that in 2001, Baycol®, a popular cholesterol lowering drug, was removed from the market after 31 people died from severe muscle breakdown, or rhabdomyolysis.[5] The figure now is well over 100 deaths and 1,600 injuries.)

Another side effect surfacing now is that statins have been shown to inhibit Vitamin D production, so vital for the prevention of cancer and immune system function. Low cholesterol levels are also associated with violent behavior, anxiety, suicide, depression, bi-polar disease, post-operative delirium, (remember how critical cholesterol is to the functioning of the brain), and increased mortality from cancer. Over-emphasis on a low cholesterol diet has been strongly linked to the recent marked increases in tuberculosis (LDL is vital to removing bacteria), celiac disease, hyperthyroidism, and liver disease. Since the brain is so cholesterol dense, low cholesterol levels can actually *cause the brain to shrink!* Great. Just what we all need. Less brains.

A full 15 percent of statin users have reported cognitive impairment of some kind–the most terrifying being something dubbed "transient global amnesia" (TGA)–characterized by complete loss of memory for short or even lengthy periods of time.

One of the most well-known stories concerning transient global amnesia came from Dr. Duane Graveline, M.D., a retired family doctor and former NASA scientist and astronaut. In 1999 he dutifully took his doctor's prescription for Lipitor® for six weeks. One day, after taking a walk, he was found dazed and confused, not knowing where he was or his wife's name, and could not recognize his own house. Six hours later he "came to", was later diagnosed with "TGA", and stopped Lipitor®. One year later, on the advice of his physician who didn't believe there was a drug connection, Graveline started on a lower dose, and within twelve hours he experienced another TGA. This time he regressed to his teen-age years. He had no memory of his college or medical school years, his marriage, his four children, his medical career, or his recent past. Again he went off statins and recovered his memory. Unfortunately, some years later he noticed unusual fatigue, increasing weakness, in-coordination, and progressive disability–all the hallmarks of ALS, or Lou Gehrig's disease, and all the hallmarks of statin damage. Recently he had to give up his daily walks. Dr. Graveline is convinced that his disease is Lipitor® related. You can follow his story at www.spacedoc.net.

Today there are many patients in wheelchairs being diagnosed with Lou Gehrig's disease, a progressive and usually fatal motor neuron disease characterized by muscle weakness and atrophy throughout the body, who can trace their symptoms back to statin drug use, just like Dr. Graveline. Their numbers are growing.

Thousands of patients taking statins have written to the FDA's MedWatch program to report memory loss and other cognitive problems. All statin drugs–not just Lipitor®–have been linked to this side effect.

Unconscionably, FDA-required trials *do not even report* memory loss attributable to the use of statins. Why? In a veritable shell game, pharmaceutical companies often divide similar adverse effects into six or more different categories in order to keep their more frightening side effects under a certain number! For instance, memory loss can be divided into confusion, senility, amnesia, inability to concentrate, disorientation, etc. If you totaled the categories you would get a *big memory loss number*. (Can't let the public know that!) These kinds of numbers games are played all the time in pharmaceutical trials. Even the prestigious *American Journal of Medicine* wrote in 2004, "Based on the evidence now available, 100 percent of statins users can expect a decrease of cognitive function." [6]

Laboratory chemicals such as statins don't belong in the human body. *That is what their "side effects" are trying to tell us.* The body communicates with us in the only language it knows: *symptoms.* It gets our attention by creating uncomfortable symptoms and manifesting even more uncomfortable *dis-eases* in an effort to tell us it is unhappy dealing with substances it doesn't recognize, or know how to handle, or eliminate. Are we hearing its frantic cries?

According to current medical dogma, high cholesterol causes coronary artery disease. If true, then why do people with high cholesterol levels have *less* coronary heart disease? *Over half of the people who have heart attacks or strokes do not have elevated cholesterol levels!* [7]

If high cholesterol actually causes coronary heart disease, then wouldn't lowering cholesterol through diet and drugs parallel lower rates of coronary heart disease? One would think so, but *it does not. Older people with low cholesterol die twice as often from heart attacks compared to people with high cholesterol.* [8]

If high cholesterol actually caused coronary heart disease, wouldn't it be reflected in high heart disease rates in all populations across the board, in both males and females, in all ages, in all disease categories? It does not. *Heart disease, stroke, and atherosclerosis rates have not fallen one bit since statins were introduced twenty years ago, even though twenty million Americans now take them.* [9] (As a matter of fact, heart disease is worse than it was fifty years ago.) *Not a single study shows statins work for women,* [10] whether they have heart disease or not. Also women are 300 percent less likely to develop heart disease than men, even though on average they have higher cholesterol levels than men.

*Instead, high cholesterol continues to be associated with longevity in old people, and consistently occurs in people with the lowest mortality.* [11] *Bottom line? People with HIGH cholesterol live longer, period.*

Undoubtedly, coronary artery disease is a very deadly disease and should not be taken lightly. It causes 1.3 million deaths a year in the United States alone. It also is complicated by many variables, but reduced to its simplest terms any layman can easily comprehend how plaque forms in the arteries. It works like this:

In a nutshell, *something* first initiates tiny cracks or wounds in the delicate lining of the coronary artery, the *intima.* This causes inflammation and/or infection. In response to that injury, the immune system swings into action. In its infinite wisdom, it uses waxy cholesterol and calcium to patch up the wound in an effort to seal it off and prevent it from rupturing or leaking. Underneath that seal, cholesterol and bacteria fester into pimples that create soft plaque. If one of the pimples bursts, a clot or thrombus forms over the site which can obstruct blood flow causing angina and other symptoms. Clogging usually appears at the bends of arteries–exactly where the plumbing in your home gets clogged up. Unfortunately, sometimes clogged arteries develop rough edges, and clots break loose and travel to the lung causing a pulmonary embolism, or to the brain causing a stroke. The link between elevated cholesterol levels and strokes has never been established.[12]

We now know that inflammation is always the precursor to heart disease. Even though it has no outward symptoms, it is one of the most serious indicators of heart disease. During inflammation or infection, C–reactive protein (CRP) is secreted from the liver. Your doctor can order this test to reveal the level of inflammation in your body. Many cardiologists believe that *high levels of CRP are a much stronger risk factor for coronary artery disease than cholesterol*. A study in 2005 of two statin drugs, atorvastatin and pravastatin, found that patients with low CRP levels had fewer heart attacks no matter their LDL cholesterol levels, and they had more heart attacks if their CRP was elevated–regardless of their LDL cholesterol level.[13]

The very same results have been found for stroke risk. The same two drugs were studied on patients taking high and moderate doses of statin drugs (the PROVE study). The results showed there was *no* difference in the cholesterol levels of those who had strokes and those who didn't. *The only difference was the levels of CRP, or inflammation.*[14]

If it is true that heart disease follows inflammation, then high cholesterol may actually *protect you from cardiovascular disease* instead of causing it! Why? Because of its anti-infection and anti-inflammatory properties. Cholesterol, by constantly tamping down the fires of inflammation and repairing the damage done by inflammation, keeps infections from becoming overwhelming. Don't leave home without it!

But more important questions to ask are: *What is causing the inflammation? And what is tearing up the intima?*

The answer is… *the yeast/beast.* Oh, no…that pesky yeast/beast again?

Time for a recap: Atherosclerosis is the consequence of an inflammatory process that begins with *"something"* causing a localized injury to the intima, a thin layer of cells lining the inside of an artery. Known contributors to inflammation are recreational and prescription drugs, high blood pressure, smoking, excess insulin, easily oxidized omega-6 vegetable oils (e.g., corn, soy, peanut, safflower, canola, cottonseed), being overweight, an increased consumption of plaque-producing sugar, and *trans fatty acids.* All of these irritate and inflame the intima, creating piles of decaying cells. And guess who comes to dinner?

Yeast and fungi heard the dinner bell and come running to gorge themselves on the debris. They hurriedly set up housekeeping in the warm, moist linings of the coronary arteries, set the table, pull up their chairs, and celebrate their good fortune with a riotous feeding frenzy.

Unfortunately, in their haste and greed, the boorish ruffians have left a mess at the banquet table, even creating gashes, pits and gouges in the smooth table top–the intima. The call goes out for cholesterol to come to the rescue. Soon the injuries are patched and smoothed over. But the host, regrettably, woofed down a ham and cheese sandwich with pickles and beer for lunch, and topped it off with a Klondike Bar. The partying yeast just moved on to another site in the artery, and the whole process starts all over again. Over time, cholesterol "scabs," or plaques, build up and blood flow becomes impaired by the blockages. Eventually coronary artery disease rears its ugly head, and here comes a prescription for...you guessed it–*statins.*

True, statins do work, and do reduce cholesterol levels by blocking its formation. But what does a cholesterol test actually measure? *A cholesterol test is actually a measurement of yeast levels!* It is an indicator of *yeast statistics.* If you have high cholesterol, it means that your yeast levels are high because the yeast beasties are busy and cholesterol is needed to repair the damage and put out the fires of inflammation. Statins' greatest benefit is taming inflammation, not in lowering cholesterol.

Cholesterol does not cause heart disease any more than firemen cause house fires! Think of the body's cholesterol as firemen, racing in to save the day by putting out the flames of inflammation. Cholesterol levels rise in response to the damage *that has already occurred to the arteries* as a result of oxidation. The actual cause of heart disease and arterial damage then is oxidation or "oxidative stress" brought on by the inflammation triggered by trans fatty acids, partially hydrogenated oils, vegetable oils, high blood pressure, alcohol, smoking and *that old bugaboo–sugar.* All create conditions that invite yeast.

Elevated cholesterol is a response to an invasion by fungal mycotoxins and free radicals in the bloodstream. Our bodies brilliantly reduce the toxicity of these poisons by producing more fat in the form of cholesterol, *effectively diluting the toxins.* Cholesterol performs a heroic duty by binding fungal toxins and rendering them less harmful. Let's hear it for cholesterol!

But the icing on the cake–excuse the sugary metaphor–is that statins were *originally used as anti-fungals!* That is why cholesterol levels come down with their use. *Statins kill fungi and reduce inflammation.* With much of the fungi out of the way, less damage is done and the need for cholesterol is reduced. Voila! Lower cholesterol levels. Studies on mice with osteoporosis have shown that when given statins, the mice actually grew bone! Why? *Statins reduced the fungi that were eating bone.*

The yeast-free diet and natural anti-fungals accomplish the same thing–without the expense and without the risks–by addressing the underlying cause of high cholesterol and atherosclerosis, *which is chronic inflammation from the original arterial injuries and the ensuing overgrowths of fungi and their harmful mycotoxins.* Not many of the millions of Americans taking statins for their heart health understand that they are merely treating the symptoms of this condition and not the cause.

Remember, statins do not address the underlying cause of heart disease, which is sick, damaged arteries. Plaque does not form in healthy arteries, no matter how much cholesterol is in your blood.[15] Statins do not clean them of harmful plaque buildup. They do not protect against heart attack or prevent premature death. They also do not lower the overall death *rate* from heart disease but actually *increase* the death rate from all causes.[16] They never have been proven beneficial to women. In fact they can endanger your heart!

So what is the point of taking them? If they don't address the underlying cause of heart disease, they don't lower the death rate, and make no difference in the rate of non-fatal heart attacks, why would anyone take them and run the risk of deadly side-effects? They simply enrich the coffer$ of the pharmaceutical companie$. (The twenty million American$ who are taking statin$ today are being told to $tay on them for *the re$t of their live$.*)

Upshot? Except for a handful of people–those who have a history of heart attacks or very high C-reactive protein (CRP) levels or genetic hypercholesterolemia–statins are, in my opinion, an ineffective and harmful fraud, and a waste of your time, money…and maybe even your life. They appear to be little more than toxic band-aids.

One of the most closely-guarded secrets of the pharmaceutical industry is the NNT, which stands for "numbers needed to treat." It is a crucial health statistic you probably never heard of and that pharmaceutical companies conveniently leave out of their ads. It states the number of patients that would need to be treated with a medical therapy to *prevent one bad outcome*. To put it another way, it is the number of persons that would need to be treated *before one person gets good results.* The NNT for Lipitor® has been determined to be 100; meaning one hundred people must be treated with Lipitor® to prevent one heart attack![17] The other ninety-nine receive no benefit whatsoever, but instead are put at risk for liver damage, muscle wasting, etc. and even death–for years–for nothing!

*Business Week* (January 28, 2008) reported that the *average* NNT for statins was a whopping 250. Two hundred fifty patients have to take statins for years, showing no measurable improvement (while risking deadly side-effects) *before one person actually benefits!* Other statins have NNTs of 500 and higher.[18] Quite a deal for Big Pharma, wouldn't you say?

Please consult with your physician to find out the NNT for *any* drug being prescribed before you take it. It is the only way to learn your true odds of receiving any benefit from that drug. He or she may be reluctant to do so, but it is your right to know.

Also, be extremely wary of recent so-called studies claiming to prove that statins reduce the risk of heart disease by reducing cholesterol. Pharmaceutical companies continuously manipulate numbers in their favor. And the proof of this can be found in their own research!

Recently in the ASCOT-LLA study used to promote Lipitor®, 3 percent of the control group experienced heart attacks, while 2 percent of the Lipitor® group did, making the actual risk reduction one percentage point. But Pfizer reported a 34 percent reduction. How did they do that? *By manipulating the math. Two percent is 34 percent less than 3 percent!* If it had reported the one percent reduction, the trial would have been rightly deemed a failure. Instead, sales of Lipitor® skyrocketed. AstraZeneca® pulled the same trick with their latest trial on Crestor®. They claimed a 50 percent reduction when the actual reduction was a measly 0.41 percent.[19] Of course, sales went through the roof.

More and more medical and research experts are beginning to suspect that cholesterol has little or nothing to do with heart disease, as more studies are coming out that do not support–and even *contradict*–the cholesterol hypothesis. A long-awaited study on Vytorin®, a cholesterol fighter by Merck, revealed recently that the drug failed to meet its main goals of improving outcomes, citing no significant difference between patients receiving Vytorin® and those receiving placebos. (Higher incidents of cancer were noted, however.)[20]

So why lower cholesterol if it's NOT the cause of heart disease?

Recently researchers at Texas A&M University were caught off guard when they discovered that lower cholesterol levels actually *reduced* muscle gained from exercising! They also found that those participants who ate diets that were higher in cholesterol-containing foods had the highest muscle strength and gain.[21] *Recalling that cholesterol builds muscles and statins tear them down...duh!*

In the meantime, the lunacy continues as statin manufacturers are lobbying hard to get statins added to our public water supply just like fluoride. They also are pushing for statins to be sold over-the-counter while urging doctors to prescribe statins to *children as young as eight. That type of advice completely ignores the risks to their immune systems, or the potential damage to their growing muscles, nerves, brains, etc.*

Incredibly, to date no long term studies have been done as to the safety and efficacy of statins in children. Soon statins will be marketed and prescribed as a way to "prevent" heart attacks. *"Prevention through drug use" will be the new mantra of the pharmaceutical industry.* Millions of new, gullible victims will succumb to the hype and also risk succumbing to an early and painful demise. Statin mania is reaching new heights as Big Pharma's integrity seems to be falling to new lows.

So, you can see that cholesterol, particularly high cholesterol, has gotten a bum rap for many years. It has become the "fall guy" for heart disease. But it is neither a reliable sign of an impending heart attack, nor is it the cause of heart disease. Cholesterol is actually your friend.

Recent technological advances in the use of x-rays, electron beams, and ultrasound have proved this to be true by showing *little association between the amount of cholesterol in the blood and the degree of heart disease.*[22] For decades, saturated fat has been blamed for the buildup of arterial plaque, but that assumption was thoroughly discredited in 1994 when investigators analyzed plaque and discovered it contained more than ten different compounds, *none of which consisted of saturated fat.*[23] Yet doctors prescription pads are still smoking with prescriptions for statins.

In the 1950s Dr. John Gofman, a medical physics professor at the University of California, discovered that, in general, the triglyceride level–not the cholesterol level–was associated most closely with heart disease and atherosclerosis. And what is the major regulator of triglycerides in our bodies? *It is not fat, but sugar and carbohydrates!* Yeast feasts!

The sudden and unexpected death in 1984 of marathon runner Jim Fixx may illustrate this fact. The running enthusiast and author of books on running, dropped dead of cardiac arrest when only fifty-two years old during a race. A subsequent autopsy revealed he had severe coronary artery disease–three of his main arteries were dangerously blocked. His heart showed signs of at least one heart attack and also was slightly enlarged. Knowing what we know now, his heart disease could have been initiated by "carbo loading" which was so popular among runners and athletes during the 1980s and is to this day.

Another excellent example refuting the theory of a direct cause-and-effect relationship between cholesterol levels, heart attack, and strokes is our thirty-fourth president, Dwight D. Eisenhower. At the time of his first heart attack, Ike's cholesterol level was 164 mg/dl – a level considered ideal by today's standards. His cholesterol was checked ten times a year; he eliminated all saturated fats from his diet; ate only supposed "heart-healthy" food such as margarine, vegetable oils, etc.; followed his cardiologist's orders to the tee; and yet he suffered several more heart attacks and eventually died of heart disease.[24] (The real damage to his arteries probably was the result of his smoking four packs of cigarettes a day for many years.) None of his doctors addressed the underlying reason for his heart disease—inflammation and the yeast that followed to gorge on the debris.

Statins are now being shown to neither prevent nor reduce heart disease. This was reflected recently in a medical journal that concluded: "No tightly controlled trial has ever conclusively demonstrated that LDL cholesterol reductions can prevent cardiovascular disease or increase longevity."[2] *So far 900 studies have shown statin drugs to be dangerous!* [26] Finally the cholesterol theory of cardiovascular disease is slowly unraveling and being disproven, and soon this whole misguided fixation is bound to go the way of bloodletting and lobotomies.

Remember, the actual cholesterol level (mg/dl) itself is not the most important risk factor. What actually matters is the ratio between the total cholesterol number and HDL. The ideal HDL/cholesterol ratio should be higher than 25 per cent, and in most cases, the higher the better.

Thirty years ago, the cholesterol level of 300 for a male was considered normal. Anything over that was met with a prescription for statins. *Ka-ching.* Twenty years ago it was lowered by the "experts" to 240 for men *and* women. *Ka-ching, ka-ching.* Now it is being lowered from 200 to 180 and being prescribed for children. *Ka-ching, ka-ching...JACKPOT!*

The lower the number, the higher the profit$. Million$ more pre$cription$ can be written, leading to more vi$it$ to the doctor and more te$t$ to run.  Ju$t what the doctor and Big Pharma ordered.  Billion$ more to be made.

**There are safer, simpler, easier, cheaper, and more effective ways to normalize total cholesterol levels into the 200-240 range without the use of dangerous statins.**

1.  Follow the yeast-free diet.

2.  Normalize insulin levels by eliminating refined sugars and cutting down on most grains.

3.  Consider one of the many yeast fighters found in health food stores.  Caprylic acid, olive leaf extract, oregano oil, grapefruit seed extract, and Taheebo tea are all excellent. It is good to rotate them.

4.  Consider supplementing with omega-3 fatty acids, CoQ10, Vitamins C, D, B complex, flax oil and curcumin.

5.  Use sparingly omega-6 oils vegetable oils (once dubbed "heart healthy") such as canola, safflower, sunflower, peanut, and corn.  They are associated with inflammation.

6.  Add more omega-3 rich foods to your diet, including avocados, nuts (walnuts especially), seeds (pumpkin and sunflower), fish (salmon, tuna, sardines), fish oils, flaxseed and flax oils, and 2 ounces of unsweetened pomegranate juice daily to help clear arties.  Knudsen's Just Pomegranate is excellent.

7.  Check with your healthcare practitioner about using 1,500 mg. of non-flush niacin (niacinamide) daily to bring down high cholesterol levels.

8.  All arterial plaque contains cholesterol, but unfortunately lowering your  cholesterol levels *does not clean out your*

*arteries.* One of the best cleaners of arterial plaque is lecithin, found in your health food store. It literally melts away hardened cholesterol plaque. (Normally HDL cholesterol scrubs arteries clean because it contains much more lecithin than our LDL particles!) And guess what is one of the most readily available sources of lecithin. *The yolk of the poor little, much-maligned egg!* There is actually more lecithin in the yolk of an egg than is needed to emulsify the fat *in* the yolk! Egg protein is of such high quality that it is used as the standard by which all proteins are compared. God doesn't make mistakes. One or two tablespoons of lecithin granules a day, sprinkled on cereals, soups, on salads, in soups, stews or smoothies is recommended. *Caveat*: Make sure the lecithin you buy is made from *non-GMO soybeans.*

If you've given up cholesterol-rich foods like bacon, eggs, and butter for fake eggs, margarine, and imitation bacon–all of which increase your risk for cancer–you can consider going back to eating real food if you want to live long and well. (I recommend eating turkey bacon only, please.)

I am reminded of a line from the classic 1973 movie, *Soylent Green,* a futuristic sci-fi movie that depicts overpopulation and a planet running low on food and natural resources. Edward G. Robinson's character, Sol Roth, said, "You know, when I was a kid, food was food! Until our scientists polluted the soil and decimated plant and animal life. Why, you could buy meat anywhere. Eggs…they had real butter! Fresh lettuce in the stores!"

Those were the days. Let's bring them back for our children and grandchildren. Because it seems that the true cause of atherosclerosis isn't cholesterol, a virus or bacteria, or caused by genes.

In the words of Professor A.V. Constantini, M.D., retired head of the World Health Organization Collaborating Center for Mycotoxins in

Food, *"There is a known cause of atherosclerosis and that cause is fungi and their mycotoxins."*[27]

I couldn't have said it better myself.

**Chapter 19**

---

# Vaccines:  Prescriptions for Disaster

*"If people let the government decide what food they eat and what medicines they take, their bodies will soon be in as sorry a state as are the souls of those who live under tyranny."*

...Thomas Jefferson

If you were going to make a list of all the controversial topics in the world, vaccines would have to be near the top.  After all the research I have done on the subject, all I can say is that I wish I could go back and "unvaccinate" our three children.  Fortunately, when they were young, only three or four were recommended, and I never took them back for "boosters."

Today, children and adults are facing a massive, invasive assault against their health and well-being, and it begins from the moment they are born.  From the totally unnecessary and dangerous Hepatitis B vaccine given at birth to the end of life, more than 150 vaccines are now recommended for the public.  Human beings have become human pincushions.

In the past thirty years the number of doses of government recommended vaccines has tripled.  In 2007 the Centers for Disease Control and Prevention (CDC) Mandatory Vaccine Schedule required thirty-six shots containing **121 vaccines** be given to children by age 6.  Forty before age one!  That is a 400 percent increase over the CDC's last vaccination schedule update.

When I was growing up, that was not the case.  I received only one vaccination, (for smallpox).  At that time there were no vaccines for common childhood diseases, like measles, mumps, whooping cough, and chickenpox. I remember "measles parties" and "chicken pox parties" where parents deliberately exposed their children to the germs in hopes they would contract the diseases while they were young, when the effects tend to be relatively mild. (Today, these "parties" are becoming popular again as parents are attempting to immunize their children the old-fashioned way.[1])

All my friends and I dutifully contracted these diseases and, of course, fully recovered. There were NO horrifying epidemics of children dying from measles, mumps, whooping cough or chicken pox. I don't remember *even one* of my friends ever developing serious complications or dying from any of those diseases.

Today too many doctors and pediatricians would have you believe that none of our children would have survived to adulthood without their magic inoculations. But look at the real facts as shown in the graphs at the end of the chapter.

1. The death rate in the United States from measles had already fallen 97.7 percent from 1900 to 1960–*before* mass vaccination programs began in 1963. The same was true in Great Britain.

2. Whooping cough death rates had fallen by 75 percent *before* mass vaccination programs began – in both countries.

3. The death rate from polio was well on its way down *before* the polio vaccine was introduced.

Government agencies and vaccine manufacturers boastfully want to take credit for these falling death rates, but the simple truth lies elsewhere. *Better sanitation, cleaner water and better nutrition, especially in the cities, account for most of the improvement in death statistics.* According to the British Association for the Advancement of Science, between 1850 and 1940 the incidence of childhood diseases decreased almost 90 percent, closely paralleling the increasingly better hygiene and nutrition practices–well before the implementation of mass immunization programs.

Today we really have no comprehension of the filth and sewage people routinely lived with for centuries, contributing to low life expectancies and early childhood deaths. There were 200 cemeteries within the city limits of London in the 1700s. Raw sewage from animals and human waste literally flowed through city streets in shallow ditches– if it flowed at all–where people walked and children played. It was said you could smell London from twenty miles away. No wonder people died like flies.

If you look at graphs of epidemics (see graphs at end of chapter) you will see that outbreaks and epidemics seem to chart their own natural courses, each with a beginning, a middle or leveling point, and a natural end. Even the two great plagues that swept through Europe in the Middle Ages, appeared, did their damage, and eventually vanished on their own. Of course this was centuries before the advent of vaccines. And since nutrition and sanitation have been greatly improved, plagues and massive outbreaks of communicable diseases have not returned. Also worth noting is that the European countries that refused immunizations for smallpox and polio watched as the epidemics ran their courses on their own, clearly indicating that vaccines had little to do with the outcomes.

Even more interesting to note is that virtually *every case of pandemic death followed on the heels of a period of widespread malnutrition.* (The influenza pandemic of 1917 occurred following the devastation of World War I, and the plague epidemics followed two periods of global cooling, when crops were wiped out and people were severely malnourished.)

Most people assume that taking a vaccine confers the same level of immunity as getting the disease. But science proves just the opposite. Actually, *getting the disease itself has proved to provide superior protection.* Natural immunization is a complex interactive process involving many organ and body systems which cannot be replicated by the artificial stimulation of antibodies!

The supposed intent of vaccination is to assist the body in building immunity to potentially harmful organisms that can cause illness and disease. Most of these disease-causing organisms gain entry through the mucous membranes of the nose, mouth, lungs or digestive tract–not through injections. These mucous membranes have within them their own specialized immune system called the IgA. This is a totally different immune system from the one activated when a vaccine is injected into the body.

The IgA immune system is your body's first line of defense, its job being to fight off invading organisms as they knock on the door, reducing or even eliminating the need for calling out the big guns–your global immune system. However, when a virus is *injected* into the body it is a different story, especially when combined with adjuvants for stimulation. Your natural and protective IgA immune system is *bypassed,* and your body's immune system kicks into full throttle in response to the vaccination.

Adjuvants added to vaccines, such as squalene and aluminum, cause your immune system to go *one step further* and *overreact* to the organism you are being vaccinated against. The subsequent hyperstimulation and overreaction of the immune system cause a chronic activation of the microglial cells in the brain. (The microglia are the immune cells that protect the brain and central nervous system when needed, and act like phagocytes by cleaning up waste products.) This continuous prodding of the immune system from vaccines triggers the release of powerful inflammatory cytokines and excitotoxins, *which inflame the brain and cause continuous damage to brain tissue,* creating a kind of smoldering encephalitis. Inflammation anywhere in the body, as we know, is a perfect invitation for a yeast-feast and resulting disease.

We can only be left to deduce that the whole scenario of injecting organisms into the human body to provoke immunity is contrary to common sense–and contrary to nature, while carrying with it enormous potential for damage.

However, when someone contracts a disease the normal way–measles for instance–the immune system is naturally stimulated, swings into action, destroys the virus and immediately goes back into its resting state, thereby affording you immunity to that disease–in most cases–*for the rest of your life.* No over activation of the immune system, no damage from inflammation. *No yeast-feast.* Lifelong immunity is achieved easily. And no booster shots needed!

Compare that to vaccines.

The length of immunity estimated for many vaccines is only two to ten years, which means booster shots are required. But booster immunity lasts for even shorter periods! To make matters worse, many of the vaccines, such as measles/mumps/rubella (MMR), haemophilus influenza type b bacteria (Hib), and multiple dosed vaccines such as DTaP, *suppress* the immune system for weeks and even months, and actually *increase* the risk of children developing asthma, allergies, eczema, and even juvenile diabetes.

Dr. Harris Coulter, co-author of *A Shot in the Dark*, and many other experts insist that allergies and vaccines are clearly connected. What is an allergic reaction? It is the body reacting swiftly when exposed to a substance to which it is allergic. Vaccinations actually make you allergic to whatever bacillus, etc. you have been vaccinated against, in the sense that your body will respond very, very quickly if exposed to them a second time.

Forty years ago teachers rarely heard of allergies in their students. Now incoming students brings *lists* of what they are allergic to: peanuts, eggs, milk, wheat, antibiotics, gluten, etc. What has happened to the health of our children in the intervening years? Why are they having so much trouble learning? Why are so many of our children and young people less vigorous, less hardy, less resistant to disease than former generations? Why are they so sick?

Today the CDC admits that one child in six in America is developmentally delayed, and the National Vaccine Information Center (NVIC) reports that one child in six is learning disabled, one in nine has asthma, one in one hundred develops autism, and one in four hundred fifty becomes diabetic. And *for the first time in our history Americans are being warned that the currant generation probably won't live longer than their parents.*

What is causing so much ill health? Could it possibly be vaccines? I thought they were supposed to be good for us. I was told they would make us stronger, not weaker. I was assured they were safe and effective. Have we been wrong? What exactly are vaccines?

My dictionary (Webster's Third New International Directory) defines a vaccine as: "a preparation of killed microorganisms, living attenuated (weakened), or living fully virulent organisms that is administered to produce or artificially increase immunity to a particular disease." They work on the principle of protection by artificially stimulating the immune system to produce antibodies (small protein molecules that attack the invading organism) to overcome disease.

The MMR, smallpox, Sabine polio, and chicken pox vaccines contain *live* viruses. Even though the manufacturers weaken the viruses so that the vaccines confer immunity rather than cause the actual disease, scientists are beginning to question the safety of these attenuated vaccines. *Live viruses wreak havoc on brain cells.*

When two or sometimes four live viruses are given together, the risk of catching any opportunistic germ a person is exposed to, or developing a chronic lifetime infection *increases dramatically.* The MMR vaccine contains two live viruses that are known to suppress the immune system for months.[2] (Vaccines have *not* been safety tested in combination with each other–only individually–nor have the effects of the *entire cumulative load* of vaccines ever been safety tested!)

In some people the virus isn't killed off, but instead takes up permanent residence in a person's internal organs. Autopsies routinely find live measles viruses embedded in organs and even the brain. The worst way to take a viral vaccine is through "mists" or nasal swabs. *You don't want a virus in your brain!* The LAIV (Live Attenuated Influenza Virus) vaccines are administered via the nasal route, and are particularly dangerous to both the person taking them and to people around them because they cause "shedding" of the virus. In other words, people who receive LAIV viruses easily infect or "shed" the virus to those around them. This is of great concern to virologists who note that these viruses can easily re–assort, or mutate, and go on to trigger completely unrelated diseases, such as multiple sclerosis, Crohn's disease or degenerative brain diseases. Doctors are at a loss to explain the dramatic rise of these diseases.

So far, five vaccines have been linked to diabetes[3], which is approaching epidemic proportions in this country:

1.  MMR
2.  DTaP
3.  Pertussis
4.  Hepatitis B
5.  Pneumococcal (PCV)

Read the package insert that comes with the MMR vaccine. It lists Diabetes Mellitus as *an adverse reaction!* In other vaccines, Sudden Infant Death Syndrome (SIDS) *is listed as an adverse reaction.* Read the literature. Anaphylactic shock, foaming at the mouth, grand mal convulsions, coma, and paralysis are some of the startling descriptions used to describe other adverse reactions.

What exactly is *in* vaccines that could be causing such devastating reactions? You may be surprised.

Aside from the viral and bacterial DNA or RNA, (plus other species' DNA), vaccines can contain fillers or adjuvants. Adjuvants (the word comes from Latin *adjuvare,* meaning to help) are *amplifiers* that make the body react more intensely to the vaccines. They all create inflammation, especially in the brain. Adjuvants are also added to *stretch* the vaccine–allowing pharmaceutical companies to use less vaccine in each dose in order to manufacture *more* vaccines and make *more* profit. And all are added without public knowledge or consent!

## *VACCINE FILLERS AND ADJUVANTS*

1. **aborted fetal cell lines**–human cells from aborted fetal tissue and human albumin (in polio, MMR vaccines and others)
2. **ammonium sulfate**–suspected gastrointestinal, nerve and respiratory poisons
3. **genetically modified yeast and yeast protein,** animal, bacterial and viral DNA which can be incorporated into recipient's DNA–causing unknown genetic mutations. Potent allergens
4. **human diploid lung cells** (diploid means cells originated from aborted fetal tissues)
5. **dry natural latex rubber**–can cause life-threatening allergic reactions (who knows if a newborn or very young child is allergic to latex?)
6. **chick embryo** culture
7. **glutamate** (as in MSG), a known excitotoxin–a neurotoxin, being studied for mutagenic, teratogenic, and reproductive effect[4], and a suspected carcinogen
8. **dog and monkey kidney cells**
9. **aluminum hydroxide**–a suspected factor in Alzheimer's and implicated as a cause of brain damage, dementia, seizures, and comas
10. **formaldehyde**–commonly used to embalm corpses; poisonous if ingested; probable carcinogen; suspected gastrointestinal,

liver, immune system, nerve, reproductive system, and respiratory poison;  linked to leukemia, brain, colon and lymphatic cancer; removed from children's cot mattresses when linked to "cot death"

11. **cowpox pus**
12. **pig, sheep and horse blood**
13. **sorbitol and sucrose**–sugars
14. **embryonic guinea pig cell cultures** (*is there a metaphor here?)*
15. **antibiotics**–fungal metabolites–allergic reactions can be mild to life-threatening
16. **rabbit brain**
17. **gelatin**–produced from calf and cattle skins, de-mineralized cattle bones and pork skin;  allergic reactions have been reported
18. **phenoxyethanol (antifreeze)**–toxic to all cells and capable of thwarting immune response
19. **polysorbate 80**–an emulsifier and known carcinogen in animals
20. **beta-propiolactone**–a known carcinogen and suspected gastrointestinal, liver, respiratory, skin and sense organ poison
21. **glutaraldehyde**–poisonous if ingested; causes birth defects in experimental animals
22. **tri(n)butylphosphate**–a detergent; suspected kidney and nerve poison
23. **live and killed micro-organisms**–viruses and bacteria or their toxins.  The polio vaccine was contaminated with a monkey virus now being found in human bone, lung-lining, brain tumors, and lymphomas.
24. **sulfites**–used in foods and alcoholic beverages; known to cause diarrhea, headache, vomiting and severe cramps; still present in some flu vaccines
25. **egg proteins**–small amounts leftover from egg mediums used to grow vaccines; can cause allergic reactions
26. **benzoic acid**–when injected into rats causes tremors, convulsions and death

27. **Triton X-100**–a detergent made by Dow Chemical; recommended for   household    and industrial use
28. **thimerosal**–a preservative that is almost fifty percent mercury. In 1998 it  was banned in over-the-counter drugs because "safety and efficacy have not been established for the ingredients." It inhibits phagocytes, one of the most vital immune defenses in the blood.  Still present in DPT, DTaP, Hib, Varicella, and Inactivated Polio Vaccine (IPV). Flu vaccines containing thimerosal contain 250 times above the level identified as hazardous waste!  Known to induce breaks in DNA.
29. **mercury**–one of the most poisonous substances known. Minute amounts can cause nerve damage. Is toxic to central nervous system and not easily eliminated from the body. Has an affinity for the brain, gut, liver, bone marrow, and kidneys. (Symptoms of mercury poisoning are similar to those of autism.)  Mercury also kills beneficial bacteria in the gut stimulating the growth of yeast, and rapidly crosses the placental barrier and accumulates in a fetus *at even higher levels than the mother!  There is no safe dose for mercury in a human being.*
30. **recycled animal tissue**–contains building blocks of Mad Cow disease
31. **squalene**–an adjuvant so toxic that a single dose injected into rats causes them to develop rheumatoid arthritis
32. **peanut oil** –a hidden and non-stated ingredient in children's vaccines.[5] Have you ever wondered where all the peanut allergies are coming from these days? Aflatoxin, a dangerous mycotoxin produced by *Aspergillus flavus* mold, is often found on peanuts and can cause *anaphylaxis.*

All are TOXIC to the human body.

Would you let your children EAT this stuff?  Then why allow it to be *injected* into their bloodstreams?  *Why allow a foul concoction of live*

*viruses, toxic substances, aborted fetal cells, and diseased animal matter
to be forcibly inserted into the arms of innocent, HEALTHY children?*

How many parents would allow their children to be vaccinated if
they knew the vaccines were manufactured with aborted human cells?
Vaccine manufacturers have made no attempt to hide this fact. Just read
the package inserts (also known as WARNING labels!). You can go to
http://www.vaccinesafety.edu/package_inserts.htm to read them all.

Merck's MMRII insert states right on the first page: ("Rubella
Virus Vaccine Live), the Wistar RA 27/3 strain of live attenuated rubella
virus propagated with WT–38 human diploid lung fibroblasts, 1,2."
Translation? (First be aware that the development of the rubella vaccine
in the United States involved not one, but 28 abortions – 27 to isolate the
virus and one to culture the vaccine.) The vaccine's strain is called *RA
27/3, meaning R=Rubella, 27=27$^{th}$ fetus tested, 3=3$^{rd}$ tissue explanted.*
We know the single aborted human was a girl.

So far, at least 10 vaccines in the United States are manufactured
from cell lines made from aborted human cells. All are listed as such in
the inserts. They are:

- Varivax (chicken pox)
- Havrix (hep–A)
- Vaqta ( hep–A)
- Twinrix (hepA/hepB)
- Poliovax (polio)
- Imovax (rabies)
- Meruvax II (rubella)
- MR–VAX (measles/rubella)
- Biavax II (mumps/rubella)
- MMR II (measles, mumps, rubella)

Has your doctor ever mentioned this to you? Has he or she ever
told you that these cell lines have never been studied, or that they were
collected and replicated as research, not as proven science? Human trials

were never run before using them, and to this day, no double blind, longitudinal study has ever been run to study their impact on the body or to reveal adverse consequences. Zero. We continue to assume vaccines are safe and safely made.

Wrong on both counts. DNA from a large range of diseased animals is often used in vaccine formulas. The May 7, 2010 *Wall Street Journal* reported that actual *fragments of pig viruses* were found in Merck & Co.'s Rotateq® and GlaxoSmithKline's Rotarix® vaccines against the rotavirus. One of the viruses is lethal and causes wasting and death in baby pigs. Tests found DNA from the viruses in the master cells used to make the vaccines. Scientists have no idea how they got there or what the consequences may be. There should have been a recall, but the FDA said "no problem". Business as usual. The actual risk of a child dying of a retrovirus is extremely small, but in 2009 Big Pharma made nearly a billion dollars from rotavirus vaccines. Business as usual, indeed.

In many ways the vaccine industry operates more like a cult than a scientific organization. Anyone who doesn't worship at the alter of the cult's beliefs or questions its dogma is swiftly branded a heretic and publicly denounced.

The Amish, who have never allowed their children to undergo vaccinations, have extremely low rates of any diseases or autism. Yet the government refuses to fund any research comparing rates of diseases of unvaccinated children with those of vaccinated children. They don't dare open that can of worms. They *know* unvaccinated children are healthier, and they will never fund science that will make them (government agencies) and vaccine makers look culpable.

Even though toxic mercury is no longer in most vaccines, (actually it was never removed from vaccines but phased out over several years, allowing existing thimerosal-laden vaccines to be used up), it is still present in multi-dose flu vaccines to the tune of 25 mcg! The flu vaccines contain the equally damaging additives or fillers listed above, which are often more dangerous than the viral component of the vaccine!

Of particular concern is aluminum, which many regard as even more toxic than mercury. High concentrations of this neurotoxin were added to vaccines after mercury was removed. Today a two-month old infant receives 1,225 mcg of aluminum from vaccines–a whopping fifty times higher than established safety levels![6] Vaccines that contain aluminum adjuvants are: DPT, DTaP, some Hib, pneumococcal conjugate vaccine, Hepatitis A and B, human papilloma virus vaccine, anthrax, and rabies vaccines. (Isn't it odd that physicians are warning expectant mothers to forgo eating fish while pregnant because of the small amount of mercury they may carry, but have no problem with shooting them up with mercury and aluminum-laden flu vaccines?)

Even *Pediatrics*, the official journal of the American Academy of Pediatrics, admitted that aluminum is implicated as interfering with a variety of cellular and metabolic processes in the nervous system and other tissues. As far back as 1996, in a policy statement entitled "Aluminum Toxicity in Infants and Children," they said flatly: "Aluminum is now being implicated as interfering with a variety of cellular and metabolic processes in the nervous system and in other tissues."[7] We've gone from bad to worse, and our helpless little ones are paying the price.

But grown-ups are paying a price as well. For instance, systemic lupus erythematosis (or lupus for short), so rampant today, is one of the innumerable recognized side effects of multiple vaccinations.[8]

And speaking of price, vaccines are not only harmful to your body, they are harmful to your pocketbook. *The New York Times* reports that in 1980 it cost about $23 (or $59 adjusted for inflation) for the seven shots and four oral doses needed to immunize a child. Today, if a child receives all the recommended vaccines, the cost would be more than $1,600–an incredible amount of money to pay, especially when so little is known about their safety, efficacy, and long-term side effects.

Have you ever thought about how vaccines are manufactured, or what medium vaccines are grown on? In the past, most vaccines were grown on *decaying, putrefying, rotting egg yolks.* Today the flu vaccine is still grown using egg mediums, but in order to speed up the process, the trend is now to use cell lines for other vaccines.

Making a flu vaccine is a slow, labor-intensive and cumbersome process requiring 500,000 fertilized chicken eggs per day for up to eight months.

In a nutshell:

1.  When a chick embryo is eleven days old, a tiny tuberculin needle is used to punch a hole through the shell into the egg white and deliver the viral-containing solution. The eggs are sealed with a spot of glue and are maintained for several days in a controlled temperature between 91.4°F and 93.2°F. During that time the viruses infect the lungs of the developing chicken embryos and begin to replicate quickly.

2.  Several days later they are placed in coolers overnight, then the shells are chipped open and the gooey suspension is removed and centrifuged to remove as much of the chicken blood and tissue solution as possible.

3.  After the viruses are separated from the egg, they are inactivated (killed) with formaldehyde (a known carcinogen), treated with Triton X (a detergent), sugar, sodium phosphate-buffered isotonic salt, gelatin, antibiotics, and many of the additives listed above.

4.  Lastly, dangerous preservatives are added and the "chemical soup" is ready to be placed into ampoules for sale to health professionals and the unsuspecting public.

To produce a "live" vaccine such as MMR (measles/mumps/rubella), the virus is passed through animal tissue several times to reduce its potency. Measles virus is passed through chick embryos, polio virus through monkey kidney, and the rubella virus through the *dissected organs of aborted human fetuses*. Killed vaccines are inactivated through the use of heat, radiation or chemicals, and then strengthened with drugs, antibiotics and toxic disinfectants.

In addition to deliberately planned additives, *unanticipated* matter has been found to contaminate vaccines. Foreign genetic material from animal DNA and RNA can transfer to the vaccine recipient, carrying with it the potential for *changing our genetic makeup!* Undetected animal viruses have been found to jump the species barrier from animal to human.

This happened in the 1950s and '60s when millions of people were injected with a polio vaccine that was contaminated with a hybrid monkey virus called Simian 40, or SV-40. The virus grew unnoticed in the organs of rhesus monkeys which were used in the preparation of the vaccine. (They were later replaced with green monkeys.) SV-40 is a powerful immunosuppressor and proved to be the trigger for HIV–human immunodeficiency virus–or the AIDS virus, and one of the worst scourges in history was unleashed. By 1963 it was estimated that 98 million people were inoculated with the tainted vaccine. Unfortunately, this virus is still active in the human population and is being found today inside human cancers, especially bone and lung, and even blood samples and sperm fluid taken from healthy individuals.[9]

Is it any wonder that these repugnant, toxin-laden swills, being directly injected into the bloodstreams of precious newborn babies, children, and adults, which bypass the natural cellular immune systems that constitute *half* of our protective immunity mechanisms, are causing such disastrous and life-altering reactions?

A case in point is the Hepatitis B vaccine given to most newborns within hours of taking their first breaths. It is the first genetically engineered vaccine we've ever had, and it was "safety-studied" for a grand total of five days. Since 2002 it has been added to the recommended immunization schedule and contains *250 mcg of aluminum!* It is given routinely, and in most cases without the knowledge or permission of parents. It is directly linked to autoimmune disease, neurological disorders, rheumatoid arthritis, diabetes, and chronic fatigue.[7]

It is supposed to protect against Hepatitis B, a virus that causes inflammation of the liver. The virus itself is very difficult to contract, requiring some kind of blood or sexual contact before it is transmitted. It is spread mainly by unprotected sex and contaminated drug needles. (Even so, less than five percent of those who contract Hep B become chronic carriers of the infection, so the risk to a newborn is extremely low.)

The groups that are more prone to contract Hep B are I.V. drug users, homosexual men, prostitutes, promiscuous adults, prisoners, dialysis patients, and health care workers –in other words people whose lifestyles reflect *high risk behavior.* So why in heaven's name are we injecting Hep B, with all the risks and side effects inherent in vaccines, into innocent and defenseless newborns? *They don't even know what high risk means!*

Because it is available and so far has generated over a billion dollars in sales for the manufacturers, in my humble opinion. (And while medics are at it, why don't they slip identification chips into newborns in case they are kidnapped, since the risk of kidnapping is actually thousands of times higher than the risk of being exposed to Hep B.)

But wait. It gets worse.

*Unbelievably, absolutely NO safety studies have ever been run on the Hep B vaccine on newborns.* None. They are innocent little guinea pigs. One of the latest studies to come out has revealed that giving Hep B to newborn baby boys more than *triples* their risk of developing an autism spectrum disorder.[10] There is absolutely no logical reason for its inclusion in the immunization schedule. Wouldn't it make more sense to screen all mothers-to-be for Hep B instead of vaccinating *all* newborns? France no longer mandates Hep.B. Shouldn't we follow suit?

Big Pharma wouldn't come out ahead, but our babies would.

You can try to make sure your newborn will not be inoculated with the vaccine (and the equally useless vitamin K shot) by filling out a waiver form before birth, and even that is no guarantee. You will be going up against the powers-that-be.

In 2009 global drug giant GlaxoSmithKline sponsored a clinical study in Argentina (still ongoing) to test an experimental pneumonia vaccine that recruited children from poor families. The Argentine Federation of Health Professionals, or FESPROSA, said families, many of whom are illiterate, "are pressured into signing 13-page consent forms" they could neither read nor understand, and "this occurs without any type of state control" and "does not comply with minimum ethical requirements." The families also were never told the vaccines were experimental.[11]

Dr. Ana Maria Marchese, a pediatrician who works in a hospital where the studies are being conducted, said, in referring to GlaxoSmithKline, "Because they can't experiment in Europe and the United States, they come to do it in third-world countries." How does this comply with *any* ethical requirements?

In the course of the trials, at least fourteen infants have died in the first year, but GSK declined to end the trials, saying that fourteen deaths was an acceptable number considering the hundreds that might be saved by the vaccine. This is always the pharmaceutical companies' fall back position on the efficacy and safety of all their drugs–*a few must be sacrificed for the many*. What is the number of deaths and injuries that will be acceptable to the public in return for the use of a drug? What are the risk/benefit ratios that are acceptable to parents? How far can they push the envelope? This is all valuable information gleaned from drug trials and used as they formulate newer drugs.

In another instance of pharmaceutical companies using third world countries as venues for experimentation, Pfizer and the Nigerian government recently settled in a long-running dispute over allegations that children there were harmed in a 1996 Pfizer study on 200 patients of an *experimental* antibiotic called "Trovan" during a meningitis outbreak. Again, the families had no idea the drug was experimental. Eleven children died during the two week test, and many others were left with brain damage, paralysis, blindness or slurred speech. The settlement calls for a $75 million payment by Pfizer, almost half of which will go to victims. The original suit sought more than $5 billion.[12] In a surprising turn of events, $35 million of the compensation has been refused by victims' families who have called a halt to the payments. The suit is going to be heard by the U.S. Supreme Court.

Continuing studies of parental attitudes toward vaccination show that, if given the choice, most parents, when pressed, would prefer that their children die from an actual disease, rather than from the side-effects of vaccines. I am betting that the parents of the fourteen children in Argentina would agree. I am also betting that most adults, if given the choice, would rather die of any disease rather than die of the side effects of a vaccine or drug.

One of the recurring themes in the Old Testament is the theme of "uncleanness." God, through Moses, told the Israelites never to put anything of an unclean nature into their bodies, on their bodies, or in their minds. There were strict laws regarding "clean" and "unclean" foods that were taken, of course, directly into the body.

Many of our vaccines are made using aborted fetal cell tissue, blood from diseased humans and animals, and decomposed, unsterilized animal parts. *You cannot get any more "unclean" than that.* These are injected directly into the bloodstream, which feeds all cells in the body.

Is it any wonder the human body recoils in horror and sickens?

Most parents believe that their children will not be admitted to school if they are not vaccinated. Not true. Almost all states provide religious, philosophical, and medical exemptions. Even though the AMA and Children's Healthcare.org are actively promoting abolishment of exemptions, there is still a totally safe and effective alternative to vaccines that parents can vie for instead.

First, go to your pediatrician's office and ask for a vaccination record book. They will give it to you. Take the record book to a naturopathic or a homeopathic physician who will vaccinate your children homeopathically against childhood diseases. Fill out the record book as you vaccinate. You can then give that record to the school and most will take it! It's at least worth a try.

Keep in mind that there have never been any long-term safety studies done on any vaccination or immunization. Safety studies have been limited to short time trial periods only—usually several days to several weeks. Many of the diseases we are seeing as a result of vaccinations take months or even years to surface.

Unbelievably, vaccines themselves have never been proven effective in preventing disease because it is unethical for researchers to deliberately expose test subjects to any disease in order to run trials on drugs to treat them. Many children contract the diseases they were immunized against anyway, so those children aren't reliable either. More and more we are seeing the return of many childhood diseases in children who have been fully vaccinated *after several generations.*

Sadly, 6,000 infants die every year in the United States alone from vaccines![13] Six thousand heartbroken families. Yet the AMA, CDC, FDA et al, continue to insist that vaccines are safe and effective. (It is worthy of note that most of the studies funded by the pharmaceutical industry conclude they are safe, whereas *independent* studies continue to find serious flaws and raise unnerving questions concerning their safety and efficacy.)

In the vast majority of cases, childhood diseases are benign and self-limiting. A child's immune system is *actually strengthened* by the diseases and thereby learns how to "flex its muscles" and perform. Usually, *lifelong immunity* is conferred, whereas only *temporary immunity* is conferred with vaccines. This temporary immunity can create much more dangerous scenarios in the child's future. Here's why.

If a vaccine has an effectiveness of six to ten years, that means the child will be near adulthood when he or she becomes vulnerable again to the disease. Unfortunately, *most of the childhood diseases are much more virulent and deadly in adults!*

Another important consideration is that in order to create immunity, the body needs to experience a full inflammatory response to viruses or bacteria. Vaccines do not allow this to happen. Instead they create a chronic condition that suppresses the immune system–just what waiting yeast want–and sets the stage for so-called "autoimmune diseases," such as the paralyzing Guillain-Barre syndrome, to surface later.

We know that live virus vaccines such as chicken pox, measles, mumps, rubella, and oral polio can survive and remain latent for years in the host's body, waiting for opportunities to erupt into more serious diseases such as rheumatoid arthritis, MS, lupus, and cancer when the host is stressed, a phenomenon known as *provocation disease.* We also know that as vaccinated children grow into adulthood with this artificially created and inadequate immunity, they have *no placental immunity* to pass onto their children, putting babies at risk for contracting measles, etc. at an age when they would normally be protected by maternal antibodies! Our future generations will be paying a huge price for this misguided immunosuppression of their parents via vaccines.

Even so, at the moment researchers are frantically working on creating over 200 *more* vaccines, treating everything from birth control to obesity to sheep flatulence! Some of the prices are outrageous. On May 4, 2010, the FDA announced the approval of a prostate cancer vaccine, which doesn't prevent cancer but extended the lives of men with the disease by *four months*. Price? $93,000 for three doses.

Today scientists are getting very creative in their search for new vaccine delivery systems, experimenting with nasal sprays, fruits from genetically modified plants, and even mosquitoes! No kidding. *Mosquitoes! How do you control doses with mosquitoes?*

Most people do not realize that vaccines literally attack and alter our DNA. Note that *yeast* and *yeast proteins* are included in vaccines. *Note also that fungus is one of the few things known to have the ability to damage or break a strand of DNA.* Disease appears only when DNA strands have been broken.

Fungi possess genetic flexibility virtually unsurpassed by any other organism. They can actually alter the genetic code of another species, making fungus the *most mutagenic organism in the world.* (Cancer patients have altered DNA.) Fungal DNA has the ability to impregnate human DNA and create a *hybrid DNA.* This hybrid DNA is not recognized as "enemy" by the immune system because of its newly acquired human characteristics. The immune system is fooled into thinking all is well by these human characteristics now appearing in the hybrid DNA and never swings into action to eliminate the upstart "enemy." With the immune system asleep at the switch, fungi spread rapidly and disease takes hold. Many people report becoming sick from some opportunistic bug after receiving a vaccine. Some even get sick from the vaccine itself.

This very personal and difficult issue needs to be brought into the public forum and debated, so that whatever decision a person makes regarding vaccines, at least it will be an informed one. Check the National Vaccination Information Center website (www.NVIC.org) and help Barbara Loe Fisher in her fight to keep us educated and join in the fight *against* all mandatory vaccines and *for* informed consent. At the moment she is trying to fund trials that will compare the health of unvaccinated children with vaccinated children. The government isn't interested in funding these trials, for obvious reasons.

All parents, and anyone else receiving a vaccine, *should read the vaccine package inserts.* Furthermore, they routinely should be told beforehand the risks and possible side effects that may occur as a result of taking *any* vaccine. Rarely is this done in doctors' offices today. *Informed consent* is not only logical and reasonable, but moral and ethical. Demand it. It's your right.

In the meantime, you can keep your immune systems pumping by eating a nourishing yeast-free diet (especially no sugar), supplementing with natural anti-microbials and anti-fungals such as olive leaf extract, elderberry extract, oregano oil or leaves, caprylic acid, grapefruit seed extract, cinnamon, garlic, and natural vitamins and minerals, Vitamin D$^3$, getting adequate sleep and exercise, and routine hand washing. It is the health of our cells and tissues that keep us healthy, not vaccines. In other words, tissue is the issue, not germs!

The bottom line is that vaccines are *not* the "magic bullet" we have been led to believe they are. Instead they have uncaged the yeast/beast, which has turned on us, and is now hunting us down. We are tiring and it is getting closer. What can we do before it overruns us?

*God gave us immune systems and placed us in a garden.* He also gave us phenomenal minds and common sense to figure out that our immune systems are nourished and fueled by what grows in that garden.

When we rediscover and reclaim Eden, we will find we have little need for toxic, synthetic concoctions created in a laboratory.

GRAPHICAL EVIDENCE SHOWS VACCINES DIDN'T SAVE US

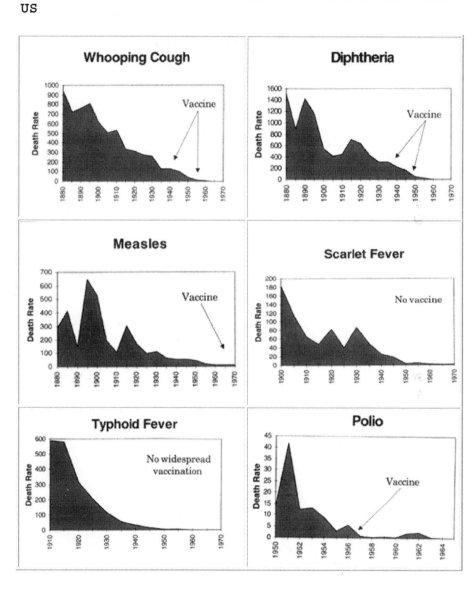

The above graphs, based on the official death numbers as recorded in the Official Year Books of the Commonwealth of Australia, represent the decline in death rates from infectious disease in Australia. They clearly show that vaccines had nothing to do with the decline in death rates. (Note: Graphical evidence on the decline in death rates from infectious disease for USA, England, New Zealand, and many other countries shows the exact same scenario as above.)[14]

So what were the true reasons for this decline? From his book *Health and Healing,* Dr. Andrew Weil best answers it with this statement:

*"Scientific medicine has taken credit it does not deserve for some advances in health. Most people believe that victory over the infectious diseases of the last century came with the invention of immunisations. In fact, cholera, typhoid, tetanus, diphtheria and whooping cough, etc, were in decline before vaccines for them became available– the  result of better methods of sanitation, sewage disposal, and distribution of food and water."*

**Chapter 20**

# *Autism*…A Sign of the Times?

*"A major cause of the Roman Empire's decline, after six centuries of world dominance, was its replacement of stone aqueducts by lead pipes for the transport and supply of drinking water. Roman engineers, the best in the world, turned their fellow citizens into neurological cripples. Today our own 'best and brightest', with the best of intentions, achieve the same end through childhood vaccination programs yielding the modern scourges of hyperactivity, learning disabilities, autism, appetite disorders and impulsive violence."*

…Harris Coulter, PhD.

Something terrible is happening to our children.

Thirty years ago hardly anyone heard of autism. In the 1980s the incidence was recorded as 1 in 10,000 births. Today it is recorded as 1 in 100 and still climbing. What could possibly account for this stunning rise?

Ask any heart-broken parent of an autistic child (or children) and most will say they had bright, normal, healthy children *before* they received vaccinations, and neurologically damaged children *after* being vaccinated. They insistently trace autism's appearance to the vaccinations (especially the Measles-Mumps-Rubellla vaccine or MMR) their children received starting at two months of age.

Known as Autistic Spectrum Disorder (ASD) or Pervasive Development Disorder (PDD), autism affects the way the brain processes information and subsequently the way a person communicates with the outside world. Symptoms can begin to appear a few days to a few months after vaccine exposure, and can range from mild to severe. For instance, Asperger's Syndrome is a milder form of autism that exhibits no significant delay in language development and affects mainly boys. Rett syndrome affects only girls.

Autism is a complex, *lifelong* developmental disorder, which manifests in varying degrees of difficulties with language, social interaction, communication, and behavior. It causes a severe and pervasive impairment in thinking, feeling, and expression of feelings. A few children are autistic at birth. Originally it was called "Cold Mother Syndrome", since the babies and children didn't seem to interact and bond with their mothers. Currently there is no known established cause or cure, but many causal pathways are being explored, including genetic predispositions, infections, metabolic errors, and environmental factors.

Indicators of autism can include:

1. Child doesn't babble, point or make meaningful gestures by age one.
2. Child doesn't speak one word by 16 months.
3. Child doesn't combine two words by age 2.
4. Child doesn't respond to name.
5. Child loses language or social skills.
6. Child has little or no eye contact.
7. Child doesn't seem to know how to play with toys.
8. Child exhibits repetitive and obsessive-compulsive behavior.
9. Child doesn't smile.
10. Child appears deaf at times.
11. Child exhibits extreme sensitivity to sound and touch.
12. Child is developmentally delayed in fine and gross motor skills.

Parents of autistic children have had to watch helplessly as their *formerly healthy and developmentally normal* children regress and lose their ability to communicate, become withdrawn and behaviorally difficult. Some exhibit head-banging and other forms of self-injury such as hair pulling and arm biting. Teeth grinding and hand flapping are common. Many withdraw into their own worlds, unable to relate to others or the world around them.

Even though vaccine proponents continue to deny the connection between vaccine use and the subsequent development of autism, the evidence linking the two is compelling. For instance:

1. Autism is almost non-existent in Amish communities that claim religious exemptions from immunizations.
2. In China, the disease was virtually unknown until thimerosal-laced vaccines were introduced in 1999. Now news reports indicate there are more than 1.8 million autistics in China.[1]
3. In Iowa–also in 1999–after the vaccine schedule was greatly increased, there was a 700 percent increase in autism![2]
4. Today autistic disorders also appear to be soaring in India, Argentina, Nicaragua, and other developing countries where vaccines have been administered.
5. Cases of autism, attention deficit disorder, speech delays, and other neurological disorders seem to increase exponentially with vaccine use.
6. The disease was unknown until 1943, when it was identified and diagnosed among eleven children born shortly after thimerosal was first added to baby vaccines in 1931.[3]

It is a revealing fact that most autistic children were progressing normally prior to vaccination. It is even more revealing that the prevalence of this disorder has significantly increased *coincident with the trivalent (triple dose) MMR vaccine introduced in the 1980s.*[4] Unbelievably no vaccines have ever been safety tested *in combination* with one another!

How often have you seen a child get three diseases at once? Nature always gives recovery time between diseases in order for the body to make natural antibodies to those diseases and repair and rebuild the immune system. This process is totally thwarted by combining vaccines. Prior to triple-dosing, measles, mumps and rubella vaccines were always given separately. The practice of "multiple dosing" has proved to be very problematic as it appears that each component interferes with the actions of the other, leading to unpredictable and unintended consequences. And one of those consequences, many researchers and parents believe, most surely is autism.

Another dangerous practice besides multiple dosing is that many vaccines are administered at very close intervals, e.g., weeks apart. There is little or no time for immature, developing bodies and brains to adapt, adjust, and cope with each toxic invasion.

Consider the fact that just one vaccine injected into a 13-pound, two-month-old infant is the equivalent of ten doses of the same vaccine in a 130-pound adult! This constitutes a full assault on an innocent child's sensitive and immature body systems not yet strong enough to fight back or detoxify. Add to that load multiple and too frequent dosing, and soon their fragile systems become overwhelmed and lapse into neurological and immune system disorders such as autism spectrum disorder.

According to Dr. Russell Blaylock, M.D., retired neurosurgeon and author of the *Blaylock Wellness Report* (March 2009), the link between the vaccine schedule and autism spectrum disorders is the "chronic activation of the brain's special immune system, the microglial, by repeated, closely-spaced vaccinations during the brain's most active period of formation– that is, during the first two years after birth." The repeated doses of vaccines cause extensive and widespread activation of the brain's microglia, which results in extensive and widespread *inflammation.* The consequent release of inflammatory cytokines, free radicals, and excitotoxins *disrupt the normal development of the brain.* As we have learned, chronic inflammation always leads to an invitation to yeast and the development of disease.

A scenario for the development of any of the autism spectrum disorders could read like this:

1.  A mother-to-be is advised by the CDC and the American Academy of Pediatrics to get a flu shot during pregnancy. She follows orders. The flu shot contains mercury, aluminum, and other toxic adjuvants, which cross over the placenta into the developing fetus. This activates the microglia in the developing *fetal* brain, a process known as *priming.*

2.  Mother-to-be takes antibiotics for a bacterial infection. Fungi destroy DNA strands in the cells of the developing brain.

3.  When born, the baby receives a hepatitis B vaccine. This causes a massive overreaction of the brain's microglia, producing inflammation and excitotoxicity.

4.  At two months of age, baby receives *six vaccines during one office visit, exposing him or her to six doses of powerful immune adjuvant plus six doses of neurotoxic aluminum, and possibly some mercury.*

5.  At four months of age, baby receives five more vaccines.

6.  By the age of one, the child will have received 26 vaccines containing 26 doses of powerful immune adjuvants and 26 doses of neurotoxic aluminum–all during the brain's most critical period of forming neurological pathways. Chronic inflammation of the brain and the ensuing hordes of yeast and their mycotoxins make it almost impossible for normal brain development, and autism is the apparent result.

Unfortunately very few pediatricians know much about how the brain develops and the interactions between repeated vaccination and brain inflammation. And as long as pharmaceutical vaccine manufacturers continue to have enormous influence on the American Academy of Pediatrics in promoting vaccine policy, nothing will change and autism rates will continue to rise.

At some point the purpose of vaccines switched from eliminating "*deadly* childhood diseases" to just "childhood diseases" in general. With parameters expanded, vaccine sales soared. Instead of receiving 3 vaccines in 1989, suddenly children were scheduled to take 12. The toxin load intensified–as did neurological problems for children.

Hundreds of peer-reviewed scientific/medical articles from some of the top universities have implicated thimerosal, a mercury-laden preservative, as the causal factor in cases of autism. (You can read a list of 22 scientific citations at www.thinktwice.com) Baby teeth of children with autism have been found to have twice as much mercury than the teeth of normal children, and a published study by researchers at Harvard found twice as much mercury and oxidative stress in the brains of autistic patients than in normal brains[5] So far over 2,000 studies have found that mercury has serious effects on the brain–most especially the developing brain. [6]

Mercury is a fat soluble heavy metal. Since the brain consists of 60 percent fat, it is a favored site for mercury storage. It passes easily through both the placenta and the blood-brain barrier, and with each new vaccine dose another increment is added to the previous doses stored there. In other words, mercury is an accumulative poison. Mercury is also the second most toxic substance known, exceeded only by the radioactive plutonium, one molecule of which will cause cancer in a human being. No amount of mercury is appropriate in any vaccine because no amount of mercury is safe.

The U.S. House of Representatives Government Reform Committee in 2003, after a three-and-a-half-year investigation, concluded "there is no question that mercury does not belong in vaccines." The committee report also said "manufacturers of vaccines have never conducted adequate testing on thimerosal," and "the FDA has never required manufacturers to conduct adequate safety testing of thimerosal and compounds," and "studies and papers documenting the hypoallergenicity and toxicity of thimerosal have existed for decades."[7]

The congressional committee then went on to accuse the FDA and other health authorities of being guilty of "institutional malfeasance" in covering it up. Yet the media spin coming from public health officials (usually citing studies authorized by vaccine industry consultants and paid for by thimerosal manufacturers) and others still insist that vaccines are harmless. Parents of autistic children know otherwise.

Incredibly, it is becoming apparent that government and public health officials knowingly may have allowed the pharmaceutical industry to injure and poison an entire generation of American children and then engage in a massive cover up effort. If true, it would constitute one of the biggest scandals in the annals of American medicine, so you can understand all the efforts to sabotage litigation, suppress investigations and, in general, downplay the harmful effects of vaccines by Big Pharma, et al.

A case in point occurred in June, 2000, when a meeting was convened in Norcross, Georgia, at the Simpsonwood Conference Center. It was held by the Centers for Disease Control, and was attended by 52 government officials from the CDC, FDA, top vaccine specialist from the World Health Organization, and a representative from every vaccine manufacturer, including GlaxoSmithKline, Merck, Wyeth, and Aventis Pasteur. The official title of the conference was: "The Scientific Review of Vaccine Datalink Information."

The meeting was held in secret. There were no press releases, and all participants were warned that all the scientific data reviewed was strictly "embargoed." No photocopying of documents was permitted and no notes or papers were permitted to leave after the meetings. In wording worthy of super-secret CIA files, each page of the study was stamped in bold: "Do Not Copy or Release" and "Confidential."

The Simpsonwood conference was called to discuss a disturbing new study that was bringing into question the safety of childhood vaccines. The records of 110,000 children in the CDC's massive database had been analyzed, and a significant correlation between thimerosal exposure from vaccines and the dramatic increases in the rates of autism, speech and language delays, tics, ADD, ADHD, and hyperactivity was found.   In nine years the numbers of autism had increased *fifteenfold, from one in every 2500 children to one in 166.* It was a bombshell, prompting one attendee (a pediatrician whose daughter-in-law had just given birth to his grandson) to say, "I do not want that grandson to get a thimerosal-containing vaccine until we know better what is going on."[8]

The study ceded that, indeed, the cumulative exposure to mercury in vaccines was exceeding guidelines set by the FDA and other agencies, and recommended thimerosal be removed as quickly as possible. But instead of doing the right thing and alerting the public immediately about the findings and taking immediate steps to remove thimerosal from vaccines, the participants spent the next two days in "damage control" mode discussing how to suppress the damning information. Under the Freedom of Information Act, transcripts were obtained that clearly disclosed how alarmed many participants were–not about the effects of thimerosal–but about the effects on their companies' bottom lines if the damaging revelations were made public.[9] (You can read an in-depth review entitled, "The Truth Behind the Vaccine Cover-up," of the Simpsonwood conference by Dr. Russell Blaylock at http://www.whale.to/a/Blaylock.html.)

To make matters worse, in order to minimize the damage, the CDC paid the Institute of Medicine to launch a new study to minimize the effects of thimerosal, even ordering researchers to "rule out" the chemical link to autism. Then, in an effort to circumvent the Freedom of Information Act, it handed over the database of 110,000 vaccine records (developed largely at taxpayer expense) to a private company, intentionally rendering it off-limits to researchers![10] So much for truth and transparency from FDA.

Thimerosal was never *removed* from any vaccines. Instead, the existing stocks were allowed to run out before new thimerosal-free vaccines were ready.  In the meantime, tens of millions of babies continued to receive the old tainted vaccines. Then, CDC and FDA, in a shocking lapse of ethics and morality, sped the process up by buying up the tainted vaccines for *export to developing countries.*[11] Huh? It's not safe for American children but okay for children in poorer countries? The CDC and FDA said yes, and still allow drug companies to use thimerosal in some American vaccines such as children's flu shots and tetanus boosters. It is even allowed in many over-the-counter medications.

Mark Baxill, Vice President of Safe Minds, a non-profit organization concerned about the role of mercury in vaccines, wrote on his website, "The CDC is guilty of incompetence and gross negligence. The damage caused by vaccine exposure is massive. It is bigger than antibiotics, bigger than tobacco, bigger than anything you have ever seen."[12]

It is impossible to calculate the scope of damage to our country– and our global campaigns to eradicate diseases through vaccinations–if Third World nations begin to realize that America's highly touted foreign aid initiatives are actually poisoning their children. Any proven links between vaccines and autism would force authorities to admit that hundreds of thousands–perhaps millions–of children have been irreparably harmed by our government's policies. The backlash and retribution could reach epic proportions. The loss of trust in America in general and American medicine, in particular, would be devastating.

In 2009 the head of the U.S. Department of Health and Human Services, the federal agency that oversees the Food and Drug Administration and the Centers for Disease Control and Prevention, finally conceded in the Hannah Poling case that, indeed, vaccines can trigger Autism Spectrum Disorders. That was a long-awaited victory for those parents who have testified in Congress and are bringing class action suits against vaccine manufacturers. It was the first of three cases chosen (out of thousands) that alleged thimerosal in childhood vaccines significantly contributed to a child developing autism.[13]

Hannah was a healthy, normal 18-month-old when she received *nine* immunizations at a regular check-up, two of which contained thimerosal. She became ill within hours of receiving the shots, and within three months she began showing signs of autism. This story is echoed over and over by loving parents who thought they were doing the right thing by vaccinating their children, and then had to stand by helplessly as they watched their formerly healthy children regress into an array of symptoms of neurological damage.

Hannah's parents and the parents of many vaccine-damaged children have only one recourse to redress their grievances–that of filing suits against vaccine manufacturers in what is called "vaccine court." Since 1986, a federal law prohibits suits against vaccine manufacturers in an effort to "insure an adequate vaccine supply."(Translation: A deluge of lawsuits could bankrupt pharmaceutical companies.) That same law set up a special "vaccine court" to handle disputes. It is essentially a kangaroo court where all the evidence is stacked against the litigants. *It is run by government attorneys, who defend a government program, using government-funded science, before government-appointed judges!* Most suits are simply rejected.

How can any parent expect to find justice there? Only if and when these suits are tried in civil courts will justice be found and the truth be told. There is hope that this may come to pass. In March, 2010, the *Supreme Court* finally agreed to hear an appeal from parents of an allegedly vaccine-injured child who sought to sue Wyeth Laboratories (now owned by Pfizer, Inc.) over the serious side-effects their daughter suffered as a result of their DPT vaccine. All eyes will be on the court in the fall of 2010 as they decide whether parents can sue vaccine manufacturers directly. Parents of vaccine-damaged children deserve to be heard in real courts.

In February, 2010, this same "vaccine court" declared mercury in vaccines do not cause autism, even though the Hannah Polling case mentioned above, plus another case known as the Bailey Banks case, admitted vaccines CAN cause autism. The government continues to be completely inconsistent on this issue. It is like saying "vaccines never cause autism, except when they cause autism." They can't have it both ways. Meanwhile there are nearly 5,000 cases like Hannah's still pending in "vaccine court."

Even though high amounts of thimerosal are no longer in children's vaccines, autism rates continue to rise. One reason for this is infants are still being exposed to thimerosal in *flu shots*. Mercury's negative effects significantly increase in the presence of aluminum–*found in all vaccines*. Most parents are unaware that vaccinations still contain aluminum (also highly neurotoxic to the brain), formaldehyde, animal viral antibodies, and all the other toxic ingredients listed in chapter 19, creating inflammation and inflicting damage. Inflammation is still the culprit.

So far the Vaccine Compensation Act has compensated over 2,000 litigants who proved they were harmed by vaccines, and *over two billion dollars* have been paid in settlements. More will be forthcoming.

Today, thimerosal is banned in Denmark, Austria, Japan, Great Britain, all the Scandinavian countries, and restricted in seven states in the U.S. Russia banned it from children's vaccines twenty years ago. *Unbelievably, thimerosal-containing flu vaccines are still recommended by doctors for pregnant women and infants.* Little or no warning about the presence of this known neurotoxin is given to patients in the United States.

But, take heart, there is hope. There are many good options for treating autism naturally. Many parents report that their children improved quickly when gluten and dairy products were removed from the diet. (Actually, the children weren't reacting to gluten per se, but to the yeast mycotoxins in grains. Probiotics help immensely here.) Chelation therapy, although expensive and time-consuming, has produced remarkable results. So far most of the evidence is anecdotal.

Chelation therapy was developed in the 1940s by the U.S. Navy to treat personnel who developed lead poisoning after painting the hulls of ships. Using intravenous drips, heavy metals such as lead, arsenic, mercury, and excess heavy minerals are successfully chelated–drawn out of the body–and excreted in urine.

Even though it is approved by the FDA today as the favored treatment for lead poisoning in adults and children, mainstream medicine generally regards chelation as a borderline 'quack' treatment for anything else such as cardiovascular disease. (Can't have anything competing with their precious statins!)

If clinical trials prove that chelation successfully treats autism in children who received thimerosal-laced vaccines, then the current stance that thimerosal is not the cause of autism will crumble and heads should roll. Also, lawsuits against vaccine manufacturers would be greatly strengthened by research that clearly demonstrates chelation therapy to be effective against autism. It would be years before government and the medical profession could pick up the pieces. So, sadly, it may be a long time before chelation therapy receives FDA research it deserves.

But there are products you can use at home that are getting rave reviews and wonderful results. Two are: Kids Chelat™ Heavy Metal Cleanser and Kids Clear™ Detoxifying Clay. You can find them at www.evenbetternow.com. Read the testimonials. The Kids Chelat™ is a liquid internal chelating dietary supplement. The Kids Clear™ Detoxifying Clay bath is a bentonite clay added to bath water. Both are natural and will safely pull out (chelate) and detoxify children from harmful toxins and heavy metals found in vaccinations. It's good for adults, too. Be sure to consult with the child's doctor if the child is taking any medications. Bentonite clay can also draw out (chelate) any prescription drugs the child is taking, so monitoring is needed.

There also is a strong yeast/fungus link to autism that cannot be ignored. Many parents and pediatricians have noted that when autistic children ran fevers, their symptoms abated. That is because *heat kills and burns off fungi* (but not their mycotoxins). Pediatricians also have noted that when autistic children take Nystatin®, a prescription drug that kills yeast, autistic symptoms lessen immediately. I hope you remember that vaccines contain both antibiotics (*fungus)* and genetically modified *yeast and yeast proteins.*

In the final analysis, it appears that vaccines initiate damage to the developing brain and nervous system and introduce fungi into the body. The immune system always takes a dip following immunizations. Yeast proliferates rapidly when the immune system becomes compromised, inflicting even more damage. The combination of vaccine damage and yeast-fungi-mycotoxin proliferation results in the wide spectrum of developmental disorders known as autism.

This is where the yeast-free diet can play a huge role in its treatment, and even its healing. It should be a top priority. Many parents of autistic children report miraculous turnarounds after just a few days. The diet goes a long way in lessening toxic loads on children's bodies, clearing their brains of fungi and stimulating their immune systems. In addition, it is critical that *probiotics, natural anti-fungals, and natural multiple vitamins and minerals* be added to the regimen.

A growing percentage of parents is beginning to say NO to the incredible barrage of childhood vaccinations, a trend that mainstream medicine and the government don't want to see. Both will continue to thwart any research that could undermine their prevailing mindset–even if that research could help thousands of autistic children lead more normal lives.

What we desperately need is independent research with well-designed clinical trials–but don't hold your breath. One thing is for certain–those trials won't be run by the pharmaceutical companies. So far, only the MMR vaccine has been studied in association with autism. Where are the studies of *all the other* vaccines in relation to autism? We also need rigorous studies on the *cumulative effect of all vaccines children receive from birth through high school years.* This has never been done.

Autism truly is a sign of our times. I see it as a symbol for loss in all of our lives. We are living in an age where daily we are losing rights that, at one time, we took for granted: The rights our Founding Fathers referred to as inalienable–life, liberty, and the pursuit of happiness. They are part of our being, part of being human and are, therefore, natural to man. We are not granted those rights by the state, federal government, the United Nations, or a king, or bureaucrat. They were recognized by our Founders as coming from God alone.

Through no fault of their own, too many of our beautiful children have lost all three–the right to a life in the real world, the right to a life lived in freedom instead of isolation, and the right to pursue their own avenues to happiness.

It is an axiom of Natural Law that each individual has the full right of determination to his own body, to make his own life decisions, and to be the determining factor in decisions made within his own family, including his children. No parent in the United States should be forced to vaccinate his children if he honestly and sincerely has concluded that the risks far outweigh the benefits. Government should not be allowed to usurp parents' rights. Unfortunately, that is what happened in Nazi Germany. We can't allow it to happen in the United States.

Slowly our rights to individually determine our own destinies through personal choices concerning food, supplements, pure water, and immunizations are being eroded and taken away by federal and state governments, federal agencies, bureaucrats, and international agencies at an alarming rate.

One of the most chilling statements attesting to this fact came out of the mouth of Dr. Donald Berwick, the new director of Medicare and Medicaid for the Obama administration. He said "The primary functions [of health regulations is] to constrain individual decision-making and weigh public welfare against the choices of the private consumer."[14] Are we all becoming the proverbial "boiled frog?" A nation of sheeple? Or, is there still time for us to find our voices.

In the past ten years, the number of autistic children *has risen by 200 percent in every state in the U.S.* It has been estimated that between 500,000 and 1,500,000 children in the United States now suffer from autism, and pediatricians are diagnosing 40,000 new cases each year.[15] *Something terrible **is** happening to our children.*

Children are a gift from God. It is the duty of every parent to nurture and care for these gifts to the best of his or her knowledge and abilities. If parents thoughtfully and prayerfully decide against vaccinating their children (or limit them), they should be allowed to do so without intimidation or recrimination from government or society. It is a question of individual rights and conscience.

This controversial subject needs to be debated openly and fully– and soon. The time for transparency and large-scale, unbiased studies, overseen by those without conflicts of interest, has come. Truly this is a moral crisis that is crying to be addressed.

That is the very least we owe–not only our autistic children–but children everywhere.

**Chapter 21**

---

# H1N1: The Pandemic That Didn't Pan Out

*"And there came unto me one of the seven angels which had the seven vials full of the seven last plagues, and talked with me…"*
                                                                 …Revelation: 21:9

In the fall of 2009 the so-called "swine flu," or H1N1, a generally benign strain of flu, made its way around the globe and the fear mongering began. *One month* after revising the old definition of pandemic: a pandemic requires "enormous amounts of deaths and illnesses" to a new definition: a pandemic only applies to "new viruses which spread easily between people, and the population has little or no immunity to it", the World Health Organization implemented the new definition and declared swine flu a global "pandemic."

*One day* after WHO declared swine flu a global "pandemic", pharmaceutical giant Baxter International, Inc. announced it was "fast-tracking" its new swine flu vaccine! Baxter claimed it had patented a new technology that reduces the normal vaccine development time from twenty-six weeks to thirteen. You can bet your bottom dollar that probably did not include time for safety and effectiveness studies. Even more frightening is that our children may have been the first guinea pigs in this experiment.

This virus has virologists literally scratching their heads. The April 30, 2009 issue of *Nature* quoted one virologist as saying, "Where the hell it got all these genes we don't know." Comprehensive analysis of the virus found it contained *two* viruses–the 1918 H1N1 flu virus, the avian flu virus (bird flu), plus two new H3N2 virus genes–from Eurasia. What is new about this virus is that it has a mixture of DNA from animals, birds, and humans! This doesn't happen in nature–only in the laboratory–and debate is heating up over whether swine flu is a genetically engineered virus. And if so, whether there was a diabolical reason for creating it. Stay tuned.

Since the 1980s the government has protected vaccine makers against lawsuits from the use of vaccines. Here again the government is shielding vaccine makers and federal officials from any lawsuits resulting from injury or death from the new vaccine. No one will be held liable if this vaccine turns out to be a health disaster. Early evidence is mounting that senior citizens who took flu shots for five consecutive years have a marked increase of Alzheimer's disease.[1]

Along these same lines, another major bombshell is brewing in the wings. It has long been feared that vaccines could be used as potent and deadly biological weapons–and be used as weapons of population control. In August, 2009, several Czech newspapers began questioning whether Baxter International *intentionally* sent 72 kilos (158 pounds) of a lethal mix of flu vaccine and unlabeled H5N1 (the human form of bird flu) to an Austrian research company, which then sent it on to eighteen countries, including the Czech Republic, Slovenia, and Germany. Only when researchers at a Czech laboratory injected ferrets with the vaccine, and they *all abruptly died* was the contamination discovered. Fortunately a worldwide disaster was averted.

Consequently newspaper reporters are investigating whether the contamination was part of an orchestrated attempt to start a pandemic (from which the pharmaceutical companies would reap astronomical profits). Baxter refused to reveal how the "accident" occurred, claiming "trade secrets" and calling the event a "mistake" and chalked it up to "human error." But vaccines makers follow extremely stringent protocols in the manufacture of vaccines. In this case, Baxter International operates on something called BSL3 (Biosafety Level 3), a set of laboratory safety protocols so foolproof that mixing a live virus with vaccine ingredients is *virtually impossible.* But it happened. How? Why?

It has happened before.  Many scientists are convinced that the 1977 Russian flu outbreak could be traced back to a virus leaked from a laboratory, and in 2006 it was revealed that in the 1980s Bayer sold millions of dollars worth of a blood clotting medicine to Asian, Latin, and some European countries that they *knew* had been tainted with the AIDS virus. Another scandal occurred in 2006 when hemophiliac components were contaminated with the HIV virus.  They were subsequently injected into tens of thousands of people, including children. Unbelievably, according to reports, Baxter continued to release the HIV contaminated vaccine even after the contamination was discovered.

In July 2009, an Austrian investigative journalist named Jane Burgermeister filed criminal charges with the FBI against the World Health Organization, the United Nations, several high-ranking government and corporate officials, Baxter AG and Avir Green Hills Biotechnology of Austria for manufacturing and unleashing live bird flu virus, charging it was a *deliberate act to both cause and then profit from the ensuing pandemic.* (Vaccine manufacturers are hoping to make 2 billion doses for a $5 profit each, amounting to a $10 billion total profit, and WHO was investigated for influence peddling as the organization received policy advice from people who stood to make millions of dollars when a pandemic was declared.)

Burgermeister claims to have definitive proof and is literally charging them with bioterrorism and attempts to commit genocide!  She points out that the new strain of flu is a synthetic structural recombinant containing genes from birds, humans, and pigs from different continents! It is a reasonable assumption that it came out of a lab–most specifically a bioweapons lab. (The U.S. government has classified both the bird flu and the swine flu vaccines as bioweapons in its own export regulations.)[2]

You would think *a story of such importance would be one of the hottest headline stories of the year,* but the mainstream media has been shockingly silent. The blackout is not hard to understand when you realize the media is, in large part, bought and paid for by pharmaceutical industry advertising. The Internet is what is keeping this story alive and in the public eye.

No matter the final outcome of this story, the most pressing matter facing us now is the looming possibility of universal forced vaccinations. At the moment there are enough legal provisions in place to make a mandated vaccination program a shocking reality–starting with our most vulnerable citizens, the very young and the very old. (Australia in 2010 banned the seasonal flu vaccines for children under the age of five after an unusually high number of children suffered serious side effects.)

The World Health Organization (WHO) declared a "Level 6" pandemic in mid-June 2009, and the CDC and WHO are forecasting that the H1N1 "swine flu" may return in a new and more virulent strain. More "angst campaigns." More fear mongering. Levels and numbers have nothing to do with how virulent a pathogen is. It is merely a reflection of how *fast* it is spreading. If a "pandemic *emergency*" is declared, federal, state, and local officials are poised for action, with draconian policies we would have never thought possible, ready to be implemented.

In the event that WHO declares a "pandemic emergency," the United States Emergency Medical Powers Act and Federal legislation (the Patriot Acts 1, 11 and 111, BARDA and others) provide for *mandatory vaccinations for all citizens.* No religious or philosophical or medical exemptions will be allowed.   It is hard to believe, but those who refuse Swine flu and regular flu vaccinations (called "vaccine refusers" or "vaccine resisters") could be fined, jailed, or moved ("involuntary transportation", a.k.a. kidnapping) into quarantined FEMA camps! Certain agencies will even be given the authority to use deadly force to ensure compliance if necessary.[3] We can only pray that Americans will never tolerate such a basic usurpation of our most basic rights, and this worse case scenario will never be implemented.

Swine flu has been hysterically over-hyped by WHO and health agencies around the world, (WHO forecast that the virus would affect 2 billion people worldwide) and in the process has been blown out of all

proportion to the actual threat it carries. It seems the vaccine may prove
more deadly than the virus itself. Even WHO admitted recently they
jumped the gun, as the "epidemic" proved very mild. More people died of
the seasonal flu than H1N1. As a result, many governments have been left
holding the bag with millions of dollars of stockpiled vaccines that are
deteriorating and therefore useless. In the United States alone, a
whopping 40 million doses worth over $260 million have expired and will
be burned. If the remaining swine flu vaccine is allowed to expire, more
than 43 percent of the total supply will have gone to waste.[4]

Your chances of being struck by lightening are 2,300 percent
higher than your risk of catching and then succumbing to H1N1. So far the
H1N1 has killed around 12,000 people *worldwide. Malaria kills one
million people every year.* Where is the panic? Where are the calls for
forcible mandatory malaria vaccines? Where are the quarantine camps?

Flu shots in general have neither cut the death rate from flu, nor
have they reduced hospitalization rates. They appear simply to enrich the
coffers of Big Pharma, (Novartis, another swine flu vaccine maker,
announced that it won't be giving any vaccines away to the poor.
Everyone must pay!) and make us more vulnerable to disease. Canadian
researchers in 2009 found that getting a regular flu shot increased a
person's risk for H1N1 disease by 68 %![5]

As of summer 2010 the flu vaccine program is still basically
voluntary. Unfortunately New York and a few other states have tried to
mandate (but fortunately was rescinded after public outcry) that health
care workers be vaccinated or face termination. According to a report in
*Time Magazine*, this mandate would have covered not only health care
workers, doctors and nurses, but also would have been expanded to
include housekeeping staff and food service personnel[6] If that ever
becomes law, could forced, mandatory vaccination for all be far behind?

If we don't protect our rights now, we may be in trouble in the
future, just like Dominic Johansson in Sweden. On June 25, 2009,
Swedish police forcibly took the seven-year-old from his parents and

placed him in foster care.  There was no warrant, no laws were broken, there were no charges made, and there was no evidence of Dominic's being harmed or abused.  His crime?  He was being home-schooled (legally) and *his parents had declined vaccinations.* Swedish authorities did not believe homeschooling or declining vaccinations are acceptable ways to bring up a child, insisting the government could do a better job. (Since when?)

The Swedish government, in a disgraceful abuse of power, exercised its authority under the U.N. Convention on the Rights of the Child, or UNCRC.  UNCRC is an international human rights treaty that has been open for signatures since 1998.  So far all members of the United Nations have signed except Somalia and the United States.  If the Senate ever ratifies the UNCRC, the right to home-school children here will be in great jeopardy.  UNCRC will automatically supersede all state laws and U.S. judges will be forced to follow all the provisions of the treaty, moving us ever closer to a one-world government.

Dominic is allowed to see his parents one hour every five weeks, and the traumatized family is desperately fighting to be reunited and correct this outrageous injustice. The Swedish Parliament is reviewing what is essentially a ban on homeschooling–and the subsequent right to refuse vaccinations. Other home-schooling parents in Sweden are beginning to fear widespread persecution from authorities. This could very well happen here. All parents have the right and authority to make decisions concerning their children's care and education without government interference.  Follow the story at http://www.dominicjohansson.blogspot.com

Edward R. Murrow was so right when he said years ago "a nation of sheep will beget a government of wolves."

A movement is now underway to protect our right of refusal, called Self-Shielding.  Under a Self-Shielding Law we would be able "just say no" to forced immunizations and voluntarily self-quarantine at home if an emergency is declared–a reasonable and rational option. You can support the proposed Protecting Americans' Self-Shielding bill by letting your congressional and state representatives know your feelings. Believe it or not, they do listen. Follow this story as it unfolds at www.healthfreedomusa.org.

A growing chorus of concerned parents, investigators, researchers, reputable scientists, and self-educated people is demanding to be heard on this very troubling subject. They want answers to their questions now, the big ones being:

*Are we all being used in a huge public health experiment that has brought about devastating unintended consequences? Are we in fact bearing witness to a tragedy of historical proportions? Are vaccines, in effect, a modern-day Trojan Horse, camouflaging and delivering lethal fungi and mycotoxins inside the walls of the human body?*

And equally tragic, could it be that *the seven vials containing the seven last plagues alluded to in Revelation are VACCINE vials,* all of which are described as being *"full of the wrath of God"?*

Our futures may depend on the answers to these questions.

**Chapter 22**

---

# Gardasil®:  Guarding Whom?

*"The chances of your daughter dying of cervical cancer are already VERY LOW, and the possibility of Gardasil sparing them from cervical cancer is so RIDICULOUSLY LOW that no reasonable person could argue for this HPV vaccine if they knew all the facts."*

... Dr. Joseph Mercola

The Gardasil® vaccine catastrophe is just getting started.  Gardasil® is a relatively new vaccine purported to protect young girls and women from the human papilloma virus (HPV), which is linked to cervical cancer. You have probably seen Merck's powerful ad campaign scaring women to become "one less" victim to cervical cancer by getting vaccinated with its much-ballyhooed vaccine.

It contains a *live* mutated virus and a whopping 225 micrograms of reactive aluminum in one shot.  It is a three shot regimen, which means one girl will receive a total of *675 micrograms of toxic aluminum.  One microgram of aluminum is considered toxic to a human being.*  Aluminum is routinely found in brains of Alzheimer's patients and is linked to M.S. (multiple sclerosis), Parkinson's, and other neurological disorders. Gardasil® also contains Polysorbate 80, which has been linked to infertility in mice, and sodium borate, *the main ingredient in roach killer!*

As of early 2010 there have been over 18,000 adverse effects reported to VAERS (Vaccine Adverse Event Reporting System) and 68 deaths since Gardasil® was introduced in 2006.  However, by the CDC's own admission, adverse effects are grossly under-reported. Only between one percent and 10 percent are ever reported, meaning the true number of injuries could actually be in the range of 150,000 to 1.5 million!

The adverse effects read like a catalogue of horrors, including 68 deaths, 45 cases of miscarriage and spontaneous abortions, 78 outbreaks of genital warts, 6 Guillain-Barre cases, plus serious internal bleeding, rashes, digestive disorders, vasculitis, pancreatitis, inflammation of the spinal cord, blood clots, stomach pain, and swelling in the joints. (Go to Medications.com and read 50 posts from real women about their experiences with this vaccine. Visit www.truthaboutgardasil.org to keep informed on the subject and the NVIC website is also excellent.) Recently I saw a report of a thirteen year old girl who became paralyzed shortly after receiving Gardasil®.[1]

Gardasil® can damage the immune system, and as 68 grieving families have learned, may lead to death. The most common causes of death include blood clots, acute respiratory failure, cardiac arrest, and "sudden death" due to "unknown causes" soon after being vaccinated. Eleven deaths occurred within two weeks of receiving the vaccination, and seven within two days, so whatever precipitated the deaths, it was quick and effective. Other side effects include facial warts, warts on hands and feet, anaphylactic shock, loss of consciousness, grand mal seizures, coma, and paralysis.

It is very interesting to note that Gardasil® is not recommended for women who are prone to yeast infections! That is because yeast products are in the vaccine, causing a worsening of existing yeast infections. That fact alone is reason enough not to take it.

Not long ago, Dr. Dianne Harper, an obstetrician and gynecologist who helped Merck run Gardasil® clinical trials and who has served on Merck's advisory board for the vaccine, admitted in an interview on CNN, "Gardasil® is not without risks. It is not a freebie." In another interview on ABC, Dr. Harper said, "Although the number of serious side effects is serious and rare, they are real and cannot be overlooked or dismissed without disclosing the possibility to all other possible vaccine recipients."[2]

Unbelievably, Gardasil® targets only 4 types out of 127 strains of HPV. (If you get any of the remaining 123 types, better luck next time.) Now the stage is set for newer and more virulent strains to emerge.

This three-shot regimen costs $125–$165 *each*, making it *the most expensive vaccine on the market*, generating a multi-billion dollar goldmine.

Even more absurd is the fact that Merck, in an effort to expand vaccine sales, has filed for FDA approval to *vaccinate young boys* (who, of course, do not have the required body parts!), to protect them from genital warts. I kid you not. Merck isn't happy with the over $2 billion it made in 2008 on Gardasil® sales. It's going after boys now.

HPV affects only 4,000 women a year–out of 150 million in the USA, so there is no real health crisis or epidemic to warrant a vaccine in the first place. And remember, we are talking about the human papilloma virus only–not cancer. *Contracting the virus does not mean you have or will get cervical cancer.* But the advertising for this drug implies that Gardasil® is a-cancer preventive drug. It is not. It is an *HPV preventive vaccine.* Even the National Cancer Institute says: "It is important to note...that the great majority of high-risk HPV infections go away and *do not cause cancer.*"[3] (emphasis added) HPV simply is not the scary monster Merck is portraying. In my estimation this is just another example of the deception and fear mongering coming from Big Pharma.

Cervical cancer used to be the leading cause of cancer deaths in women in the United States. In the last forty years the number of cervical cancer cases and deaths has steadily *declined,* a fact attributed to women getting regular Pap smears and early treatment for any pre-cancerous lesions that may be found. Just as the polio rates declined long before polio vaccines were introduced, Merck's Gardasil® is hitting the market at a time when cervical cancer rates are at their lowest. But never mind the facts. Watch Merck in the future try to take credit for the declining rates.

To date Merck has not even evaluated Gardasil®'s potential carcinogenity or genotoxicity (the ability to alter genes or the genes of your future children). Its safety has *never* been proven, as it was fast-tracked and pushed through the approval process without proper long-term trials. Even Merck readily admits that the long-term consequences are anyone's guess. We have no way of knowing this vaccine's effects on a young girl's fertility, cancer risks, immune systems, or its relationship to birth defects. We don't know its effects on pregnant women. We don't know if it passes through breast milk and damages a nursing baby. But we cannot sue Merck if there is a bad outcome or a child dies. Vaccine manufacturers are immune –pardon the pun–from prosecution.

Even so, the American Cancer Society estimates about 3,870 women died of cervical cancer in the U.S in 2008. It usually develops in the mid-twenties to late thirties. The protection period for Gardasil® is only five years, which means young girls and women will need *two to four booster shots to cover them through their thirties.*

Two to four more times they must expose themselves to the risks and side effects of Gardasil®. Two to four more times they must shell out to Big Pharma.

And don't forget that Gardasil® does not protect against all types of HPV. You can still get cervical cancer even if you have been vaccinated. The CDC itself states: "About 30 percent of cervical cancers will not be prevented by the vaccine." On top of that, if a female already has cancer cells in her cervix, the vaccine actually *increases* the cervical cancer rate! [4]

So, basically what they have created is a drug to treat a disease that most of the time is spread through promiscuous sex and probably will encourage more promiscuous sex! This creates more immune system overload and failure, and more chance for yeast to thrive. Great. Now what!

But here is the big picture. Hang in there with me, folks.

1.  U.S. statistics show there are 30-40 cervical cancer cases per
    year per one million females between the ages of 9-26. (The
    exact age bracket Gardasil® targets.)

2.  According to Merck, Gardasil® has been shown to reduce pre-
    cancers by 12.2% -16.5% in the general population.

3.  Again according to Merck, instead of having 30-40 cases of
    cancer per year per one million women (in the 9-26 age
    bracket), the HPV vaccine can potentially reduce it to 26-35
    cases of cervical cancer.

4.  *This means you would have to vaccinate one million girls to
    prevent (?) cervical cancer in 4-5 girls!*

5.  Further, only about 37 percent of women who develop cervical
    cancer die from the disease. *So vaccinating one million girls
    and women would prevent only 1-2 deaths a year, for the rock
    bottom, closeout, red tag, giveaway price of only $360 million
    a year![5]*

6.  The CDC's own website admits that in 90 percent of females
    infected, HPV clears up and disappears on its own within two
    years *and does NOT lead to cancer.* Even the vast majority of
    abnormal Pap smears clear on their own within two years.

So why do we even need Gardasil® when our own bodies are more
than capable of eradicating HPV?! In addition, according to the *New
England Journal of Medicine*, the use of condoms reduces the incidence of
HPV by 70 percent, *offering a far better protection than Gardasil®'s
measly 12.2 percent to16.5 percent.[6]*

All of this to treat a disease that females have less than a one
percent chance of contracting and is 100 percent preventable through

lifestyle choices! The entire campaign seems totally irrational for a vaccine that is mostly ineffective, potentially dangerous–if not life threatening–and a colossal waste of money.

Merck spent millions in lobbyist fees to influence government agencies to mandate all girls ages 9–12 receive the Gardasil® vaccine. The attempt failed. Then Texas tried to mandate it, but after an overwhelming backlash, that attempt failed. (Eighteen states are debating mandating it now in 2010.) Then Merck declared that women up to age thirty-five take the vaccine. Few takers. Overseas became the next target, but most countries are also leery of the vaccine. Let's see. Hmm. Who's left?

Aha! Unsuspecting immigrants! In July 2008 it was United States immigration law that female immigrants between the ages of 11–26 be mandated to receive the vaccine or they wouldn't be allowed citizenship, even if they have lived here on visas for years!

How could this happen when it isn't mandated for existing female American citizens? HPV is communicated only through consensual sex, or in other words through human behavior. Children and the public at large are not at risk. What public health issues are being addressed? How un-American can you get?

Such enforced immigration policy was a violation of their rights as women to make choices for their own bodies and amounted to making them human guinea pigs against their will. This government intervention into policing the bodies of immigrant women is unconscionable. Fortunately, as more and more people protested, this outrageous and over-reaching policy finally was  rescinded, but it just goes to show you how far pharmaceutical companies will go to further their bottom lines.

Fortunately the word about the dangers of Gardasil® is slowly is getting out. In June 2009 a teen-ager in Britain died  shortly after receiving a competitive HPV vaccine Cervarix® made by GlaxoSmithKline. (Our FDA is holding off approving Cervarix® for sale in the U.S. "pending review.") In 2009 authorities in Spain withdrew nearly 76,000 doses of

Gardasil® after two teenagers had to be hospitalized for seizures shortly after receiving the shots. Spanish health spokesmen reported the vaccine had been distributed country-wide during a government vaccine program. [7] Wouldn't you think that the United States would issue a recall of Gardasil® after 68 deaths, when Spain issued a recall after only two *injuries*? In April, 2010 clinical trials using Gardasil® and Cervarix® vaccines were *halted* in India after 6 girls died after being vaccinated.

In a similar vein, Toyota issued a $2 billion recall after 52 deaths were attributed to unintended accelerations in their vehicles. Why not recall Gardasil® after 68 deaths and untold injuries (in the United States alone) were attributed to the vaccine? Not as long as the powers-that-be have their way. It will remain on the market.

The bottom line is that instead of becoming "one less" victim to cervical cancer, more and more girls and young women are becoming "one more" victim of a dangerous, apparently worthless vaccine and money-hungry pharmaceutical companies.

Tom Fitton, President of Judicial Watch, said it best: "Given all the questions about Gardasil®, the best public health policy would be to re-evaluate its safety and to prohibit its distribution to minors. In the least, governments should rethink any efforts to mandate or promote this vaccine for children."

Currently, the NVIC is petitioning President Obama and Congress to investigate Gardasil® vaccine deaths and injuries. If you wish to support NVIC in their efforts, go to the website and sign the *Petition to Investigate Gardasil® Vaccine Risks Now!* They need our help.

The same Dr. Dianne Harper mentioned earlier in this chapter said in an interview on ABC what many perceived to be an explosive comment: "The rate of serious adverse events is greater than the incidence rate of cervical cancer."[8] Yikes!

*Meanwhile Merck is marketing Gardasil® in over 100 countries.*

**Chapter 23**

_____

# Antibiotics and Their Legacy

*"The focus of the marketing of drugs is mainly on the benefit side. Doctors are historically under informed about the risks of drugs."*
...Dr. Sidney Wolfe, M.D.

One of the greatest discoveries in the history of medicine is, undoubtedly, the antibiotic. In lifesaving situations its use can be nothing short of miraculous. Untold numbers of lives have been saved since their introduction in the 1940s, and none of us would want to live in a world without antibiotics. They are major players in a physician's arsenal, as they should be.

The use of molds in the treatment of disease dates back thousands of years. An Egyptian physician in 1500 B.C. quoted in the *Ebers Papyrus* (the ancient Egyptian hieroglyphic scroll that contains over 700 remedies), stated "if a wound rots…then bind on it spoiled barley bread." Twenty-five hundred years ago the ancient Chinese routinely used moldy soybean curds to treat boils, carbuncles, and other skin infections. But it wasn't until the twentieth century that purified forms of antibiotics were isolated and created to treat human disease caused by bacteria.

Antibiotics were discovered in 1928 when Scottish biologist and pharmacologist, Alexander Fleming was working on an experiment in his lab and discovered a fungus had accidentally contaminated a colony of bacteria he had been culturing. When he examined the dish closely he saw that the area around it was cleared of bacteria. The fungus had produced a substance he would later call *penicillin*. In the years to follow a class of drugs known as antibiotics was born.

Introduced in the 1940s, today there are hundreds of different types of antibiotics on the market. Nearly 160 million antibiotic prescriptions (or 25,000 tons!) are written by U.S. doctors each year to ambulatory patients and 190 million doses are administered daily in U.S. hospitals. [1] Pediatricians prescribe over $500 million worth of antibiotics *annually to treat one condition*–ear infections! The pharmaceutical industry spends $21 billion per year on marketing them, and over $3 billion per year on direct-to-consumer ads.[2] They have become one of the most sacred of the sacred cows of conventional medicine.

Now, after over sixty years of use, we are beginning to reap what we have sown.

Once hailed as the "savior" of mankind, antibiotics now are revealing their dark sides. We are seeing devastating side effects and the exacerbation of many diseases from having taken too many of them too often. These side effects and links to so many diseases are making us take second and third looks at this miracle of modern medicine.

First of all it is important to understand the basic differences between the two major types of organisms that make us sick–bacteria and viruses. Even though they can produce similar symptoms, the ways they multiply and spread illness are different.

Bacteria are *living* organisms that exist as single cells. Some are beneficial, such as the three-to-four pounds of lactobacillus and other good bacteria which live in our intestines, helping us digest food and making B vitamins. Others are harmful, such as *staphylococcus* and *streptococcus*, which cause illnesses by invading the body, multiplying and interfering with bodily processes.

Viruses, on the other hand, are *not strictly alive and not strictly dead*. They are tiny bundles (so small they can only be seen by the most powerful electron microscopes) of genetic material–either DNA or RNA– encased in a hard shell called the viral coat, or capsid. They exist for one purpose–to reproduce–but cannot reproduce by themselves. They must invade and hijack living cells in order to take over the cells' replicating abilities. Once inside, they use their own DNA and start makings copies of themselves and transform the commandeered cells into virus factories. When mature, the self-assembled new viruses leave the host cells, either by "budding" or bursting through the cell walls, as new infectious particles. They can infect nearly every living thing.  Even bacteria can get viral infections!

There are a growing number of researchers who are convinced that *viruses are really microfungi*–miniscule pieces of fungi. If you re-read the paragraph above, the similarities between how cancer (fungal cells) grows and how viruses operate are striking. Both are efficient parasites. Both enter and hijack cells, alter DNA, and replicate wildly. Both have hard, protective outer shells. Both reproduce by budding. Both harm or kill cells. The list is long and further underscores my contention that most of our diseases are really fungus in disguise.

There has been a long-standing controversy over whether there is a viral connection to cancer. If a virus is really a fungus and fungus is really cancer, this could illustrate that connection. Also, if a virus is really a fungus, then that would explain why antibiotics have no effect on viral or fungal infections.

Antibiotics, in essence, are poisons that are used to kill. They kill bacteria. They are so toxic only licensed physicians are permitted by law to prescribe them. Antibiotics are dangerous mycotoxins or fungal metabolites. Never forget that an antibiotic actually is the waste product of a *live fungus colony*. It literally means *anti-life*.

From what you learned in preceding chapters, it will not be hard to understand why researchers are discovering how widespread the damaging side effects of antibiotics are.

Here are the major hazards:

1. **Antibiotics can contribute to cancer.** In 2008 two carefully run studies on a large number of people were published in very reputable journals. One involved three million people that were divided into three groups. One group took no antibiotics in a two-year time frame; the second group took two-to-five prescriptions for antibiotics in the two years; and the third group took more than six prescriptions in the two years. The participants were followed for six years. Those who had taken the two-to-five antibiotic prescriptions showed a *27 percent increase* in cancers compared to those who took none. Those who took six or more prescriptions had a 37 percent increase in cancers.[3]

In addition, a National Cancer Institute study found the incidence of breast cancer *doubled* among women who took more than 25 antibiotic prescriptions or took antibiotics for more than 500 days over 17 years.[4]

2. **Antibiotics can create allergic reactions.** Antibiotics contain sugar, chemical dyes, and other harmful additives that trigger allergic reactions in sensitive individuals.

3. **Antibiotics are destructive to our delicate intestinal flora.** Our immune systems are very dependant on the proper balance of micro flora in the gut. Wide spectrum antibiotics are especially notorious for upsetting this critical balance. That leads to parasitic invasion, vitamin deficiencies, loss of minerals through diarrhea, inflammation of the gut, malabsorption syndrome, and the development of food allergies.

4. **Antibiotics lead to immune suppression**. They literally hamstring our immune systems. Clinical evidence shows that people taking antibiotics are more prone to repeated infections than those who are not. Antibiotics do not aid the immune

system but actually make the immune system response weaker. We all need stronger immune systems, not weaker!

**5. Antibiotics stimulate overgrowths of Candida.**
Antibiotics *ignite* yeast, leading to all the associated miseries outlined in this book. When friendly bacteria in the intestines are destroyed, we become vulnerable to rampant yeast overgrowths, salmonella, cholera, the bad E. coli, inflammation of the colon, and colitis.

**6. Antibiotics are intimately connected to Chronic Fatigue Syndrome.** Antibiotics are one of the major risk factors for this disease. Vitamin B-12 is destroyed by antibiotics, contributing to fatigue.

**7. Antibiotic use has led to the development of mutant, drug-resistant super bacteria.** Antibiotics, as a result, are becoming increasingly ineffective as germs become more resistant and stronger. As diseases become antibiotic-resistant they are much more difficult to treat–a direct result of over-prescribing antibiotics. The flesh-eating staph infections such as MRSA killed more people in the United States last year than AIDS, and the numbers are rising.[5] MRSA has become such a huge problem in Ireland that physicians across the country are cutting back on antibiotic usage. In the final analysis, it seems antibiotics have created a situation far worse than the original condition.

Additionally, look at the range of side effects and hidden dangers of antibiotics. All can be attributed to the ever-voracious yeast/ beast.

- Anaphylactic shock
- Angina
- Angioedema

- Antibiotic use in early life increases the rate of asthma in later life
- Burst intestine
- Cerebral thrombosis
- Constipation
- Dermatitis
- Fevers and chills
- Gastrointestinal bleeding
- Heart attack (In one study, the rate of sudden death from cardiac causes among patients on erythromycin was twice as high as compared to those who had not taken antibiotics.)[6]
- Heart murmur.
- Heart palpitations
- Hyperactivity –listed as one of the side effects of Amoxicillin® in the PDR!
- Irritable bowel syndrome
- Jaundice
- Liver failure
- Lupus
- Skin rashes
- Sudden death on first dosage
- Swelling of lips, eyes and face
- Tendon tearing (The FDA has received over 2,250 reports of tendon disorders and 775 reports of tendon ruptures from patients taking fluoroquinolones, a class of antibiotics which includes Cipro® and Levaquin®.)
- Ulcerative colitis
- Vasculitis
- Vomiting
- Weight gain

Adverse effects from antibiotics led to more than 142,000 emergency room visits in the United States *annually* during 2004 and 2006.[7]

Because bacteria multiply so rapidly, they are able to evolve and adapt to their new environments in the twinkling of an eye. That is why doctors warn their patients to finish the prescriptions for antibiotics instead of stopping them when they feel better. They are aware that *whatever bacteria escape and aren't killed off MUTATE.*

Treatment with antibiotics results in the survival of the fittest organisms. When weaker bacteria succumb, the stronger, more resistant bacteria that can tolerate the drug survive and are the ones left standing. These renegade variants multiply, increasing their numbers a million fold in just one day. With no natural beneficial bacteria to balance them (having been killed off by the antibiotic), the mutated superbugs replicate wildly, thumbing their noses at the old antibiotics and the scientists who created them, jeering "catch me if you can." Now, as older antibiotics are losing their power, doctors are getting desperate in the search for new treatments against these superbugs. One of the most recent and popular group of "super-antibiotics" is known as fluoroquinolones such as Cipro®. Over 280 million prescriptions have been written to date and is so toxic it carries a skull and crossbones on the label! Survival of the fittest, one of the most basic precepts of Mother Nature, has come back to teach us again that, try as you might, you really cannot fool her.

Even though we try to fool her, she carries no grudges. Mother Nature has provided us with many options when looking for natural products that kill bacteria. Herbs, such as garlic, golden seal, and astragalus, Vitamin C, colloidal silver, grapefruit seed extract, olive leaf extract, and oregano oil have excellent anti-microbial effects. Do not use Tylenol® or aspirin to reduce fever (fever burns up the bugs) as they actually slow down the fever reaction and can prolong the illness. *All anti-oxidants are anti-fungals, and all vegetables are strongly anti-fungal–* asparagus, broccoli, cauliflower, and brussels sprouts in particular. The yeast-free diet encourages you to eat them for that reason.

Anyone who has been prescribed antibiotics MUST take PROBIOTICS (meaning FOR life) in order to replenish the good bacteria the antibiotics destroyed. The rule of thumb is: take probiotics in a day to week ratio. If you take antibiotics for *four* days, you should take probiotics for *four* weeks, etc. Probiotics are critical to the recovery from almost all diseases. The immune system is dependent upon a healthy gut terrain.

In the 1880s there was a famous running debate that took place between the French chemist, Louis Pasteur, and his colleague, Andre Beauchamp. Doctor Pasteur argued that germs were the cause of disease. Doctor Beauchamp insisted that the health of the host was more important, stating that the "environment" or terrain in which cells live was more important than germs themselves. On his deathbed, Pasteur is reported to have capitulated and admitted, "The host is everything. The germs are nothing." In other words, a healthy body (terrain) and immune system trump any and all germs. If you have a healthy immune system, you don't need to be concerned that much about germs.

Unfortunately, orthodox medicine chose to embrace Pasteur's germ model and ignored Beauchamp's immune system model, and the rest is history. What a different world we would have today if scientists had chosen the other path. Perhaps we are ready now to focus on the status of a person's immune system rather than the germs that bedevil him.

The legacy of antibiotics is still being written. In the future perhaps we will find a way to isolate and harness only the beneficial aspects of antibiotics and eliminate the harmful. But for now we will have to continue to live with both.

In 1979, Dr. John I. Pitt, M.D., well-known physician and author, wrote in his book, The Genus *Penicillium*: "It is ironic that this humbled fungus, hailed as a benefactor of mankind, may, by its very success, prove to be a deciding factor in the decline of the present civilization."

A scary prediction to say the least, but we can see his prophetic vision unfolding around us every day.

Doctor Pitt tried to teach his colleagues (and us) that antibiotics should be used as a last resort, not the first.

Right now they are being handed out like candy.

## Chapter 24

# The Demise of Big P(harm)a ?

*"One of the first duties of the physician is to educate the masses not to take medicine."*

...Sir William Osler

At the outset let me make it clear again that there are times when conventional medicine and prescription drugs are necessary and appropriate, even beneficial. I am not advocating that anyone stop taking prescription medications cold turkey. If you decide to go off meds, it should be done slowly and under your physician's supervision. Your body has become dependent upon chemicals, and should be weaned carefully as the body balances.

If you do not have a physician who is open to your attempts to go more "natural," then find one who is. There are many wonderful and caring doctors and health care providers who will support you and monitor your progress. You might have to search a little.

In the last few chapters we learned a little about the history of the rise of the colossus known as Big Pharma. Let's look now at some of the failures, fiascos, and disasters that have been left in its wake.

In the last fifty years there have been innumerable instances where the use of drugs has resulted in injury and death. Below is a short and very incomplete overview of 26 benchmarks of note. There are many more.

1. In 1937 scores of people died from taking the antibiotic sulfanilamide, which had been dissolved in a lethal liquid.

2. In 1942 hundreds of troops contracted deadly hepatitis B from a yellow-fever vaccine.

3. In 1955 an incorrectly prepared vaccine was responsible for an outbreak of polio.

4. In 1960 thalidomide, a drug given to many pregnant women for morning sickness, was discovered to be the culprit in thousands of tragic birth defect around the world.

5. In 1971 I.V. fluids contaminated with bacteria caused hundreds of hospital patients to develop blood poisoning.

6. In the early '70s, 2.6 million women took the drug DES to prevent miscarriage. Soon doctors began to discover many of the female children born to those mothers developed vaginal cancers. In addition, male children had a higher rate of testicular cancer, and the mothers themselves had a markedly increased rate of breast cancer. Even more tragically, later studies showed that DES did little to prevent miscarriages and over 80,000 women ended upwith cancer or pre-cancerous changes in their reproductive organs.

7. The Swine flu debacle in 1976. After a flu outbreak the government called for every man, woman, and child to be inoculated, However, after 40 million Americans received the swine flu vaccine, the program was halted after ten weeks. Thousands of people developed Guillian Barre syndrome, a supposedly incurable disorder that ravages the protective sheathing of nerves affecting the brain and spinal cord. It can cause death and disability, or even paralysis to the point that patients must be put on respirators to breathe. The pandemic never unfolded and only 200 cases of flu and one death were

reported. *But more than 25 died from the vaccine!* [1] Claims
totaling $1.3 billion were filed by victims.

8.  In 1982, a new drug called benoxaprophen, which was used to
    treat arthritis, was recalled when 61 people died from
    complications in England. Lethal kidney and liver damage had
    not been observed in the testing done in the USA.

9.  Between 1980 and 2007 over 30 drugs *formerly approved* by
    the FDA have been *withdrawn from the market* after causing
    widespread injury and death. Some of the more familiar ones
    are: OxyContin®, Propulsid®, Baycol®, Redux®, Seldane®,
    Zelnorm®, Lotronex®, Phen Phen®, and Vioxx®, after 60,000
    people died of heart attack and stroke.( In March, 2010,
    Merck&Co. made its final payment to the Vioxx® settlement
    fund: $4.1 Billion!) Vioxx® had been "fast-tracked" without a
    full safety testing or an analysis period taking place.  A number
    of drugs, such as Zetia®, have been declared simply
    ineffective.

10. In recent years the FDA  issued recalls and/or warnings on
    many widely-used drugs, including: Lipitor®, Prozac®,
    Paxil®, Fosamax®, Bextra®, Avandia®, Celebrex®,
    Crestor®, Meridia®, Prempro®, Neurontin®, Ketex®, Ortho
    Evra® and Cipro®.  Many others are coming under scrutiny.
    Tamiflu® (a drug that reduces symptoms of flu *only 1 ½
    days*), has been discontinued in Japan because of the "sudden,
    serious psychiatric disorders" that appeared in users.[2]
    Tamiflu® has contaminated rivers downstream of sewage
    treatment facilities and researchers are becoming alarmed that
    birds that ingest these toxic residues might develop and
    spread stronger and more drug-resistant strains of various
    types of flu. Tamiflu®'s side effects include nausea,
    vomiting, diarrhea, headache, dizziness, fatigue, and cough.
    *Why take a drug that mimics the flu itself; may kill you; is
    banned in Japan; and costs over $100?!*  Even so, many

governments are currently stockpiling it as "bird-flu insurance." The damage done to internal organs and immune systems by all these drugs is incalculable, and many have died from their use. Now Tamiflu-resistant strains of flu are appearing. "Scami-flu" is a more descriptive term!

11.  As of early 2010, a number of anti-depressants, pain killers, and drugs containing phenolpropanolamine are being investigated as more deaths and injuries are being reported every day.

12.  The *Canadian Medical Journal* published the results of a scientific study on four popular anti-depressants used to treat depressed American children. All four–Paxil®, Zoloft®, Effexor® and Celexa®–were declared unsafe and ineffective. On top of that, the manufacturer, GlaxoSmithKline, was found to be "concealing evidence" that clearly showed these drugs provided no benefit to the children in any way, but instead actually *increased their risk of killing themselves.*[3] All of these drugs had the stamp of approval from the FDA.

13.  The incredible rise in the use of vaccines seems to have created a horrifying scenario we are just beginning to unravel. We now have several generations of children damaged with ADD, ADHD, autism, Asperger spectrum disorder, mood disorders, and behavioral problems that can be traced back to "baby shots," which precious, immature nervous systems undoubtedly could not tolerate. The lives of these innocent children and their parents will never be the same.

14.  Sudden Infant Death Syndrome, SIDS, or "crib death", is highly implicated in vaccine use, especially with multiple dosing vaccines. Infant immune response is crushed under this unnatural onslaught of three diseases at once, (as in the MMR vaccine). The infant, not having a mature and

functioning immune system, succumbs: A tragedy that didn't have to happen.  SIDS is listed in pharmaceutical literature as an *adverse reaction.*

15. In 2002 pharmaceutical companies began removing mercury, (*a known neurotoxin* found in thimerosal, a preservative that is 49 *percent mercury*), from some children's vaccines after floods of bad publicity and complaints.    However, the original lots of vaccines containing thimerosal (dubbed "hot lots") *were never recalled but were allowed to run out.* Today most vaccines still contain trace amounts of thimerosal.  The much-heralded flu vaccines are among the vaccines that *still contain mercury*–each dose contains 25 micrograms, an amount considered unsafe for anyone weighing less than *550* pounds!  It is also 250 times the Environmental Protections Agency's safety limit for mercury.[4]  Is it any wonder that getting regular flu shots has increased the risk of developing Alzheimer's by ten times?![5]

16. As for adults, our soldiers in military service receive as many as 17 vaccinations in a short period of time, despite the manufacturers' warnings that they should be spaced over a one-year period.  Latest studies are now showing this overload has much to do with the Gulf War Syndrome fiasco and many of the severe health problems being faced by our veterans today. The military is the perfect place for Big Pharma to cut through the red tape on new drugs and go straight to human testing.  President Clinton signed documents that legally granted the military exemptions from both prosecution and responsibility for compensations deriving from lawsuits, and withdrew servicemen and women's rights to informed consent, specifically concerning biological/vaccination testing done on military members. Talk about courage and bravery!

17. The polio vaccine is another case in point. All cases of polio occurring after the polio vaccine was introduced were traced back to the polio vaccine itself! [6]

18. Meanwhile, we are beginning to see the recurrence of many childhood diseases previously vaccinated against (this time even more virulent than the original). Other vaccines, such as those for diphtheria and whooping cough, are showing high failure rates. These scourges have figured out how to outwit our most brilliant scientists.

    *Have we traded normal and mostly benign childhood diseases for multiple sclerosis, Parkinson's, Alzheimer's, cancer, autism, and other more cruel and dangerous diseases?* Please inform yourself with books and websites discussing this tragic and disastrous chapter in medical history.

19. The Gardasil® vaccine fiasco is just beginning, with complaints and injuries mounting. (3,500 "adverse events" were reported in the first year–*more than any other vaccine in history*.) Many state legislatures have been considering mandating its use but are reconsidering as more is being learned about its dangerous side effects and deaths. *In the meantime, maybe you should hide your daughters!*

20. It looks like the overuse and over-prescribing of antibiotics by the medical community have created a health crisis worse than they were trying to prevent. Antibiotics are now the eleventh leading cause of death in the U.S. Originally antibiotics were reserved for serious or life-threatening cases only, *as they should be*, but now they are indicated for everything from "itchy ears" to acne. Some are even being prescribed to *prevent* infections!

    All of this has led to unintended consequences of gargantuan proportions.

21. Welcome to the world of *mega bacteria*. These super bugs are the direct result of prescription antibiotics. Antibiotics have become increasingly ineffective as germs become more resistant to them. Germs actually have become more powerful. The stubborn and sometimes deadly MRSA infection seen today is one of many of these new superbugs. It is a strain of staph that has developed a resistance to broad-spectrum antibiotics commonly used to treat it. Meanwhile, drug companies are frantically trying to manufacture stronger and stronger, more costly and more toxic antibiotics to deal with the new monsters. Some have admitted reaching their limits. People are dying every day because of lack of treatment for these super-powerful pathogens.

22. In 2003 a groundbreaking report which involved a painstaking review of thousands of medical journals by Gary Null et al, called *Death by Medicine,* revealed that an astounding *783,963 annual deaths were attributed to conventional medical mistakes.* Of those, 106,000 were from properly prescribed and properly taken prescription drugs (at a cost of $280 billion). These are the *Journal of American Medical Association*'s own numbers. All drugs had been approved by the FDA. *That makes the American medical system the fourth leading cause of death in the United States after heart disease, cancer, and stroke.*[7] The recorded medical errors and deaths is equal to six fully loaded jumbo jets falling out of the sky every day, 365 days a year. Where's the outrage?! Add to that the untold numbers who suffer adverse reactions, uncomfortable side effects, and dependency addictions. Most are not even reported.

23. Most women are aware of the turnaround that has taken place in the last few years regarding Hormone Replacement Therapy (HRT) previously dubbed safe and effective by the FDA. Once touted as the savior of women going through menopause, with promises of everything from saving bones to

the elimination of hot flashes, the latest studies have proven strong links to cancer, autoimmune diseases, heart disease, and stroke. Recently HRT therapy has been found to *double* a woman's chance of dying from lung cancer.[8] That may be the final nail in the coffin for these drugs, which are already in declining use. How many women were harmed or killed by those drugs? *Hormones feed yeast!*

24. We are becoming increasingly aware of the dangers of birth control pills. They contain high levels of synthetic estrogen that trick a woman's pituitary gland into thinking she is pregnant and doesn't need to ovulate, thereby creating an abnormal cycle. Fifty years ago we were promised the hormone-laced pills were safe and effective. Now we know that they increase the risk of cervical and breast cancers, heart attacks and strokes, migraines, hypertension, gall bladder disease, infertility, benign liver tumors, thinning bones, yeast infections, increased risk of fatal blood clots–all of which are stimulated by the yeast/beast because *hormones feed yeast!* Birth control pills have wreaked havoc in the bodies of millions of American women and many are seeking safer alternatives as studies continue to bring the truth to light.

25. More than 700,000 people visit emergency rooms in the U.S every *year* due to adverse reactions to drugs. The total number of people having in-hospital adverse reactions to prescribed drugs is over 2.2 million per *year.* The number of unnecessarily prescribed antibiotics annually for viral infections (antibiotics kill bacteria only, not viruses) is over 20 million per *year.* The number of unnecessary medical and surgical procedures has been estimated at 7.5 million per *year,* and the number of people hospitalized unnecessarily is estimated at 8.9 million per *year.*[9] Incredible statistics.

26. Many people 'trip out' on or go berserk on properly prescribed medications. Anti-psychotic and anti-depressant drugs have

been implicated in almost every school shooting in recent years, including the massacres at Columbine, Virginia Tech, and Ft. Hood. Even the chimpanzee that ripped off a woman's face had just been given a dose of Xanax by his owner, according to CNN news.

Are we fighting a wrong war on drugs? Illegal drugs like cocaine and heroin are responsible for between 10,000 and 12,000 American deaths per year. *A paltry number compared to the 106,000 deaths caused by pharmaceuticals.*

Is this any way to heal? Are pharmaceuticals and enormously costly research our only options to find cures for diseases that continue to plague mankind? How can we continue to pay exorbitant amounts of money for drugs that only mask symptoms and don't cure us, all in the name of funding research for future drugs?

Next time you hear about or are asked to join in or contribute to a charity or fund raiser for any disease, such as a "walk for MS" or a "run for breast cancer," etc. ask where the money is going. You may be surprised to learn that most of the money will go straight to a drug company for "research," or to a so-called independent lab that happens to be owned or controlled by a drug company. In all probability no great breakthroughs will ever be announced to the waiting world.

In the past twenty-seven years, over $1 billion has been raised to fund research and "find cures". Not one cure has ever been found for cancer, cardiovascular disease, diabetes, M.S., muscular dystrophy or any other disease. *Not one!* These diseases are now reaching epidemic proportions with an estimated 5,000 Americans dying every day. Annually, that's roughly the equivalent of a city the size of San Francisco! We should be incensed. It seems researchers are more interested in protecting their jobs through garnering a constant supply of grants and research money than they are in truly finding a cure.

At last count, almost all personal bankruptcies in the United States involve exorbitant medical bills.[10]  Insurance premiums have doubled for struggling families in the last ten years as medical costs continue to spiral out of control and bureaucracies to administer them multiply like fungi.

*Big Pharma plays a key role in this litany of suffering and sorrow.*

And their way–the way of synthetic, toxic chemical drugs–will never bear the fruit of true healing.  Here's why.

Drugs are essentially "one-dimensional," which makes it easy for pathogens, (microorganisms that cause disease) to evolve around and outwit antibiotics and anti-virals.  On the other hand, herbs and other natural anti-pathogens are multi-dimensional, often containing a myriad of biochemicals that present a scenario so complex that microbes find it almost impossible to evolve around them.  That leaves you with a stronger immune system rather than a weaker one. Chemical drugs force your body to do something unnatural, *thereby making the immune system weaker.*

When it comes to management of the most mundane to the most catastrophic of our illnesses, medical doctors seem to remain clueless. They merely treat symptoms, run tests and more tests, push test numbers up and down, and prescribe drug after drug. That is what they were trained to do.

You really can't blame them.  They are just reflecting what they were taught in medical school, i.e., *disease and drugs.*  What they were NOT taught in medical school is *health and nutrition.*  On average medical doctors spend a grand total of 6-8 hours *in their entire careers* studying nutrition.  Many of their patients know more about natural healing than they do!

If you really want to understand how woefully ignorant the medical profession is about food and healing, just walk into any hospital and you will see sick patients being fed steroid-laden hamburgers on yeasty buns, sugar-filled ice cream, Jell-O® and soft drinks, and juices full of artificial flavors and colorings, all under the watchful eye of the hospital's Registered Dietician. Yeast and fungi are gleefully feeding, multiplying, and promoting more disease, right under all the professional's noses.

So much for Hippocrates, who implored us to let our food be our medicine and our medicine be our food.

As I wrote earlier, conventional medicine is responsible for 783,936 deaths per year at a cost of over $280 billion dollars. By contrast, in the field of alternative medicine–the use of diet, herbs, supplements, homeopathics, and other natural remedies, has averaged *less than 5 confirmed deaths per year over the past 25 years!* Adverse side effects are extremely rare.[11] It makes you wonder who the true quacks are here.

Herbs and natural supplements are incredibly safe. They have been around for millennia. Millions of people have been taking them successfully for generations. People around the globe have found them to be dependable and effective. There have been *zero* deaths reported from cultural medicines, such as Ayurvedic, Asian and others using herbs, etc., and none reported from the use of phytoestrogens, glandulars, blue-green algae, or homeopathic remedies. A handful of deaths was reported in the late 1980s from *genetically modified* L–tryptophan, manufactured in Japan, not the USA. It was removed from the market and recently was allowed back on the shelves in its natural form.

Herbs, even the dried varieties, with their vitamins and minerals, are living food. They are made in God's laboratory–Nature–and cannot be patented. They have a consciousness, and know where to go in the body in order to heal. Vitamin C "knows" to go to every cell in the body; hawthorn "knows" to go to the heart and circulatory systems; red raspberry "knows" to go to female organs; lobelia "knows" to go to the lungs and respiratory system; saw palmetto "knows" to go to the prostate; etc. (If you don't believe this principle, I invite you to take a couple cascara sagrada the next time you are constipated. It certainly doesn't go to your elbow!) Herbs also work to heal at the very deepest level–our

DNA. They transfer information to our genes, which greatly benefits our health at the genetic level, and then are harmlessly eliminated after their jobs are done.

Drugs, on the other hand, have no consciousness, but are dead synthetic chemicals that work by forcing the body to do something unnatural, either by speeding up or slowing down body processes, creating uncomfortable and sometimes dangerously high complication rates (euphemistically called "side-effects") along the way.

Since pharmaceuticals are notoriously difficult to excrete, most take up residence in organs and glands, and wait to appear at a later time in the guise of another disease! (For instance, antibiotics cause a disruption to the intestinal flora, which then causes you to develop Irritable Bowel Syndrome or other intestinal diseases.)

Yet, Big Pharma's continual mantra is *"no one can be well or get well without our chemicals."* (Womb to tomb: a customer for life). As we know, nothing could be further from the truth.

But truth can be elusive in the medical/pharmaceutical world. Dr. John Abramson, M.D. made this clear in his excellent book, *Overdo$ed America*, when he wrote: "Rigging medical studies, misrepresenting research results published in even the most influential medical journals, and withholding the findings of whole studies that don't come out in the sponsor's favor have all become the accepted norm in commercially sponsored medical research."

Drug companies actually conduct studies on their own products–a huge conflict of interest. Researchers routinely take money from drug companies that fund their "research." Since they own the results of those studies, they can choose what they want to publish, effectively hiding studies that find their products ineffective or dangerous. At the same time they continually hammer away at many alternative remedies that threaten their bottom lines. Big Pharma can't stand competition.

One example of deception is a study by a pharmaceutical company that attempted to discredit the efficacy of the herb called St. John's Wort, which treats depression among other things. It was later determined that the test participants were given an *inactive* form of the herb. Of course the results were skewed and incorrect, but they were published, nonetheless.[12]

Another example is the way the media covered a study that claimed Fosamax® cut the risk of osteoporosis by 50 percent. What they didn't mention was the fact the trials were *100 percent funded by the makers of Fosamax®*. And the whopping 50 percent decline of hip fractures? The decline in hip fractures actually went from *two percent to one percent,* (thus the 50 percent decline).[13] Hardly worth getting excited over. Yawn.

Also, the drug manufacturers conveniently left out the fact that the one percent of the "success group" now had a 160 percent increased risk of developing gastrointestinal problems serious enough to require medical attention! Now there is evidence that Fosamax® actually increases the risk of bone fractures by making bones more dry and brittle, and people are being advised to stop the drug if they develop osteonecrosis, or rotting of the jawbone![14] It is becoming so common now that dentists are calling it "Fossy Jaw." Great drug.

Such antics go on all the time in an industry that has become media savvy. It is reminiscent of the litany of denials, evidence manipulation, suppression of research and stonewalling by the tobacco industry when they knew for years that smoking was harmful and caused cancer.

For the first time in history, many pharmaceutical companies are projecting negative growth in 2011 and a decline in sales in the following years. Shrinking pipelines, increased competition from generics, increasing costs, job cutbacks, blizzards of lawsuits melting their profits, and a slew of patent expirations are putting them in precarious financial positions. The leading pharmaceutical companies are expecting to lose between 14 and 41 percent of their existing revenues as a result of patent expirations between 2010 and 2012.[15] They are desperately scrambling to invent new drugs and branching into emerging markets (global initiatives) to stem the tide.

Also, pharmaceutical companies are increasingly being tried in federal courts as a result of their exploitation of Medicare. AstraZeneca had to pay more than $340 million in penalties for "coaching" doctors to cheat Medicare.[16] (Passed on to you and me.) The world's largest drug manufacturer, Pfizer, Inc., has agreed to pay at least $400 million in order to settle civil charges in regard to kickbacks they employed to encourage doctors to prescribe the anti-epileptic drug, Neurontin®, *for other purposes* in order to increase their bottom lines.[17] More lawsuits are on the way.

Another branch of natural healing that is gaining popularity around the world and threatening pharmaceutical companies' bottom lines is *homeopathy.* This elegant and simple therapy was devised by the respected German doctor and chemist in the 1800s, Samuel Hahnemann. Most of the early homeopaths were originally traditional physicians (allopaths) who switched to homeopathy when they found that Dr. Hahnemann was more successful in treating cholera, diphtheria, influenza, yellow fever, and other epidemics so prevalent at that time.

In the United States, homeopathy had achieved strong acceptance by 1840. In retaliation, the American Medical Association (AMA) was formed specifically to discredit the practice. Its charter even forbade its members to associate with homeopaths or their medicines! As a result, many doctors were expelled for non-compliance. (Good old boys clubs have been around for eons.)

Homeopathy is based on a single law of therapeutics, the *Law of Similars.* This law states that *a substance that can cause the symptoms of disease can also CURE it.* The word homeopathy means: similar (homeo) and suffering (pathy). For instance, one of the best remedies for insomnia is a remedy called *Coffea Cruda* (made from a tiny amount of coffee). Even though coffee can cause sleeplessness, a tiny drop of it balances the body and cures the symptoms of insomnia.

There are thousands of substances that homeopathic preparations are made from, most are natural, a few are toxic in their original form, and a few can be made from chemicals. All are based on the basic concept of "like cures like." Many conventional doctors use homeopathic principles without knowing it. Ask one why Ritalin®, which is a drug that would normally *cause* hyperactivity, can calm down children *with* hyperactivity. They don't know, but any homeopath will tell you "it's the law of similars." All preparations are ultra-diluted to the point that not a single molecule of the original molecule can be found. Only the *electromagnetic energy* remains to heal–with almost no side effects!

This whole concept of an unseen electromagnetic energy confounds and perplexes orthodox medicine, practitioners, and Big Pharma. No wonder they are afraid of what could happen if expensive drugs could be potentized into homeopathic remedies, creating billions of effective doses at a fraction of the cost of a pharmaceutical drug–with little or no side effects. Drug companies are running scared and quaking in their boots at the thought.

Homeopathy has the potential to decimate the whole medical model and industry as we know it. Big Pharma would then collapse into the ash heaps of history–where it probably belongs. A true David and Goliath story is in the making. In the meantime, find a good *classical* homeopath who will work with you to find remedies that fit your particular needs. Homeopathy is one of the best investments in your health you'll ever make.

So, it seems that alarming cracks are beginning to appear in the foundations of the drug cartel. The whole edifice is slowly beginning to crumble–and its members are scared witless. They can see the handwriting on the wall, and will be fighting dirty as people are waking up, asking questions, and demanding alternatives.

Don't forget that it was *years* before drug companies revealed their own studies linking Cox-2 inhibitors to heart attacks, and it was *decades* before they finally admitted that *hormone replacement therapy could trigger cancer*. Their "cash cow cures" were just too lucrative.

Do not expect them to declare their drugs and vaccines a "ghastly mistake" as they rightfully should. Do not expect them to proclaim *"mea culpa"* and contritely ask our forgiveness. The stakes are too high and the odds are too slim that they would survive.

Expect, instead, a mixture of lies, deceit, cover-ups, and defensive moves to explain away their flops, fiascos, and faux pas. Expect bolder steps to push more drugs on physicians and the public. Watch for moves to mandate vaccines and eliminate all the competition–the alternative and holistic physicians and health care providers, and the herbs, vitamins, and remedies they employ.

Be prepared to fight for the right to choose the type of health care you want. Write your congressmen/women and tell them "hands off" our supplements and homeopathics; and "no" to mandating vaccines in the land of the free; and "no" to the mandating of chemotherapy if parents of children do not want to choose that route. The tyranny of the state and those in authority is fast approaching.

Please bear in mind that the yeast/beast dines happily on all the drugs and synthetic, toxic garbage you can swallow. The more you take, the more they grow. The more they grow the more miserable and sick you become. The more miserable and sick you become, the more doctor visits you make, and the more doctor visits you make, well… you know the drill. And it's just what Big Pharma ordered. It's their dream scenario.

The bottom line is that much of the care and treatment of disease by "modern medicine" is a massive, dismal failure. In the last twenty years the United States has dropped from eleventh to fiftieth place in life expectancy, even though we have the highest per capita health care spending in the world. Medicare in going broke. Almost two million Americans are forced into bankruptcy every year due to medical bills. In fact, the system's excessive medical bills have become the *number one cause* of personal bankruptcies in the U.S. and are threatening our country's solvency.[18]  For all our efforts we are discovering that one-half of our population is obese, and our rates for diabetes, cancer, heart disease, and other diseases are soaring.  We are taking more and more medications and we are not getting healthier. We are getting sicker.

The sad tragedy is that we are spending trillions of dollars on disease management which has been focused mainly on drugs and surgery. Our return on this investment has been poor at best.  The only way to stop the slide into medical bankruptcy and eventual socialized medicine is for all of us to take responsibility for our own health with nutrition, supplements, and lifestyle changes. We trusted Big Pharma but our trust was misplaced.

Big Pharma has lost consumers' confidence.  With death from prescription drugs now being listed as one of the leading causes of death in the United States, the time has come to change direction.  We have become unwitting pawns in a huge public health experiment, and our faith in "better living through chemistry" has brought us a brave new world we can no longer tolerate.  This medical tyranny has reached its tipping point, and modern medicine as we know it is dying.  It is moving into its terminal phase, and the demise of Big Pharma seems underway.

The disease that is killing modern medicine and Big Pharma is being caused by a toxin-laden vaccine of another kind–one of their own making. They have created and injected themselves with a sleazy witch's brew of negative, harmful ingredients called: conflict of interest, greed, doctored research, cheating, fraud, corruption, pretentiousness, massive egos, armies of misguided drug reps, politicians, and state regulators, etc. It is imploding from its own internal toxicity. And so it should.

Albert Einstein said years ago, *"A foolish faith in authority is the worst enemy of truth."*

It is time for us to make way for a more enlightened, humane, and less expensive approach to regaining and maintaining true health. It is time for us to educate ourselves in the search for truth, to "just say *no*" to synthetic or chemical drugs, to think "outside the pillbox," to take responsibility for our own health, and return to natural, time-honored, effective and non-toxic therapies for healing our diseases.

They never left us.  We left them.

**Chapter 25**

---

# The Future of Food

*"And the serpent said unto the woman, Ye shall surely not die: For God doth know that in the day ye eat thereof, then your eyes shall be opened, and ye shall be as gods, knowing good from evil....And when the woman saw that the tree was good for food, and that it was pleasant to the eyes, and a tree to be desired to make one wise, she took of the fruit thereof, and did eat, and gave also unto her husband with her; and he did eat....And the Lord God said unto the woman, What is this that thou hast done? And the woman said, The serpent beguiled me and I did eat."*

...Genesis:3

The more research I did on the subject of food the more I became convinced of one thing:  We should all be afraid...we should be very afraid.

What is going on behind our backs and without our knowledge in the world of agribusiness will make your hair stand on end.  It is a scary sci-fi scenario with huge, far-reaching implications for our future food supplies and our future health.

For the past ten years, untested, unlabeled, patented, genetically engineered foods have quietly slipped onto the shelves of grocery stores in the United States.  Millions of unsuspecting shoppers have been purchasing and serving food to their families that have been "modified" by the insertion of foreign genes into plant cells.  The inserted genes come from species including viruses and bacteria which have never before been found in the human food supply. They are referred to as GMO (genetically modified organism) foods, or GE food (genetically engineered), or simply,

GM food. (I use all three terms interchangeably.) Soybeans, corn, strawberries, canola oil, cottonseed, and squash are a few of our "altered" crops. It has been estimated that 75 percent of processed foods in our grocery stores now contain genetically modified ingredients! Tortilla chips, soft drinks, drink mixes, taco shells, veggie burgers, muffin mixes, high fructose corn syrup, corn flour, dextrin, soy sauce, margarine, tofu, and baby formulas are just a few.

"Genetically modified food" is generally referred to as crop plants raised for human or animal consumption whose seeds and genetics have been modified in the laboratory to enhance desired traits, produce more crops, extend shelf life, or to increase resistance to pests or pesticides and freezing.

Genetic engineering (recombinant DNA technology) begins with the process of artificially modifying genes by cutting and splicing them, then forcing them into the genetic code of non-GE plants. Genetic material from one organism becomes part of the permanent genetic code of another, creating an entirely new plant with altered DNA that can be patented. Since 1996 bacteria, viruses, and other genes–never before found in human food–have been artificially inserted into the DNA of various plants in an effort to create new, "improved" life forms through scientific experiments in a kind of high-tech crossbreeding, which agribusinesses deem necessary "in order to feed a hungry world."

Farmers have used crossbreeding to improve their crops and animals naturally for thousands of years, but this new type of genetic engineering is more complex and more uncertain than crossbreeding in the past, which was confined to two varieties of the *same or similar species.*

In the inner sanctum of laboratories, scientists have discovered how to genetically engineer *between two different species– plants and animals.* For instance, genetic engineers have added genes from the flounder to tomatoes in order to lengthen the shelf life of tomatoes. *The natural protective barrier between species has been by-passed.* This "gene-jockeying" represents a huge leap into the unknown, which many see as an unnatural and dangerous step, and presents us with a basket-load of moral and ethical dilemmas.  Now the door has been opened for the spread of diseases *across species barriers,* creating problems that would never have surfaced *naturally.*

Genetic manipulation and experimentation have produced fish with cattle growth genes; potatoes with bacteria genes; a strain of "super pigs" with human growth genes; cats that glow fluorescent green; goats (called "spider goats"), whose milk produces spider silk protein which can be spun into incredibly strong fibers; corn with pig genes; safflower with growth hormones from carp; corn with jellyfish and mouse genes; potatoes with fruit fly genes; wheat with chicken genes; tobacco plants with cow genes, etc. I recently read of a woman who sliced into a perfectly formed tomato and found a perfectly formed strawberry inside!  After freaking out, she took pictures

.

A vegetarian cannot even be a vegetarian anymore! Now they are putting cow genes, fish genes, rat genes, and human genes into our vegetables!  So much for giving up meat.

In Holland scientist have put human genes into cows to make them produce "human milk."  In Canada the government is on the verge of approving the introduction of bizarre mouse/pig hybrids into the food supply.  This new "breed" was created by splicing in genes from mice *to decrease the amount of phosphorous in pigs' excrement.*  Supposedly this is much better for the environment, and the pigs have been dubbed "enviropigs."  In the United States there are plans to produce pigs with human genes in them.  These hybrid pigs will be "grown" so their organs can be used for transplants into humans.  Is any of this disturbing to you?

These creations are being patented and released into the environment at an astonishing rate.  *The gene-genie has been let out of the bottle* and it can't be put back. The use of genetic-engineering in agriculture can only lead to uncontrolled biological pollution from GE sources, threatening many microbial, plant and animal species *with extinction.* GE foods have the potential to infect and contaminate *all non-GE life forms* with new and potentially hazardous genetic material.

Last time I checked, human beings are non-GE life forms!

The biggest player in this drama is St. Louis-based biotechnology-agriculture-chemical giant Monsanto, the same company who gave us two of the most toxic substances ever known: polychlorinated biphenyls, known as PCB's, and dioxin (Agent Orange). In recent years Monsanto has provided us with aspartame (a dangerous artificial sweetener) and recombinant bovine somatotropin or rBGH (a genetically engineered growth hormone–a steroid) injected into dairy cows to force them to produce more milk (which made milking machines work harder, which made cows udders sore and infected, which created more pus, that required more antibiotics be given to the cows, which infected the milk, which gets into children and adults, which makes them sick, which calls for trips to the doctor, which means more drugs and antibiotics, which makes them sicker…and on it goes).

Once a plain old chemical company before it reinvented itself as a "life sciences" company, Monsanto is now a world leader in the genetic modification of seeds. So far it has engineered 674 biotechnology patents–more than any other company in the world. ("Biotechnology" is the new euphemism for genetically engineered patented seeds.)

Before 1980 the United States Patent and Trademark Office had refused to grant patents on seeds, regarding them as life-forms with too many variables to be patented. Unfortunately that all changed when, in 1980, in a five to four decision, the *U.S. Supreme Court* allowed for seed patents. When Monsanto began genetic engineering of seeds and plants, it claimed "ownership" of the seeds and plants because it had "created" *new life forms* and patented them. As sole owner of the very seeds needed to sustain world demand, Monsanto assumed an incredibly powerful position, and the groundwork was laid for a small number of corporations to begin taking control of the world's food supply.

Never before had life forms been patented, and, unbelievably, it happened without a vote by the people or a single debate in Congress.

When Monsanto developed GM seeds that resisted its own herbicide, Roundup®, it immediately patented them, calling them Roundup Ready® seeds. They are GM seeds that are genetically modified to survive applications of Roundup® herbicides while nearby weeds are killed. Being immune to the herbicide, they can withstand far more dangerous chemicals than normal crops.

Yippee! Monsanto gets to sell farmers their patented Roundup Ready® seeds *plus* their super-strong Roundup® herbicide that will be required to keep weeds at bay. (Roundup® accounts for half of Monsanto's revenues.) And we're supposed to *eat* this stuff? A "food" that produces its own pesticide?

It seems to me that what has really been engineered is a technological fiasco.

From the beginning of the Agrarian Age, farmers have planted their seeds, harvested their crops, and saved seeds from the harvest to replant the following year. Extra acres were planted solely for the harvest of seeds for planting the following year. Collecting and replanting seeds have been crucial steps in agriculture's historical cycle, feeding billions of people successfully through the ages. This also ensured the farmer of a profit that allowed him to live and continue farming.

But Monsanto sought to change the system for its own financial benefit. Once it legally gained patents on seeds, Monsanto began *requiring* farmers who bought their GM seeds to sign an agreement promising *not* to save seeds from their harvests for replanting, or to sell them to other farmers for any seeding purposes without the permission from Monsanto and their agents, *meaning they must buy new seeds every year from Monsanto*! Most farmers cannot afford to buy new seeds every year, and many are forced into bankruptcy, leaving their land open for Monsanto to buy and then plant with more of their GM crops.[1]

Today Monsanto has the legal capability to make life miserable for anyone who may have infringed its patents on genetically modified seeds. The company employs a cloak and dagger group of underground private investigators and agents, some posing as surveyors, who secretly infiltrate, videotape, and photograph farmers who might attempt to reuse their seeds. They spy on their meetings, watch co-ops and store owners, and gather information about farming activities. Farmers refer to them as the "seed police," and often use the words "Gestapo" and "Mafia" to describe their efforts at intimidation. They even have been known to confront farmers on their own land and try to pressure them into signing agreements giving Monsanto access to their private records![2]

It doesn't stop there.

If GM seeds or pollen from a genetically-engineered field accidentally blow or drift onto a nearby organic field contaminating that field, Monsanto can legally sue the *innocent farmer for infringement of its patent!* Monsanto has done it successfully 1,500 times so far.[3] It has become a felony to save your own seeds! To add insult to injury, traits from genetically-engineered crops can pass on to organic crops, ruining them along with farmers' yields and income. Eventually there won't be any native or natural genetic seeds left because of cross-pollination with GM seeds. (Or any farmers? Every year in the United States more than 17,000 farmers go out of business. That's one every half hour.)

In 2009 an organic farmer counter-sued and eventually Monsanto settled out of court. Incredibly, he received only the cost of having the invading biotech plants removed.[4] Go to the Organic Consumers Association website and read "A Farmers Struggle Against Monsanto" by Percy Schmeiser. He is fighting for the rights of all farmers to save their farms, their seeds, and the futures of their children and grandchildren.

One of the most alarming new innovations in GM technology (financed in large part by the United States Department of Agriculture) is *the terminator seed* being developed by Monsanto. It is genetically modified to self-destruct *after one planting*, meaning the seeds and the forthcoming crops are sterile, ensuring new seeds must be purchased for the next season. Once terminator seeds are introduced in an area, the trait of seed sterility could be passed to all crops, *rendering all crops in the area sterile*. This would mean that every farmer would have to rely solely on Monsanto for his seed supply, and if the GM traits spread, agriculture, as we have known it, could be destroyed altogether.

Can you see the implications for worldwide famine and starvation in our future if terminator seeds are unleashed globally by Monsanto?

Additionally, Monsanto is buying up seed companies at a rapid rate. If allowed to continue, it eventually could corner the market on seeds, and farmers would have no choice except to purchase Monsanto's "Frankenseeds". Monsanto provides 90 percent of the world's GM crop seeds, fulfilling its ultimate aim of controlling most of the world's food supply. Is this the company we want to be in charge of food? As a consequence, bioengineering of genetically controlled crops is threatening to destroy the agricultural biodiversity that has served mankind well since the beginning of agriculture.

The editors of *Well Being Journal* put it succinctly when they wrote: "Despite heavy advertising and PR greenwash, and despite a cozy relationship with the White House, Monsanato's image, profits, and credibility have plunged. Its aggressive bullying on "frankenfoods", its patents on the terminator gene, its attempts to buy out seed companies and monopolize seed stocks, its persecution of hundreds of North American farmers for the 'crime' of seed-saving, have made Monsanto one of the most hated corporations on earth."[5]

In recent years Monsanto has worked its way into many high-level positions in the U.S. government. The Secretary of Agriculture, Tom Vilsack, is an ardent fan of factory farms, GM crops, cloning of dairy cows, and often flies in Monsanto jets.[6] Vilsack was appointed by President Obama over the objections of 20,000 "grassroots" emails objecting to his deep ties to Monsanto. The former vice-president of public policy and chief lobbyist for Monsanto, Michael Taylor, who oversaw the creation and implementations of GMO and genetically-engineered bovine growth hormone policies and fought against special labeling for rbGH milk, *is a senior advisor for the U.S. Food and Drug Administration*! Heaven help us. How did we ever survive without their so-called cutting edge chemical tampering and manipulation?

The honeybee has been hit particularly hard in this "better living through chemistry" mindset. "Colony collapse disorder," or CCD, is a case in point. This frightening scenario raised its ugly head in the winter of 2006, when beekeepers on the east coast of the U.S. began noticing "die-offs" of their bees. Within a short period of time it spread across the United States and parts of Europe. Millions of bees vanished without a trace.

Most of the bees in an affected colony simply disappeared, going off to die elsewhere. The few remaining bees found in the abandoned colonies were riddled with disease. All were found to be carrying an enormous pathogen load, exhibiting an entirely new set of symptoms that didn't match anything in entomology books. Virtually every bee virus known was detected in the insects, *as well as fungal infections*, indicating the bees' immune systems were somehow suppressed. (Bee AIDS?)

Pesticides and herbicides are also highly implicated in this staggering decline of honeybees. They are known to affect the nervous systems, digestive systems, immune systems and brains of bees. Used in farming and on suburban lawns, they can weaken or kill bees. One of the new nicotine-based insecticides, Advantage®, clearly states on the label: "Highly toxic to honeybees" and "Do not use when honeybees are feeding in the area."

The creation of GE plants with built-in insecticides will kill insects as designed, but guess what! The bee is an insect!

Ninety percent of our fruits and vegetables depend on bees for pollination: fruit, vegetable, and seed crops worth between $8 billion and

$12 billion each year. Many beekeepers are beginning to suspect the "colony collapse disorder" that is responsible for the disappearance of *half our honeybees*, may be traced in part to the introduction of GM seeds. Some GM seeds are even pollen free! Compounding the problem, many honeybee colonies are being fed GM corn syrup and recycled hives containing more GM food residues, contributing to malnutrition in hives. (Interestingly, almost no colony collapse disorder is found in organically raised hives.)

Pollen is bee food. When bees feed pollen from GM plants to larvae, they can't process it for energy and subsequently starve to death. Eventually the colony collapses. Without honeybees we won't have fruits or vegetables to eat. No more almonds, cherries, cantaloupe, oranges, apples, cranberries, vine crops, etc. The Law of Unintended Consequences is swinging into full action. "Frankencrops" are here; "Frankenfood" is our future. The Brave New World is upon us.

FDA scientists have warned that GM food can create elusive side-effects, allergies (in the UK soy allergies skyrocketed by 50 percent after GM soy imports from the U.S. were introduced)[7], toxic reactions, new diseases, and nutritional imbalances. However, to date *GMOs do not require any safety evaluation.* No safety trials on humans have ever been published, and probably will never be done since, unbelievably, the FDA considers GMOs "substantially equivalent" to non-GMO food. The fact remains that genetically engineered foods have not been proven safe, and they have been linked to thousands of toxic reactions, uncounted sick, sterile and dead livestock, and damage to virtually every organ and system studied in lab animals.

Even laboratory mice don't like genetically-engineered food. If given a choice between natural and GM food, they leave GM food untouched. GM potatoes have been found to damage the kidney, thymus, spleen, and intestinal linings of young rats.[8] Mice injected with GM proteins from peas develop a hypersensitive skin response, and those exposed to the airborne form develop airway inflammation and lung damage.[9] You are what you eat. If it's not good for lab animals, how can it be good for us?

The catchfly plant is a good example of how fungi and genetic modification can go hand in hand. When a catchfly plant is invaded and taken over by fungi, instead of emitting pollen, the plant *begins to emit fungal spores!* Fungi entered into the nucleus of the cells, hijacked their DNA, and genetically engineered the normal pollen production of the plant to become fungus-like. Sounds like an agricultural version of Invasion of the Body Snatchers! Sounds eerily like cancer.

Now a new disease in humans is suspected of being caused by GM foods. It is called Morgellons disease.

As of February, 2009, more than 12,000 reports of this mysterious nightmare of a disease have been reported to the Morgellon Foundation's website. Reports have come from around the world, but the majority come from Texas, California, and Florida.

Patients with this bizarre and terrifying disease report feelings of bugs or worms crawling under their skin, with open lesions or sores that heal slowly and ooze blue, black, white or red fibers, some up to several millimeters long. These fibers look like pliable plastic and many can be seen coiled under unbroken skin. Many twist, bend, and divide forming parasitic lesions from what normally would be *non-living* material but somehow have assumed the characteristics of a *living thing.* Victims of this terrible disorder say it causes biting and stinging sensations, which result in what can only be described as "itching from hell." Many have been driven to suicide. Additionally, victims complain of joint swelling, fatigue, hair loss, memory loss, and brain fog. Doctors are baffled as to what it is or how to treat it. The CDC has set up a web page about the phenomenon (which they call "Unexplained Dermopathy") and has given Kaiser Permanente $338,000 to investigate this new disease.

In the interim, a research team from Oklahoma State University studied fibers that were sent to them by Morgellons patients. They were then sent to the Police Crime Lab where a search of all known fibers was conducted through the FBI's database. All were found to be remarkably similar, but did not match any *known* environmental fibers, such as cotton, wool, or synthetics. More study showed the fibers contained DNA from *both a fungus and a bacterium!*[10]

The most interesting finding came from Dr. Vitaly Citovsky, Professor of Biochemistry and Cell Biology at Stony Brook University in New York, who discovered that the fibers contained a substance called *Agrobacterium tumafaciens,* a soil bacterium capable of genetically transforming not only plants but also HUMAN cells.

Agrobacterium is also a significant plant pathogen (which means it is capable of producing disease) that *causes tumors* called "crown gall disease" common to grape vines, stone fruit, and nut trees. *Agrobacterium is a vehicle used in research labs to transfer foreign DNA into the host plant genome!* Could Morgellons disease be the equivalent of a gall disease in humans caused by the transferring of bacteria from plant to animal in the form of GM food?

We already know that genetic engineering can transfer genes across natural species barriers (plant to animal and vice versa) with unforeseen and unpredictable results. Foreign genes from viruses or bacteria artificially injected into our food supply may be responsible for this horrible modern-day plague.

To me, Morgellons disease is more likely a man-made genetically modified *fungal* disease. It is most prevalent in California (especially in the San Francisco Bay area), Texas, and Florida where humidity levels are high. Victims who treat it with yeast-free diet and anti-fungals such as colloidal silver, garlic, and oregano oil show great improvement and even cures. In the future, more research will be needed to prove that genetic engineering may have triggered Morgellons disease, as it does seem suspicious indeed.

So far there has been no independent government-supported research into the effects of genetically engineered foods on mammals, meaning *their safety has never been verified!* With no proof of their safety, there is no telling what either the short-term or long-term consequences of eating GM food will be–for both humans and animals.

One well-known fiasco in the GM world happened in the late 1980s. A well-known manufacturer of tryptophan (a natural amino acid used to treat insomnia) in Japan saw a way to increase profits by gene-splicing a bacteria into the natural product. Unfortunately dozens of people died, over 1,500 were left crippled, and up to 10,000 were afflicted with a new blood disorder from a new *incurable* disease called *eosinophilia myalgia syndrome* or EMS. Hundreds more have died since. It cost the manufacturer over $2 billion to settle claims. Of course all tryptophan was immediately taken off the market and only recently has a clean, non-GMO tryptophan been allowed back on the shelves.

This incident is an example of ONE foray into the bizarro world of genetic engineering. Can you imagine what may be in store for us if we continue along this path?

In the words of prominent biologist, Dr. Barry Commoner, "The genetically engineered crops now being grown represent a huge, uncontrolled experiment whose outcome is inherently unpredictable. The results could be catastrophic."[11] Damning evidence worldwide is piling up against the safety of GM food and feed. Farmers are finding they do not increase yields but in fact *decrease* yields– and their profits.[12] Yields and profits are down and agrochemical use is up. The "new and better" crops are creating stronger pests and "super weeds" (requiring more and stronger pesticides and herbicides) and more serious diseases similar to the way antibiotics have created "superbugs." The soils in which GE crops are grown are being grossly contaminated, and earthworms and beneficial organisms are being killed, rendering the soil "dead" for future generations.

Even though industry-sponsored research continues to claim that GM foods are safe to eat, feeding trials sponsored by scientists *independent* of the GM industry claim just the opposite, reporting serious damage to the health of animals, including damaged livers and spleens, smaller livers, hearts, testes and brains, damaged thymuses, and pre-cancerous conditions,[13]

*That makes us guinea pigs in the most enormous, unregulated, untested biological experiment in the history of mankind.*

We need to ask why the FDA is allowing GMO to move forward in the United States. We need to question why the U.S. government hasn't required that GM foods undergo the same rigorous testing required of medicines created by recombinant DNA technology, and why the industry has resisted efforts to label GM foods, as Europe requires. (The European Union previously had banned all GM food but has allowed some crops now. It is also banned in much of Africa.)

We know why. Sadly, it appears more and more that bottom line profits are trumping human health. Just follow the money. Monsanto and other giant international agribusiness companies are aggressively taking over the global food chain by overwhelming it with GMOs with apparently little or no regard for the consequences to the earth or its occupants.

A case in point is the catastrophic earthquake that hit Haiti in January 12, 2010. This provided Monsanto with the opportunity to spread its wings, by offering 475 metric tons of GM seeds, plus the pesticides and herbicides they needed, to that devastated country. The Ministry of Agriculture wisely declined the offer, but did accept tons of hybrid corn and vegetable seeds (many unsuitable for seed saving and were treated with pesticides). Many of the small, independent farmers were upset and angry, and threatened to burn Monsanto's seeds.

During the 111th Congress bill HR 875: Food Safety Modernization Act of 2009 was introduced. This bill dies in Congress

12/31/10 if not passed. It called for mandating criminality for "seed banking," prison terms and confiscatory fines (up to $500,000) for small farmers for non-compliance, and outlines what feed farmers must use, what seeds and herbicides they must use, etc. That shows how serious Monsanto, Cargill, Tyson, and Archer Daniels Midland, sponsors of the bill, are in their attempts to monopolize agriculture and eliminate organic farming. Even roadside stands and farmers markets could fall under the umbrella of this legislation if passed, effectively eliminating them. Keep yourself informed on this very important subject.

But while you and I may be branded criminals for "seed banking" our own seeds, the Bill and Melinda Gates Foundation, the Rockefeller Foundation, and the United Nations (under a group called Global Crop Diversity Trust) have funded the construction of a massive *natural seed bank* dubbed the "doomsday seed vault." It is officially called the Svalbard Global Seed Vault and houses over *3 million varieties* of non-hybrid, *non-GMO seeds* from all over the world. This ultramodern facility is located on Spitsbergen Island in the Barents Sea, halfway between Norway and the North Pole. It is 425 feet deep inside a mountain and is surrounded by permafrost–a veritable frozen Garden of Eden. It has dual blast-proof doors, motion sensors, two airlocks, and walls of steel-reinforced concrete one meter thick, built to withstand earthquakes, climate change, natural disasters, or a nuclear strike. It was constructed ostensibly "so that crop diversity can be conserved for the future."

The largest users of the seed bank are Monsanto, Dupont, Syngenta, and Dow Chemical Companies, all major players in the production of GMO foods. Why are they stockpiling natural seeds and not wanting anyone else to do the same? Aside from natural disasters, what future could the seed bank's sponsors foresee that would jeopardize the availability of current seeds? A potential GMO disaster perhaps?

We do know that one characteristic of GMO crops is that they cross-pollinate with natural plants, rendering their genetic structure forever altered. Eventually all crops will become genetically modified. Plus the use of "terminator seeds" could easily create that disaster scenario. Another real fear is that the development of patented seeds for much of the world's sustenance crops, such as rice, corn, wheat, and feed grains, could even be used as a grisly form of biological warfare.

Both the Gates and Rockefeller Foundations support the proliferation of GMO patented seeds and terminator seeds, and at the same time invest tens of millions of dollars to preserve every natural seed variety known to man in a frozen repository in the Arctic Circle. What do they know that the rest of us do not?

Activist groups against GM foods and Monsanto are beginning to form, reflecting a growing, world-wide resistance against Monsanto and other multi-national agro-businesses. In May, 2010, 40 people gathered outside Monsanto's seed company outside Rotterdam, the Netherlands, chained themselves to both gates and prevented personnel from entering in an effort to stop Monsanto from manufacturing GM seeds. They implored Monsanto get out of the seed market and demanded an end to patents on seeds and living organisms. Even though the plant was closed for a short time, there will be more activism in the future.

Another way we can fight back that is not so dramatic, is with our pocketbooks. We can "just say no to GMO." If we are careful not to buy the stuff, demand will fall and stores will be unable to sell them. This can be a bit tricky as the *FDA is not allowing GMO food to be labeled!* Why? *Every country except the U.S.A. requires GMO foods to be labeled.*

Consider boycotting GM products, buy local, and eat organic (Food that is certified organic must be free of all GM organisms, produced without artificial pesticides and herbicides or from an animal raised without the use of antibiotics, growth promoters or other drugs.) Look for grass-fed organic beef, as they will not have been fed GM corn feed or alfalfa. Download a list of safe food to buy at www.nongmoshoppingguide.com. Plant a garden. Eat as little processed food as possible. Watch the DVDs "Food, Inc." and "The Future of Food." Cook from scratch. Support sustainable farming everywhere. Write your congressmen/congresswomen. Read labels. Pressure your local markets, produce sellers, dairies and health food chains to provide full disclosure if they sell GM food. *Demand that Monsanto and other GM companies stop the cultivation of all GM crops NOW.* The Organic Consumers Association is fully updated on this subject. Their website is http://www.organicconsumers.org.

You can also learn to avoid GM foods by studying the stickers you find on fruits and vegetables before you buy them. The PLU code for *conventionally* grown produce consists of four numbers (for example, a conventionally grown banana would be 4011). The PLU code for *organically* grown produce has five numbers prefaced by the number 9 (for example, an organic banana code would be 94011). A *genetically engineered* product carries a 5-digit code starting with the number 8 (for example, a genetically engineered banana would be 84011). A good way to remember this is to say: *"Hate eight" and "nine is fine."*

Another good defense we all have is to start buying non-hybrid heritage and heirloom seeds. They are old lines of seeds saved for hundreds of years by home gardeners and farmers worldwide. They are genetically pure and uncontaminated. They are just as Nature made them. No one owns them or has patents on them. You will be eating food that reproduces "according to its own kind," by its *own* seed, not an artificially concocted one. You can find them in health food stores, co-ops, organic nurseries, on the Internet (go to www.survivalseedbank.com or www.newhopeseed.com) or buy them from organic farmers.

Be very aware in the future of what the FDA is doing to restrict our access to the kind of food we want. On April 26, 2010 the FDA finally made its food-rights policy very clear when it submitted a response to a lawsuit filed earlier in the year by the Farm-to-Consumer Legal Defense Fund (FTCLDF). In the response the FDA made its position on the issue of "freedom of food choice" a part of the public record. A few of the more frightening statements are:

- "There is no absolute right to consume or feed children any particular food". (p.4)

• "There is no deeply rooted historical tradition of unfettered access to foods of all kinds." (p.25)

• "Plaintiffs' assertions of a 'fundamental right to their own bodily and physical health, which includes what food they do and do not choose to consume for themselves and their families' is similarly unavailing because *plaintiffs do not have a fundamental right to obtain any food they wish."* [emphasis mine] (p.26)

If this doesn't send a chill up your spine, I don't know what will. This could mark the beginning of an end run around the outlawing of GM foods. The FDA may be trying to establish a legal precedent that Americans do not have the right to their own bodies and health. If we have no rights to our own bodies and health, then GM foods can literally be shoved down our throats! *We will not have the right to refuse something we do not want!*

The United States Constitution's Fifth Amendment states "no person shall be deprived of life, liberty, or property without due process of law." It is inconceivable that our fundamental freedom to choose the food we want and *do not want to eat*, so inherent to life, liberty, and property, would not be protected, but the FDA thinks otherwise. Americans overwhelmingly oppose the genetic modification of food.

After 30 years of experimentation and 15 years of cultivating genetically modified crops, *2009 witnessed a record amount of starvation around the world.* GM seeds are providing neither increase yields nor profits, but do increase our chances for horrendous unintended consequences. In India, according to the National Crime Records Bureau, more than 182,900 Indian farmers took their own lives between 1997 and 2000 as a result of failed GM crops. With failed crops, the inability to save seeds to replant and spiraling debt, farmers are hopeless. It is estimated that 46 farmers commit suicide every day in India today. This is only one country. Instead of opening a can of worms, have we opened a crate of snakes?

The symbol of the serpent in this chapter is appropriate on several levels. As you know, the caduceus is the symbol of American medicine. It consists of a single staff around which two serpents are entwined, topped with a pair of wings. The symbol's origins can be traced back nearly 3,000 years to Mesopotamia, and is thought to be used in Atlantis and Ancient Egypt. It originated as a willow wand with intertwined ribbons that later evolved into snakes. There are several references to a caduceus-like symbol in the Bible (see Numbers 21: 9). In Greece it was an ancient astrological symbol of commerce and is associated with the god, Hermes, the messenger of the gods, the conductor of the dead, and the protector of merchants and thieves! During the seventh century the caduceus became associated with the practice of medicine based on Hermetic principles of the astrological influences of planets and stars.

In 1902 the symbol was used by the U.S. Medical Corps as a logo on their uniforms, and eventually was adopted by the medical profession as its official symbol.

Even though the two snakes coiled around a staff somehow is supposed to be comforting, I personally react like most people react to a snake—with horror and disdain. God cursed the serpent (a metaphor for Satan) in Eden, and told him he would henceforth be doomed to slither on the ground and eat dust for the rest of his days for his transgression. Adam and Eve were then banished from the Garden for their transgression of listening to the lying, deceiving serpent. Is this really a suitable symbol for the healing profession?

On another level it seems the snake may be appropriate as a symbol of the "snakes nest" of Big Pharma, the AMA, Monsanto and other agribusiness giants, the FDA and others whose directives continue to swallow whole (like a snake) so many people's lives, their pocketbooks, and their health. It is no accident that many of the pharmaceutical companies that comprise Big Pharma also manufacture pesticides. Monsanto is particularly "intertwined" with the pharmaceutical industry.

In 2000 the Pharmacia Corporation was created when Pharmacia and Upjohn merged with Monsanto and its G.D. Searle unit. Toxic products created by chemical giants cause illness and disease, which mean drug companies must create drugs to treat them. One is feeding the profits of the other. Corporations that profit in *both* pharmaceuticals and pesticides besides Monsanto include: American Home Products, AstraZeneca, Aventis, BASF, Bayer, Dow Chemical, Dupont Chemical, Merck and Syngenta (previously Novartis).

An additional "intertwining" is the link between doctors and Continuing Medical Education (CME) courses, courses doctors are required to take in order to maintain their licenses and continue to practice medicine in the United States. Who provides grants for most of these courses? The pharmaceutical industry. It appears that without the pharmaceutical industry doctors couldn't practice medicine, and without doctors the pharmaceutical industry would in all likelihood disappear.

Snakes bite…even the non-poisonous ones.

It is time to remind ourselves of God's warning to mankind not to succumb to the wily serpent who tries to seduce us into eating the fruit from the Tree of Knowledge of Good and Evil. Are we stepping into uncharted territory we were warned never to enter? History shows us that man and his brain are capable of making extraordinary mistakes, even honest ones. Surely we will create lives of misery and pain if we proceed unfettered to tinker and tamper with nature's original design.

In May, 2010, scientists proudly announced the birth of a "synthetic cell." It was created by injecting a bacterium with genetic material created from scratch. Man-made DNA can now power a live cell, as scientists inch ever closer to creating life. Artificial life is almost here, and the door to the unknown has swung open wide. I, for one, do not want to venture through that door.

Evidently we have opened that door before. In the ancient book of *Jasher*, (4:18) written 3,000 years ago before the Flood, (around 2300

B.C.) we read: "and the sons of man in those days took from the cattle of the earth, the beasts of the field, and the fowls of the air, and taught the mixture of animals of one species with the other, in order therewith to provoke the Lord." Also the ancient book of *Enoch* (7:14) tells us: "and they began to sin against birds, beasts, reptiles, and fish, and to eat their flesh one after another, and drink their blood." So, not only were they "mixing" animals together, they were eating them too, *just like we are today*. We don't know if or how they were genetically engineering, but it seems they did, and God was not pleased with the corrupting of His creation. Mankind was severely rebuked by the Flood.

We need to consider carefully how far we dare go in the pursuit of knowledge and science. The pursuit of such knowledge has wrought many blessings. Honest and transparent scientific research should continue to further our knowledge and understanding. But there are limits to how deeply we should delve into the mysteries and workings of the universe. Ethics, morality, and a sense of propriety should always be our guides as we continue our journeys of discovery.

In Ecclesiastes we are warned: "As you do not know the path of the wind, or how the body is formed in a mother's womb, so you cannot understand the work of God, the Maker of all things."[14]

In these Orwellian days of "octo-mom," cloning of animals (are humans far behind?), embryonic stem cell research, "designer" babies, nanotechnology (the process of manipulating matter at atomic and molecular levels), and the genetic engineering of food and seeds, and plants and animals, are we on the precipice of a tragedy of our own making? A tragedy of unintended consequences? How many times do we have to re-learn "You can't fool Mother Nature?"

These are pressing and important questions we should investigate individually and as an advanced civilization.

Biblical prophecy has warned us that a worldwide famine and food crisis was in the offing if mankind didn't follow specific guidelines when raising crops. With seeds such as terminator seeds and GM crops we could be *sowing the seeds of our own destruction.* Even as far back as 1994, warnings were issued concerning genetic modification. Norman Braksick, president of Asgrow (a subsidiary of Monsanto) was quoted in the *Kansas City Star*, March 7, 1994, as saying "If you put a label on genetically engineered food, you might as well put a skull and crossbones on it."

I believe the creation of GM foods and seeds in the laboratory is the result of our listening to our dark side–the side that whispers we, too, can play God, making new creations and knowing all. Are we playing God, or playing the devil?

Either way, it can only result in tragedy.

The serpent beguiled us and we did eat.

Don't forget. **The serpent lied.**

**Chapter 26**

# *Codex Alimentarius*

*"Find out just what any people will submit to and you have found out the exact measure of injustice and wrong which will be imposed upon them."*
...Abraham Lincoln

*Codex Alimentarius.* Now there's a mouthful–pun intended. I'll bet you never heard of it. Most of our congressmen/congresswomen have never heard of it either. And that is exactly what is hoped for.

It is Latin for "food rules." It is a trade commission, which was started in 1962 when the U.N. authorized a joint venture with the World Health Organization (WHO) and the Food and Agricultural Organization (FAO), to develop a universal food code and set up regulations to control the international trade of food. One hundred seventy-seven countries are members of the *Codex Alimentarius* Commission, or the CAC.

Twenty-seven committees are studying every aspect of the food chain, but two we need to follow the closest are the Committee on Nutrition and Food for Special Dietary Uses, and the Committee on Food and Labeling.

CAC started innocently enough as it assumed a benevolent role as an international public health and consumer protection organization. Its stated purpose in the beginning was to "harmonize" dietary regulations for dietary supplements worldwide and set international safety standards and uniform regulations for the purpose of increased trade. Some of these regulations are in force today.

Sounds benign enough. Even reasonable. But as you will see, corporate interests have taken over and the actual goal of *Codex* has shifted. *Now its mission is to outlaw all health products and information on dietary supplements except those under its direct control.* Because of *Codex* guidelines, global pharmaceutical companies, food and banking giants, together with the U.N. and U.S. government agencies are now promoting GMOs over healthy food and drugs over natural remedies. It seems to be all about profits, not human health any more.

Instead of focusing on safety, its aim today is apparently to increase profits for the international pharmaceutical cartel, multi-national chemical companies, and giant agri-business companies and promote worldwide restrictions on vitamins and supplements. In doing so it will eliminate the competition from natural and alternative sources and surreptitiously gain control of the world's food supply. *He who controls food, controls the world.*

If fully implemented, *Codex* would outlaw our free access to nutritional products such as vitamins, minerals, amino acids, herbs, and homeopathics–and any information in connection with them–*on a worldwide basis*. It also would limit our free access to natural therapies such as acupuncture and natural practitioners such as homeopaths, naturopaths, chiropractors, etc. GM foods will proliferate; labeling will be banned; and food and drug giants will decide what will or will not be sold. Health food stores, nutritional supplement manufacturers, and health food manufacturers will fall like dominos as their wares are declared unsafe and illegal. The only players left standing will be Big Pharma, Big Agra, and GMO producers like Monsanto.

Even though *Codex* standards supposedly have no legal weight or standing, they are enforced through the World Trade Organization (the teeth of *Codex*) largely through *intimidation*. If a country refuses to follow the prescribed standards, it can be severely punished with withdrawal of trading privileges, huge fines, and the imposition of enormous and crippling trade sanctions. Congress has bowed to this pressure several times, as have the governments of many countries. Even though an exemption clause was created to protect U.S. laws from harmonization, it is totally ineffective and we already have lost seven trade disputes. More are in the wings. Meanwhile, the FDA, which is known to favor the pharmaceutical industry (and Big Agra) at the expense of the natural food industry, *is firmly committed to harmonizing with Codex.*

The most alarming and far-reaching aspect of *Codex Alimentarius* is that its regulations *supersede the domestic laws of the United States–* without Congress and the American people ever debating and voting on this issue. "Harmonizing" is clearly the vehicle by which *Codex* will override the sovereign health and food laws of a country. In the U.S. Constitution, Article VI, Clause 2, clearly states that *treaty law trumps domestic law.* Not only the federal government must change federal law in order to comply, but also state and local governments would be required to change their laws in order to be in accordance with international law.[1] (Or, perhaps, one-world government?) Congress has already capitulated to lobbying from multinational companies and changed U.S. law in many instances.

Sound impossible? It is not only possible, it is required by the *Codex Alimentarius* itself!

The United States is now serving the interests of the U.N., the World Health Organization, and the World Trade Organization as our sovereignty as a nation is crumbling. Right now the United States, Canada, Europe, Japan, most of Asia, and South America have signed agreements pledging "total harmonization" of their respective laws with *Codex* regulations and international standards in the future, and once in place there is no going back. *They are virtually irrevocable. Governments will be prohibited from countermanding them.*

As of 2010 this extremely powerful trade commission and its committee members formulated 4,000 guidelines and standards for anything that is sold, traded, eaten or ingested (except pharmaceutical drugs). Committee members are from countries around the world, but the most dominant country is the United States, which is the chair and wields the most influence. So it stands to reason that our pharmaceutical companies, agribusiness corporations, and chemical companies will profit handsomely if *Codex* sneaks through.

If *Codex Alimentarius* is implemented, almost every single thing you put in your mouth (excepting pharmaceuticals, of course) will be highly regulated, *including water. Codex* Vitamin and Mineral Guide, finalized on July 4, 2005, classifies nutrients as TOXINS!

**Some *Codex* goals that are being discussed and may be mandated include:**

1. No supplements can be sold for preventative or therapeutic use.

2. *All* food, including organic, is to be *irradiated*, removing so-called toxic ingredients from food (unless eaten locally and raw). The levels of radiation will be much higher than previously allowed.

3. *All* nutrients, such as CoQ10, vitamins A, B, C, D, zinc, and magnesium that have any positive health benefits on the body *will be declared illegal* under *Codex* and will be reduced to negligible amounts.

4. You will not be able to get the above-stated nutritional supplements anywhere in the world–*even with a prescription.*

5. All advice on nutrition (including written, online, journal, or oral advice to a friend, family member or anyone), even from nutritionists and naturopaths, *will be illegal.*

6. *All dairy cows* are to be treated with Monsanto's recombinant bovine growth hormone.

7.      *All animals to be used for food* are to be treated with potent antibiotics and exogenous growth hormones.

8.      Twelve deadly and *carcinogenic pesticides,* which have been banned by 176 countries, including the U.S., will be allowed back into food at elevated levels. These include Hexachlorobenzene, Toxaphene, and Aldrin.

9.       Toxic levels (0.5 ppb) of *aflatoxin* in milk products from moldy storage of animal feeds will be allowed. Aflatoxin mold is one of the most carcinogenic substances known.

10.     *Mandatory* use of growth hormones and antibiotics on all "food herds, fish, and flocks" will be implemented.

11.     Worldwide implementation of *genetically altered organisms* (GMOs) into crops, animals, fish, and trees will be initiated.

12.     Higher levels of residue from *insecticides and pesticides* will be permitted. *Codex* allows 3,275 pesticides, including those suspected of being carcinogens and endocrine disrupters.[2]

13.     Potencies for nutrients in vitamins, minerals, and herbs will be reduced to *negligible levels.*

14.     Therapeutic dosages of vitamins and minerals will become unavailable because they will be declared illegal.

15.     Prescriptions will be *required* for anything above the extremely low doses allowed, such as 35 milligrams on niacin.

16.     Common foods such as garlic and peppermint will be *classified as drugs* or put into a third category that only

big pharmaceutical companies could regulate and sell. Any *food* considered to have therapeutic effects will be considered a drug.

17.    Any new dietary supplements will be *banned* unless they jump through very expensive *Codex* hoops of testing and approval.

18.    All organic gardening will be *degraded and rendered useless by regulations.*

19.    All labeling will be restricted or removed.

20.    Herbs and other natural health remedies will be classified *as drugs.*[3]

*Codex Alimentarius'* latest outrage was announced in June, 2010. It has decided that melamine–a totally man-made, toxic, industrial chemical that is NOT food–can be permitted in acceptable levels in food, baby formulas, and baby food! Melamine is used in the production of melawares, a nearly indestructible plastic that is impossible to digest. It is found also in laminates and fertilizers. It is exceedingly dangerous to ingest as it accumulates in the kidneys and leads to kidney failure. In 2007 thousands of pets in the U.S. died of renal failure from eating dog food from China that had been contaminated with melamine. Thousands of infants in China were hospitalized with renal problems after drinking melamine-tainted formula and at least four died. Even so, the *Codex* Commission will allow melamine contamination in food up to 1.0 parts per million (ppm) for infant formulas and 2.5 ppm for adults. Why would *Codex* adopt standards of *any* substance that has been proven to harm both humans and animals all over the world?

Does this look to you like *Codex* may be out to kill us? Think of the massive hordes of yeast/beasts that would be unleashed if these new "rules" were put into place. What is going on here and how did this come about? How did nutrients, so critical to human health and co-evolutionary with humans down through the millennia, suddenly become poisons?

Because one man thinks so, and, unfortunately, he is head of the *Codex* Committee on Nutrition and Foods for Special Dietary Uses.

His name is Dr. Rolf Grossklaus, a German physician who believes *that nutrition has no role in health.* He formulates Codex's nutrition policy and has stated that "nutrition is not relevant to health". Unbelievably, he actually declared *all nutrients to be toxins* in 1994 and then instituted the use of toxicology, (the science of toxins), now called Risk Assessment, as the appropriate science to assess the maximum level of a nutrient or toxin that is needed to be ingested before any discernable biologic effect is noticed. As soon as a biological effect is noticed, the maximum "safe" limit for that substance is established. "Safe" in this case means that NO physical effect is exhibited. *Codex* has skillfully been maneuvering itself into a position to mandate the universal "safe" limits of every vitamin, mineral, herb, and supplement sold.

This is absolute insanity. Nutrients are critical to all the workings of our bodies and minds. They are essential to life. Animal studies continue to corroborate the essential role of nutrients in life. Each human being–and animal–has unique nutritional requirements. Nutrients are not–nor have they ever been–toxins. But according to *Codex,* nutrients in food and herbs are *toxins* and must be "assessed" and eliminated through toxicology, or Risk Assessment. Nutrients in vitamins and minerals are toxic, so the thinking goes, and must be "assessed" and severely restricted in order to "protect" us.

*Codex* is using "risk assessment" to create an image that it is science-based, and that *Codex Alimentarius* is a scientifically-based organization with the lofty goal of "protecting consumer health," while concurrently creating alarmism and falsehood around anything to do with nutritional supplements and unadulterated food. Unbelievably, in a blatant conflict of interest, Doctor Grossklaus is chairman of the board of BIR, a private corporation that specializes in risk assessment and advises *Codex* on this issue. BIR and Doctor Grossklaus make money every time toxicology services are needed for the assessment of nutrients.[4]

Even though Risk Assessment and toxicology are legitimate sciences, they are the wrong science for assessing nutrients. The branch of science that does that most accurately is *biochemistry*–the science of life processes. Note the word life. Everything *Codex* is doing to our foods and herbs seems to bare the hallmarks of disease and death.

Ostensibly, *Codex* is trying to "protect people from dangerous toxic nutrients." Under that mantle it is proposing through Risk Assessment to lower nutrients to ultra low, ineffective doses. When therapeutic grade supplements are eliminated from the marketplace, natural health professionals will lose the tools of their trade and we will lose our freedom to choose how to treat our bodies.

Vitamins are extraordinarily safe substances. Prescription drugs are not. They are dangerous. That's why they must and *should* be regulated. Herbs are as old as history, and have been used successfully by millions of people throughout the world for millennia. *Eighty percent* of the world relies on herbal remedies today. In some places they are the only medicinals both available and affordable.

Dr. Rima Laibow, M.D., intrepid watchdog for our health freedoms, travels all over the world attending and reporting on *Codex* meetings. She says, using WHO's and FAO's own figures and epidemiological projections, that it is reasonable to assume the implementation of the Vitamin and Mineral Guidelines alone will result in 3 billion deaths, asserting: "I believe 1 billion will die through simple starvation, but the next 2 billion will die of preventable diseases and under-nutrition."[5] *That is nearly one-third of humanity.*

This could be what the ominous passage in Revelation (9:15) may be referring to when it states: "And the four angels were loosed, which were prepared for an hour, and a day, and a month, and a year, for to slay the *third part of men*." Revelation is difficult and even inscrutable in the best of circumstances, but this is pause for thought.

*Codex Alimentarius* is a shrewd vehicle designed to eliminate the competition of natural and nutritional medicine in favor of Big Pharma, et al, by protecting them from the inevitable loss of income they will suffer due to the rapidly growing interest in natural healthcare. *Codex* plans for all natural remedies to be shifted into the prescription category so they can be manufactured, distributed, and priced exclusively by the medical monopoly and their overlords, Big Pharma.

When natural therapies and practitioners become illegal, *Codex* will go home with the trophy and the rest of us will have lost a mighty big game. The pharmaceutical industry, agribusiness corporations, and chemical companies stand to make huge profits if *Codex* is implemented, and all are busy spinning webs of falsehoods, e.g., *Codex* is harmless and the guidelines are voluntary, and disinformation campaigns to discredit natural healthcare and make consumers leery of using vitamins, minerals, and herbs. In 2001 the FTC and FDA launched a joint campaign to accomplish just that called "Operation Cure-All," supposedly waging battles in the ongoing war against "Internet health fraud." They want us to relax while they go about protecting us, hoping to lull us into complacency. Our complacency and ignorance are what they are counting on.

If you want a peek into the future of what might happen in the United States if *Codex* has its way, look at Germany and Norway where *Codex* proposals are already law. *The entire health food industry has been taken over by the drug companies.* Vitamin C is illegal over 200 milligrams, as is vitamin E over 45 IU, vitamin B1 over 2.4 milligrams, etc. Gingko and an echinacea tincture are now controlled by the Norway pharmaceutical giant Schering-Plough, and are being sold over the counter at grossly inflated prices.[6] Echinacea has skyrocketed in cost as much as nearly 1,000 percent. Germany, the home of the father of homeopathy, Dr. Samuel Hahnemann, M.D., is witnessing all homeopathics being taken off the market. They are now either unavailable or unaffordable.

In this country there are ominous signs that the same scenario may be playing out here.  Recently the FDA took several steps that could spell doom for our ability to buy supplements.

1.  Pyridoxamine, a naturally occurring form of $B^6$ found in chicken, fish, and walnuts, has *been declared a drug*.  Any supplements containing it are now considered illegal.  This powerful form of $B^6$, which has been used effectively against atherosclerosis, chronic inflammation, and diabetes, will no longer be available until a prescription version meets FDA approval.[7] *NO side effects from pyridoxamine have ever been reported.*

2.  Red yeast rice products are under attack.  Big Pharma first developed and then patented a statin drug from red yeast rice–a natural plant– then the FDA attacked many red yeast rice products saying they contained a regulated "prescription" product and quickly moved to shut down some distributors.  (I don't recommend red yeast rice either as a statin or as a natural plant, for obvious reasons.)

3.  Even Cheerios® has been labeled a drug!  No kidding.  Since oats are known to bring down cholesterol levels and treat cardiovascular disease, and Cheerios® claimed to help both conditions, the FDA proclaimed the product to be a drug.  They recently sent a letter to General Mills saying, "Based on claims made on your product's label, we have determined that your Cheerios Toasted Whole Grain Oat Cereal® is promoted for conditions that cause it to be a drug because the product is intended for use in the prevention, mitigation, and treatment of disease."[8]  They went on to say Cheerios® "may not be legally marketed with the above claims in the United States *without an approved new drug application*."  Does anyone know the lethal dose for Cheerios®?  What's next? Does this means that vitamin shop owners could be arrested and prosecuted for practicing medicine?  Can the FDA now declare that vegetable juices, probiotic yogurt, anti-oxidant teas, high-fiber, V–8 juice or raw sprouts can be

regulated as "drugs" because they might prevent, mitigate, or treat disease?  With all the truly dangerous processed foods, GMO and nano-foods, health-robbing artificial sweeteners, and diet products on the market, the FDA goes after CHEERIO'S®?  How nutty can they get?  And speaking of nuts, the FDA sent the same warning letter to Diamond Food, the world's largest walnut producer, telling them "your walnuts are drugs."  It seems the FDA has lost its marbles.

4.  The FDA's website is encouraging anonymous reports of any adverse reactions to dietary supplements "even if you are unsure the product caused the problem or even if you do not visit a doctor or clinic." Talk about a fishing expedition.  Talk about witch hunts!

*Remember, over 100,000 deaths are attributed to prescribed pharmaceutical drugs each year, while only a handful of deaths can be attributed yearly to natural supplements.*

Remember also that Big Pharma has the money and the power. They have three or four lobbyists for every congressman working tirelessly to discredit all forms of natural healing and decrease the availability of supplements. Big Pharma is out to win this one.

It is a criminal offense in parts of Europe to sell herbs as foods (agreement EEC6565) and pressure is being applied to force other European countries also into "harmonization." Many countries are racing to become compliant so they won't be hit with trade sanctions. Doctors here and elsewhere are being muzzled from even *suggesting* the use of vitamins, herbs, etc.  Several are under indictment in North Carolina for such brazen acts. California can no longer ship raw almonds out of state because of *Codex* regulations. In Canada people are being given jail terms for recommending the use of nutrients for health benefits. This could be just the beginning.

Another issue that is aligned with the food issue is the *Codex* directive to remove all labeling, claiming labels are a form of direct advertising. Such nonsense is beyond belief.  Genetically modified organisms, or GMOs, allowed and promoted by *Codex,* also will be promoted by the U.S. by making labeling them unnecessary–even though there is ample evidence to warrant a widespread moratorium on their use and most consumers are overwhelmingly opposed to eating them. Sadly, the *U.S. is the only country in the world* where unlabeled use of GMOs is permitted. Hope you like eating your rice with a human liver gene stuck in it!

The only thing we have that is protecting us at the moment is the Dietary Supplement Health and Education Act (DSHEA), passed in 1994. It is a law that appropriately classifies supplements and herbs as *foods,* which can have no upper limits on their use. It passed by unanimous consent in Congress after a massive grass-roots campaign, orchestrated by health food stores, told Congress in no uncertain terms they wanted their nutritional supplements protected. Congress got the message. DSHEA is now under significant legislative attack from pro-*Codex* forces lobbying for its appeal. So far in 2010 five bills are pending in Congress designed to gut or eliminate DSHEA.  We will be helpless without it.

There is an outside chance that *Codex Alimentarius* will fall apart from its own unwieldiness. With luck and an outraged electorate, we may be able to maneuver around it through the courts.  In any case it's time to formulate a new message to our elected officials and others in positions of authority.

Please educate yourself on this most vital issue. Watch the videos *Food, Inc.* and *The Future of Food,* and read *Seeds of Doubt* written by staffers at the *Sacramento Bee*. Go to Dr. Rima E. Laibow's www.healthfreedomusa.org website to read and sign a citizen's petition, which is a suit against the U.S. government for redress and correction of this travesty, and other websites to learn more. Write, phone, or fax your congressman or congresswoman and tell them "protect our nutritional supplements or we will vote you out of office." Tell them to vote against anything that would threaten DSHEA. Demand an end to FDA "gag rules," which are part of "HARMonization with *Codex* on health-related information. Tell them you don't want to be "HARMonized." Global criminalization of natural healthcare cannot be tolerated. *Let's "globalize" the health/freedom movement instead.* Congress has listened to–and carried out–the will of the people many times in the past. They hold the key to our health freedom, which really means *we* hold it!

A few years ago, traditional medicine vehemently denied that vitamins, minerals, herbs, homeopathics, and alternative healing methods such as chiropractic, acupuncture, massage therapy, etc. had any real value. Now, after seeing the rapidly growing trend toward natural healing in general (and the ensuing decline in their profits), Big Pharma is admitting there are indeed many benefits to them to the extent *they want global control of all of them! Codex* is the answer to their prayer.

It may take a few years for all this to become reality, but *Codex* is accelerating and expanding, and is trying to stay on track for going into full global effect by the end of 2010. Early in 2010 the alarm bells sounded and a "push back" campaign has been successful in slowing down *Codex*'s grandiose plans. (Bulgaria and a few other countries have managed to be excluded.) But don't think for a minute their supporters have given up. They don't mind if it takes a little longer. Incrementalism is their game. The longer the better, because the slower the process, the less alarmed people will be. It's the old "boil the frog slowly" story again.

In case you are unfamiliar with that phrase, let me clarify. Years ago there used to be an experiment in high school biology labs where students would drop live frogs into a pot of extremely hot water to test the frogs' nervous systems. They wanted to see if the frogs were smart enough to jump out. They always did. Then they would drop the same frogs into pots of room temperature water where they swam happily and remained unaffected by their surroundings. Lastly, students placed burners under the pots and slowly turned up the heat one degree per minute. The frogs continued swimming around, seemingly oblivious to the change. The water became hotter and hotter and the frogs eventually died. Despite the fact that the frogs were literally being boiled, they never once tried to escape from certain death. They didn't seem to notice the peril they were in. Because the change was gradual, the frogs adapted to the pain and discomfort of being boiled until they were too far gone to save themselves.

Thankfully, this cruel experiment is no longer allowed, but serves as an excellent metaphor for the situation we find ourselves in today in regard to *Codex* and our freedom of choice regarding food and nutritional supplements.

We are paddling as fast as we can, but if we don't wake up and jump out of the hot water before it's too late, we will be too brain-dead and debilitated to climb out of the pot.

The water is getting hotter.

## Chapter 27

---

# The Answer to Cancer

*"Fungus is emphatically the most invasive and aggressive microorganism that exists in nature...It seems therefore logical to assume that a cause of neoplastic proliferation could be fungus – the most powerful and most organized micro-organism known."*

...Dr. Tullio Simoncini, M.D.

Cancer, that most enigmatic and debilitating of all diseases, has been with us since the beginning of recorded time. It was documented as early as 1500 B.C. in the *Ebers Papyrus*, and description of it can be found in the ancient literature of India and Persia. It seems to have "devilled" mankind throughout history.

But today we are living in a virtual sea of cancer. All of us know many people, family members, and friends who are battling or dying from this dreaded disease. We watch and admire them as they bravely face surgery, chemotherapy, and radiation, followed by pain, nausea, hair loss, and all the other attendant miseries. We, too, suffer as we watch most of them eventually lose their battles, and their families are left to grieve and wonder why more couldn't be done.

Why, if we can get a man to the moon and back safely, are our survival statistics for cancer so poor?

It is shocking to realize that for our most common cancers, which constitute 90 percent of all cancers, the survival rates have remained unchanged for twenty-five years! At the moment the overall survival rate for all cancers hovers between 2 and 7 percent or less.[1] Despite an immense investment in all areas of cancer research, the age-adjusted death rate for cancer in the United States actually *increased* by 74 percent from the beginning of the twentieth century until its end.[2] In 1971 Congress passed the National Cancer Act and President Nixon declared "war" on cancer. Nearly forty years later the overall death rate is very close to what it was when the war was first declared. What are we doing wrong?

The answer is that we have been looking in the wrong places, both in the area of causation and in the area of cure.

**If you don't know what causes a disease, how can you possibly create a cure?**

In the early 1800s the cancer rate in this country was 1 in over 100. It was quite rare. Now it is fast approaching 1 in 3! What is behind this explosion of cancer? And what can we do to change those statistics for the better?

As far back as the late 1800s it was well-documented in medical literature that cancer was *fungal.* However pharmaceutical companies quickly focused on developing drugs and treatments for the disease, and its etiology (cause) was soon ignored and forgotten. More money was to be made in developing drugs to treat the disease than to research its cause.

Then in the early 1900s there was a meteoric rise in the consumption of dietary carbohydrates in the form of sugar and grains. When our population reached twenty million we began to store grains in silos, which created the perfect conditions for growths of mildew and mold. Consequently, almost all of our grains are contaminated today. Around World War II, antibiotics, and hormones, appeared, along with artificial colors and dyes. Birth control drugs came on the scene in the 1960s. In the latter decades of the twentieth century until today we have added to the mix countless synthetic chemical drugs, new and stronger antibiotics, more vaccines, including multiple dose vaccines, artificial sweeteners, tons of sugars and processed and fast food, *all of which yeast gobbles up hand over fist.* These factors, combined with our increasingly hectic lifestyles and accelerating levels of stress, have contributed to the skyrocketing of yeast-related diseases…including cancer.

Today, oncologists, scientists, and researchers aren't sure exactly what cancer is, often referring to it as a "mystery." The word *cancer* is a generic term that in no way describes its cause. It may be described as an abnormal swelling in or on any part of the body. One thing we do know is that this "mystery" is about to surpass heart disease as the number one killer in the United States.

Specialists look at cancer as a "cellular reproductive anomaly," meaning it exhibits exaggerated and uncontrolled cellular growth. They attribute these growths to an array of instigators from immunological dysfunctions, to viruses, to parasites, to alterations in DNA, to toxins, to dietary deficiencies, to stress, etc. In the process, many different drugs (cancer drugs now make up the second largest category of drugs in the U.S; cholesterol-lowering drugs being the first) and treatment therapies have been developed to target the different stages of different cancers. A bewildering and hugely profitable $200 billion industry has arisen to fill the "need." When you total up the costs of surgery, chemo, radiation, hospital and hospice care, it now costs on average $350,000 to die of cancer in the USA today.

Hospital cancer wings, floors, treatment centers, and hospitals (some cancer centers are actually owned and managed by pharmaceutical companies that *make* the chemotherapy drugs!) have many caring and devoted physicians who truly wish to see their patients get well. Unfortunately, in most cases their treatments only create more misery and an earlier death for those they are trying to help.

Everyone knows that traditional treatments for cancer don't work very well, if at all. We all are terrified of this disease because we know if we are diagnosed and submit to chemotherapy and radiation, we will endure pain and suffering, but pray we will be one of the few "lucky ones." In such a climate, tens of thousands of Americans flee to other countries every year in search of gentler therapies not allowed by the cancer "powers that be." The cancer "police" can't afford to let the public know that many alternative therapies are equal, or even surpass, the traditional FDA-AMA-approved therapies used today. The cancer industry would be trashed.

So far, $100 billion dollars have been spent on endless research, yet the death rate from cancer has not dropped appreciably in the last century. Why are we so stuck in a paradigm that obviously isn't working? Because it is sustained by trillions of dollars of vested interests, coupled with enormous amounts of power. Dr. Julian Whitaker, in his excellent *Health and Healing* newsletter, recently wrote: "To protect the vested interests of those engaged in cancer surgery, chemotherapy, and radiation, virtually all regulatory agencies persecute physicians who offer alternatives. This persecution is harsh, because established cancer therapies are particularly gruesome and ineffective and thus need a lot of protection."[3] He refers to our current approach to treating cancer as a "festering, non-healing sore on human culture."[4] Sadly, few oncologists have the courage to buck the prevailing orthodoxy and think for themselves, fearing ridicule, review boards, loss of license, and even jail.

Our doctors are trained in medical school to recognize the entire range of bacteria and viruses, but receive *very little training to recognize fungi.* They have been taught to recognize all the *external* manifestations of fungi, such as "fungi nail," ringworm, vaginal yeast infections, "jock itch," and thrush, but are taught nothing about how to recognize *internal* manifestations of fungi, such as cancer, heart disease, MS, irritable bowel syndrome, bi-polar disease, arthritis, etc. Even our state boards of health don't require doctors to report fungal diseases (mycoses) like they do bacteria and viruses. The lowly fungi are overlooked and ignored. So cancer treatment modalities continue along the lines of cut, burn, and poison to purge the body of–*they aren't sure what!*

Most cells in the body divide between 50 and 60 times and then die, a phenomenon known as the Hayflick limit. But cancer cells can divide forever and are *immortal,* unless they are killed by design. They have lost the ability to communicate properly with adjacent cells and receive proper control messages. As a consequence they simply do not know when to stop replicating.

Localized cancers, or single cancerous tumors, rarely kill. In almost all cases it is the cancer that has metastasized, or spread throughout the body, that kills. (Remember that when yeast morphs into fungus it spreads and attacks.) Researchers are becoming convinced that inflammation is the key to cancer growth, as many inflammatory diseases, such as Crohn's disease, progress to cancer at much higher rates. They have also confirmed that the metabolism of cancer cells is different from normal cells. While normal cells use several different fuels for survival, cancer cells are almost *totally dependent on glucose. Sugar!*

Conventional cancer treatments today approach cancer as if it were the enemy, which must be killed at all costs. Purge, purge, purge. Kill, kill, kill. Never mind the costs to your heart, your liver, your kidneys, your immune system, or even your life. Killing the enemy is paramount and cancer must be eradicated with extremely toxic chemical agents and highly destructive radiation–*now*.

Chemotherapy is poison. Period. And in no way does it make sense to make a sick person sicker in order for him to get well. Chemotherapy is toxic to cancer cells, yes, but it is equally toxic to healthy cells–including immune cells. It walks a thin and precarious line between killing the cancer and killing the patient, and in most cases only speeds up the inevitable by damaging the patient's core line of defense– the immune system. Developing cancer represents a significant failure of the human immune system. In a 2008 poll, 75 percent of oncologists admitted they would refuse chemotherapy if they ever developed cancer.[5] Even they have little faith in the tools of their trade. It seems logical that we should be *building up that immune system up* and supporting it, rather than tearing it down!

Additionally, chemotherapy is rarely effective. In December, 2004, a study was published in the journal *Clinical Oncology* that showed chemotherapy provides an average five year survival rate of just over 2 percent for all cancers![6] Yet if you go to the American Cancer Society web site you will see claims of cure rates in the 45–55 percent range. How can that be?

Don't forget that "cancer survival statistics" are for five years only (after diagnosis). This arbitrary time limit is a *five-year survival rate–not a lifetime survival rate.* If you die of cancer one day after the five years are up, you are still counted as a "cure" in the statistics department. Also, many cancers are slow-growing, giving them a very high "5-year cure rate." This is a case of deceptive statistical tricks and a statistical truth not being presented as the whole truth.

Cancer statistics are notoriously manipulated in orthodox medicine's favor. If a patient treated with chemotherapy or radiation dies of pneumonia or other infections, (acquired from lowered immune system function from the treatments), the death is not counted as a "cancer death." Why? Because doctors are required by law to enter the *final* cause of death–in this case pneumonia–not the true cause of death: cancer. Official statistics conceal hundreds of thousands of cancer fatalities this way.

Chemotherapy and radiation kill far more healthy cells than they do cancerous cells. Cells damaged and dying from these hellish treatments actually become *fodder for new crops of yeast,* which then potentially become *more cancers!* Cancer patients become more debilitated, more acidic, and more toxic from these therapies. By crippling and disarming the immune system and damaging healthy cells, *chemotherapy and radiation can cause cancer to spread wildly.* Both modalities unleash massive storms of free radicals, which make cancers invasive and deadly. It is like throwing gasoline on a fire.

Another questionable "preventive" for cancer in women is the mammogram, another cash cow for the cancer industry. Women are told by doctors they must have them every year in order to "catch it early" when cancer is "easier to cure." But by the AMA's own admission, radiation causes cancer, and low-dose radiation into a woman's breast increases her chances of developing cancer between one and 3 percent.[7]

This doesn't sound too alarming until you consider that if she follows that advice and gets a mammogram every year for ten years, her rate increases to a full 10 to 30 percent!

We know the effects of radiation are cumulative, meaning that the damage is *compounded* with each exposure, and even experts really don't know how much is too much. But we do know *the most sensitive and receptive tissue to radiation in a woman's body is the breast.*

Have you ever thought about what actually happens during a mammogram? I have never had one, but I have been told they can be very painful as breasts are mashed and squeezed between two photographic plates (until it *hurts* according to the instructions on some equipment.) in order to get the x-ray. If there are cancer cells in the breast, and if cancer is a fungus–a sac mycelium–what happens to the sacs when the breasts are compressed? Many are likely to burst, of course, and their lethal seeds or spores then squirt out into the surrounding breast tissue, free to spread and colonize new tumors elsewhere, a process know as *metastasis!*

Medical schools used to drum into the heads of medical students that breast lumps should be handled with utmost delicacy because even slight mishandling could make them rupture and spread cancer. They understood this fact years ago, even not knowing what cancer was. When did they change their minds and start recommending that women get yearly mammograms that brutalize their breasts? *When money entered the picture.*

With the creation of the lucrative mammogram industry, mainstream medicine apparently threw earlier cautions to the wind. The sensitive and delicate breast tissue became fair game for the newfangled equipment, and the old protocols were scuttled. Now they can't smash breasts fast enough.

Ionizing (penetrating) radiation in ANY dose, no matter how tiny, damages DNA and wreaks havoc on cells and their genetic codes, setting all living cells exposed on a fast-track to cancer. Dr. John Gofman, M.D.

PhD, Professor Emeritus of Molecular and Cell Biology at the University of California, Berkeley, and one of the leading experts in the world on the dangers of radiation, warns that "over 50% of the death rate from cancer is in fact induced by x-ray."[8]

The routine practice today calls for taking four films of each breast annually, which results in approximately 1 RAD (radiation absorbed dose) of exposure. That is *1,000 times greater than that from a single chest x-ray.* Even the American Cancer Society lists high-dose radiation to the chest as a medium to high risk factor for developing cancer.

In addition, contrary to what most people believe (including doctors), mammograms do *not* save lives. Recent research proves that convincingly. The fact is, *a woman's chance of dying from breast cancer are exactly the same whether she has a mammogram or not.* The National Cancer Institute recently published a report stating that adding an annual physical exam of the breast does not improve breast cancer survival rates over getting the physical exam alone.[9] Add the fact that mammograms have a very high rate of false-positive readings, which lead to countless unnecessary surgeries (plus more invasive procedures and tests, more x-rays and more emotional stress), and you have to wonder why they still are being promoted as the gold standard in detecting breast cancers. *The gold standard has become a goldmine, that's why.*

To illustrate the irony of all ironies, a friend of mine just sent me an advertisement for a baking contest organized across the country. The manufacturer promised to donate $250,000 to a breast cure organization from a percentage of proceeds garnered from products used in contestants' recipes. And where was the advertisement found? On the back of a package of yeast!

The best alternative option to mammograms is *Thermographic Breast Screening.* It measures the radiation from infrared heat from your body and translates that into anatomical images. Since cancer tissue is warmer than normal tissue, tumors stand out as bright colors. Mammography cannot detect a tumor until it has been growing–

sometimes for years–and reaches a certain size. Thermography, on the other hand, is able to reveal the possibility of cancer much sooner (sometimes even ten years sooner), because it can image the *earliest stages of angiogenesis*, the formation of the blood vessels that supply nourishment to cancer cells, a necessary step before cancer can grow into tumor size.

One interesting aside is that many chemotherapeutic drugs (Tamoxifen®️ is an example) are actually anti-fungals! Chemotherapies and radiation can and do annihilate fungi (tumors). But look at the side-effects: nausea, vomiting, hair loss, liver and kidney damage, immune system damage, etc. *Whatever happened to "first thou shall do no harm?"* It simply isn't necessary to use a shotgun to kill a mouse. It might get the job done, but look at what happened to the floor!

Animal studies have verified that certain foods make tumors grow rapidly and make them more likely to metastasize. Two of the worst offenders are processed sugars and omega-6 oils, such as corn oil. (In some animal studies, tumors didn't spread at all until the animals were *fed* corn oil!)[10] And guess which grain in the United States today is the most contaminated with mold: corn. Corn is now one hundred percent contaminated with mold. There is your clear inflammation/mold/cancer connection.

**In order for anyone to be healed from cancer, seven conditions must be corrected first. They are:**

1. A weakened immune system
2. A lack of oxygen uptake by cells
3. Excessive toxins
4. Acidity
5. Inflammation
6. Fungal overgrowths
7. Emotional distress or trauma

*All seven of these conditions are worsened by chemotherapy and radiation.* Six are caused by Candida yeast and all six can be overcome with anti-fungals and the yeast-free diet. Most cancer patients die from complications from treatments, not cancer itself.

Wouldn't it make more sense to use safe, natural, non-toxic remedies that support the immune system and kill fungi–with no harm being done to the patient? Wouldn't it be more humane and effective to treat a sick and frightened patient with gentleness and sensitivity, rather than the "shock and awe" tactics used by mainstream medicine today? Such modalities are at our disposal here and now. The yeast-free diet and anti-fungals are here now.

With a little self-education and determination, true healing is at our door.

One of the first books I read linking cancer to fungus was *The Germ that Causes Cancer* by Doug A. Kaufmann. It is a wonderful book, clearly and simply written for the layperson. In it he describes *Candida albicans* as that germ, and recommends his version of the yeast-free diet (called the Phase One Diet) and anti-fungals to cure cancer. He is the author of *The Fungal Link Books – Vols. 1.2.3, The Germ that Causes Cancer*, and *The Fungal Link to Diabetes*, in which he persuasively links fungus to *all* major diseases. He also has a thirty minute TV show Monday through Friday where he talks every day about fungal connections to disease. His show and website are called "Know the Cause". Go to his website where you can find the time his TV show is aired in your area. It is really worth your time.

In July, 2007, a new book was published, written by Dr. Tullio Simoncini, a surgeon in Rome, Italy. He specializes in oncology, diabetology, and metabolic disorders at his clinic. His astonishing and revolutionary book is *Cancer Is a Fungus*, and is the result of his thirty plus years of observation, investigating, and treating this horrible disease. He states that there is no doubt in his mind that cancer is simply a *fungal infection caused by Candida albicans*, and this simple, lowly organism can

be treated and cured with an anti-fungal program and–of all things–
bicarbonate of soda.

His thesis is elegantly simple and straightforward.  All diseases
like and grow in an acid medium.  Cancer thrives in acidity. That is why it
is important for us to keep our body pH near 7.24 –7.42 or slightly
alkaline in order to achieve and maintain perfect health. Bicarbonate of
soda changes the terrain of disease from acid to alkaline, making it
exceedingly difficult for yeast, cancer, and other pathogens to live and
grow.

Doctor Simoncini sees cancer tumors as really fungi colonizing
throughout the body, and writes convincingly that it makes much more
sense that "something" started the tumor–that "something" being *Candida
albicans*, or yeast. He totally refutes today's prevailing science that
describes cancer as a "*spontaneous lump occurrence*" of unknown
etiology.  He calls this view a "stupidity."

Doctor Simoncini is convinced that cancer begins when Candida
roots itself in the deep connective tissue of an organ or organs and begins
to attack and consume tissue.  Then, in a defensive action, the organ
valiantly encysts the Candida in an attempt to protect itself, resulting in
the formation of tumors.  Growths continue as fungi spread locally and
distantly (metastasis).  It is always the same Candida attacking different
tissue, but, because of its highly adaptive nature, it is able to mutate in
order to conform to whatever environment it finds itself–sometimes in as
little as three or four days. *This ability to morph and mutate explains the
hundreds of various and different types of tumors we find.*

Then why don't biopsies of tumors show evidence of yeast?

Biopsies, when taken, only remove part of the *outer rim of
cancerous tumors*.  This ring, or rim tissue, is the defensive reaction of the
body to the fungi, not the fungi itself.  It is the result of the body's attempt
to wall off the offending organisms in order to protect itself from further
damage.  If you go deep inside the tumor *to the core,* you will find the

original stimulus–the voracious and deadly fungi, creating inflammation and destroying tissue as it gnaws on its host in order to survive.

Doctor Simoncini brilliantly goes on to describe the commonalities between cancer and fungus (pointing out that cancer and Candida are always concurrent), and outlines his treatment protocols with "before and after" photographs of 18 clinical cases. It is a truly astounding and visionary book. If you want to watch a *very scientific* video which supports the fungus/cancer connection, go to www.grayfieldoptical.com/online_videos.html, scroll down to "Symbiosis or Parasitism: A Treatise on Cancer". You can see, thanks to the new and extremely powerful Ergonom microscope, a video of a living virus mutate into a bacteria, and then into a fungus, illustrating how highly mutagenic fungi are. (Eventually I believe we will find that viruses are actually *microfungi,* which would explain why they do not respond to antibiotics.)

I urge you to read *Cancer Is a Fungus* and share it with someone you know or love who has cancer. Doctor Simoncini makes his case with conviction, clarity, and compassion. You can order it at *cancerfungus.com.*

Even more astounding is when I first met Sylvia and started working with her in 1985, she told me, "Cancer is a fungus, as most diseases are, and we will be treating almost all of my patients with anti-fungals and the yeast-free diet."

We have been doing exactly that, and over the years I have been privileged to witness more cures than I can count–in every disease known to man. These healings have proven that the original thesis is correct: Most diseases–and cancer in particular–do indeed have a fungal etiology. Chronic irritation and inflammation are the culprits that set up tissue to invite Candida to take up residence. *With time and a malfunctioning immune system, Candida morphs into cancer.*

*The answer to cancer is anti-fungal protocols*: eating yeast-free; supplementing with herbs and homeopathics that kill fungal overgrowths;

immune system stimulators; the releasing of negative emotional triggers; and Doctor Simoncini's bicarbonate of soda treatments if needed and when possible.

Medical research already has proven that cancer cells are notorious *"sugar junkies,"* and multiply frantically when glucose is present (known as the Warburg effect.) Conversely, they self-destruct (a process known as apoptosis), when glucose is removed.[11] (When cancer patients are scanned using the new PET scanner, they are given a sugar solution to drink before the procedure *because sugar goes straight to cancer receptors!)* Cancer cells are almost completely dependent upon glucose for survival.

Glucose elimination has proven to be the Achilles heel of cancer cells and has always been the cornerstone of the yeast-free diet. (Cancer cells have 95 receptors for sugar. Normal cells have 4.) Cancer is a fermentative and inflammatory process. Since fermentation requires sugar and yeast for fuel, cancer patients should not touch any food with refined sugar, or anything else that feeds yeast, until they are totally cured. Even moderate intake of alcohol increases a woman's chance of developing breast cancer.

Along with the diet, there are both prescription and natural anti-fungals to choose from. The protocol is the same for treating yeast/fungal infections. In extreme cases, Diflucan®, Nystatin®, Sporanox® and Nizoral® can be prescribed by your doctor. Otherwise, caprylic acid, grapefruit seed extract, olive leaf extract, oil of oregano, garlic, probiotics, and Pau D'Arco tea are excellent natural fungicides found in the health food store. Immune system stimulators, such as Poly-MVA (an alpha lipoic acid concentrate) are also needed.

Emotional releasing is extremely important to the recovery of cancer patients. Emotions always make the nest for disease, and cancer is no exception. All cancer patients must go deeply within to identify and then release any and all past traumatic and stressful incidents, or memories or relationships that still lurk in the subconscious and conscious minds. They must identify and release "what is eating them" in order to heal completely (See chapter 14, The Body-Mind Connection). Negative thoughts, memories and fear all tip the body into acid mode. Acid is the medium cancer/fungus requires in order to thrive. Prayer and meditation are invaluable at this time, as they bring peace of mind and positive outlooks that tip the body into alkaline mode where cancer cannot live. (It is interesting to note that chemically tears of anger and hurt are acid, while tears of joy are alkaline!)

One of the most miraculous and revolutionary tools being taught now, which accomplishes emotional release is EFT, which stands for Emotional Freedom Technique, or simply "Tapping." It is like acupuncture, but without the needles. It involves tapping on acupuncture points while mentally focusing on an issue. Soon the issue dissolves as it is released from the body/mind. Go to www.emofree.com and download the free manual of instructions. There are DVDs also, which you can buy. I highly recommend all their programs. They are incredibly effective.

Finally, let's look at some of the amazing parallels between cancer cells and ascomycete yeast and fungi. Remember: *Candida and cancer cells show the same genetic structure.*

| Cancer cells: | Yeast/Fungi: |
|---|---|
| 1. Respire and metabolize without oxygen | 1. Also |
| 2. Excrete lactic acid (a poison) | 2. Also |
| 3. Need sugar and warm moist environment | 3. Also |
| 4. Anti-fungals kill them | 4. Also |
| 5. A tumor is like sac fungus | 5. A sac fungus is like a tumor |

| | |
|---|---|
| 6. Thrive in an acid environment | 6  Also |
| 7. Can hide and disguise themselves | 7. Also |
| 8. Can enter cells and alter DNA | 8. Also |
| 9. Cancer metastasizes (disseminates) | 9. Fungus disseminates (metastasizes) |
| 10. Can reproduce indefinitely | 10. Also |
| 11. Reproduce asexually through spores | 11. Also |
| 12. Are always white | 12. Also |
| 13. Can morph into different forms | 13. Also |
| 14. Don't just go away. They must be starved or killed | 14. Also |
| 15. Have minds of their own. Cell communication goes haywire. | 15. Also |

Many times even lab technicians and microscopists cannot tell the difference between fungal spores or cells and cancer cells in the blood. For example, histoplasmosis, a fungal infection, cannot be differentiated from cancer under the microscope.

What is cancer and how is it created?  Cancer is not a "spontaneous lump occurrence."  It does not occur because the DNA within the cells just "happen" to change. Some outside instigator enters the human body, gains entry into the cells and changes the DNA coding within the nucleus by breaking DNA strands. The vital life force of the cell becomes disabled.

This entity must be capable of multiplying inside the cells. Once inside the cells it merges with it to form a *hybrid* cell with newly "programmed" DNA. *Once hybridized, the fungal partner becomes DOMINANT.* After a while the nuclei of many cells are damaged and form into the masses and tumors we call cancer.

I believe the ascomycete (sac) fungi to be that entity. Ascomycete fungi are a class of fungi that requires a container (sac) in which to lie dormant. Upon entry into a human host, it starts to shed its hard durable sac, making it free to invade human cells, take them captive and use *them* as sacs and incubators to make spores for reproduction. The spores can lie dormant for many years, waiting to break their dormancy when immune systems become stressed or depressed.

Put another way, picture the entity as being a terrorist planning to hijack a plane (cell). After taking off its camouflage gear (sac), it bashes down the cockpit door (damages cell wall or membrane), bursts into the cockpit (nucleus) and disables the pilot (DNA), who moves over into the co-pilot's seat. The entity immediately de-oxygenates the cockpit so it can live; merges its DNA with the pilot (hybridized state); commandeers the pilot's seat, and is now in control of the cockpit and plane (fungal dominance). Then the entity rapidly starts to proliferate babies, which spill out of the cockpit and into the fuselage. It immediately clothes its babies in protective gear and parachutes (mycotoxins). When the plane encounters heavy weather (immune system stress), the entity decides to jettison his heavy load of yammering offspring, opens the cargo doors and pushes his brats (spores) out to land on new territory (organs and glands) where they regroup (metastasize) and lie in wait for further instructions. Before long, masses of cells begin to congregate and form a defensive barrier (lump or tumor) that eventually will spew out more bratty entities (spores) to hijack more cells.

*The concept of impregnated cells becoming fungally dominant* is the key to understanding how cancer works. Once fungi dominate the cells, they call the shots. Only if the immune system is strong can they be contained.

Cancer, being a fermentative process, creates lumps and tumors as they congregate. Picture a boiling cauldron and all the bubbles. Now picture a human body *fermenting with bubbles.* The bubbles are *tumors. A cancerous body literally bubbles into tumors.* (Remember the definition of yeast in chapter one?) Because cancer/fungus is a parasite, and obtains nourishment through the fermentation of sugars rather than through oxidation (as is the case with normal, healthy cells), unless there is an intervention with diet and anti-fungal treatments the body will continue to ferment (bubble tumors) and fill with mycotoxins until death.

The missing link in the search for a cure for cancer is *the study of fungi.* By studying fungi we can demonstrate and prove that fungi enter nuclei of cells and alter their DNA by breaking their strands. As stated before, fungus has the ability to damage and break DNA strands.

The aftermath of broken DNA strands is **disease.**

As far back as 1997, the medical journal *Carcinogenesis* reported that eating spinach, tomatoes, and especially carrots, decreased DNA strand breakage and the oxidative damage that led to cancer. Another reminder to eat your veggies!

Doctor Milton White, M.D., Fellow of International College of Surgeons states, "Cancer is a chronic, intracellular, infectious, biologically induced spore (fungus) transformation disease."[12] *That means there is only one type of cancer, not hundreds. That one type of cancer is fungus.* Just as fungus causes all cancers in the plant and vegetable world, fungus also causes all cancers in human beings.

The resulting, simple concept, that *cancer is an infection and an infectious process,* caused by the ascomycete group of fungi known as *Candida albicans,* could shake the very foundations of conventional medicine to its core. Huge paradigm shifts will then cause us to change both the way we view cancer and the way we treat and cure it.

For you and me, and every patient struggling with this dreaded disease, that cannot happen fast enough.

**Chapter 28**

---

# *Diabetes:* A Feast for Yeast

*"As for doctors who dismiss the idea of a cure for diabetes…remember that the fault lies not with the doctor, but with a system of medicine that is designed to maintain the status quo."*

...Doug Kaufmann

Diabetes has been part of the human scene for thousands of years. The earliest known record is a Third Dynasty Egyptian papyrus in 1552 B.C., describing frequent urination as a symptom. The papyrus also lists remedies to combat the passing of too much urine.

The word itself is a derivation of two Greek words: "διά" meaning "through" and "βάίυφ" meaning "to pass," referring to the copious amounts of fluid diabetics "pass through their bodies" in the form of urine.

But to me, the most striking part of the word is "bête", which is French for beast. How fitting that the name of a disease–that is the personification of the yeast/beast–carries within it an allusion to its genesis!

In 120 A.D. the Greek physician Arataeus gave us the first medical description of diabetes, which he described as "the melting down of flesh and limb into urine." It seemed that the body wasted into fluids from this mysterious malady until the patient eventually succumbed.

Throughout the centuries many forms of treatment have been used to treat this dreadful disease, from the oat diet and the milk diet, to rice cures, potato therapy and even the use of opium, to no avail. Up until the eleventh century, diabetes was diagnosed by "water tasters" who actually drank the urine of those suspected of having the disease. If the urine tasted sweet, the disease was confirmed. The Latin word for honey, "*mellitus*," was added to the term diabetes centuries later, alluding to the urine's sweetness. But it wasn't until 1921 when a 'de-pancreatized' dog was successfully treated with a new drug called "insulin" that scientists knew they were on the right track.

Today we are witnessing an explosion in the rise of new cases, especially since the year 2000. Nearly twenty-four million Americans suffer from this debilitating disease and millions have yet to be diagnosed. The incidence of diabetes has risen from almost nothing a century ago, to a major health issue today. Worldwide it has more than tripled in the last forty years, and is expected to double again in the next twenty-five, affecting more than 366 million people.[1] Even the U.N. recognizes it as a global threat, and has designated November 14th as World Diabetes Day.

It is now rated as the sixth killer disease in the United States. Its ravages can lead to kidney disease, heart disease, high blood pressure, heart attacks, erectile dysfunction, stroke, cataracts, nerve damage, hearing loss, memory loss, blindness, and amputations. It is a mean, nasty disease. I have personally witnessed the devastation it can wreak, as my own wonderful father died of diabetes and kidney failure at age 67. (This was several years before I met Sylvia and learned the yeast connection to diabetes.) He had all the conditions listed above, except heart attack and stroke. I'll never forget the suffering.

What is this disease, and what makes it so dangerous? In as few words as possible: Diabetes is all about sugar. In fact, it used to be called "sugar diabetes." The sugar in our bodies is known as blood sugar or blood glucose. Every cell in our body requires a constant supply of glucose in order to fuel metabolism and for use in growth and repair.

When we eat food, our digestive system converts much of that food into glucose, which is then released into the bloodstream. The hormone insulin, which is secreted by the pancreas, is like an escort that moves glucose from the blood and conveys it into cells so it can be used as fuel. If the cells are unable to get adequate amounts of glucose, they starve to death. As they do, tissues and organs begin to deteriorate from lack of nourishment. This is what happens in diabetes.

There are two major forms of diabetes: Type I and Type II. Type I (also known as insulin-dependent or juvenile diabetes) usually begins in childhood and results from the inability of the pancreas to make adequate amounts of insulin because the beta cells responsible for making insulin are disabled or destroyed. Without an escort service, not enough glucose gets to all the cells in the body. Injections of insulin are required one or more times a day to make up the difference. Also a strict low-sugar diet is usually recommended. Eighty-five percent of all patients with Type I diabetes have no family history of diabetes.[2]

Type II diabetes, (also known as non-insulin dependent or adult onset diabetes) is not classified as an autoimmune disease but rather is defined by its primary symptom–the cells' inability to absorb and respond to insulin. In years past it appeared in middle-aged and older adults and constitutes 90 percent of all diabetics. In this case, the pancreas may secrete a normal amount of insulin, but the cells don't respond to what is there.    Insulin, which acts like a key, goes to cells to unlock their doors so glucose can enter. But if the locks on the cells are faulty, the key won't work and the door remains closed. Insulin keeps banging on the door, but no one answers, so, being deprived entry into cells, it has no choice but to keep circulating in the bloodstream.

Therein lies the damage. The excess glucose (and its buddies, yeast) circulating in the bloodstream attacks and damages the eyes and nerves, kidneys, the circulatory and nervous systems, and increases the production of destructive free radicals. (Diabetes is the number one cause of gangrene and amputations.) In a heroic attempt to protect the body from this damage, fluid from cells is called forth to dilute the sugary blood, and the kidneys perform yeoman's duty to clear it from the bloodstream and usher it out through the urinary tract through excess urination. But if the sugar remains uncontrolled, the attempt is futile.

In both types of diabetes cells are left wanting of the glucose they need. Fatigue, thirst, excessive urination, weight loss, ravenous hunger, and other symptoms result from this deprivation and manifest in the "melting down of flesh and bone into urine" that Arataeus so graphically described nearly a thousand years ago. In essence, diabetes is a disease of cellular nutritional wasting brought on by excessive urination.

The entire body of a diabetic from head to toe can be affected by one fungal condition or another, both internally and externally. Doctors have known for a long time that diabetes increases the risk of fungal infection in any diabetic, both young and old. Doesn't it make sense that a diabetic, whose blood glucose is abnormally high and yeast is feasting on the windfall, would have an immune system that is necessarily not up to par? Even the skin of a diabetic is a lush medium for yeast, leading to eczema, psoriasis, "jock itch", etc. because of the sugar found in their sweat. Acne has been called "skin diabetes" because studies have shown that people with acne have elevated glucose levels in the skin.

Twenty years ago, Type II diabetes was virtually unheard of in children. Today it is approaching epidemic proportions in both children and adolescents. Type II usually occurred during middle age, but now children as young as five are being diagnosed Type II. In the early 1900s, only 3 percent of new diabetes cases in children were Type II. Now 45 percent of new cases in children are Type II, conferring a 'life sentence' for nearly all of them. Recently there have been so many children developing Type II at very young ages that the former age designations (juvenile and adult-onset) have been dropped, and diabetes is now simply classified as Type I and Type II. Truly a sign of the times.

What is going on? What has changed this scenario so drastically?

Part of the answer can be found in what we eat. Homo sapiens appeared on the scene about 40,000 years ago, and our genetic makeup today differs little from our original ancestors. For 10,000 years they lived as hunter-gatherers, eating a diet low in fat and high in plant food and lean protein from wild animals. There was no sugar, bread, or cereal, no caffeine, no alcohol. They thrived on a high-fiber menu of fresh fruit, nuts, tubers, seeds, beans, and meat.

Compared to our modern diet, their diet was much lower in fat and sodium and much higher in Vitamin C and fiber. They consumed an abundance of chromium, magnesium, folic acid, and other B-complex vitamins–all the critical vitamins and minerals that are missing from processed foods. Their food was natural, organic, and full of natural enzymes. I believe this disparity between our original way of eating and our modern day diet to be one of the major contributors to the rise of the scourge known as diabetes.

The food pyramid, that well-known triangle that is purported to embody official dietary guidelines for Americans to follow, is reflective of how out of step we are with our ancestral heritage. It has created a scenario where two-thirds of our population is overweight or obese today. Its heavy emphasis on carbs (and the fungal frenzy that follows) prompted sportscaster George DeJohn to write on his website "If you eat like the food pyramid, you'll look like the food pyramid."[3] So true.

Other major contributors to the rise of diabetes are antibiotics, steroids, a high-carbohydrate diet, hormones, and birth control pills–the very same things that feed yeast.

So, is there a connection? Could diabetes be caused by yeast and fungus? Remember, sugar is yeast's favorite food.

The hormone insulin is produced by beta cells that are located in the pancreas's islets of Langerhans. In Type I diabetes, scientists speculate that the body turns against, attacks, and destroys its own insulin-producing beta cells. They call it an "immune system malfunction" and classify it as an "autoimmune disease." They theorize that the victim's immune system incorrectly identifies its own beta cells for invading viruses or bacteria, and goes berserk in efforts to eliminate them. Other autoimmune diseases where the immune system is supposed to turn on itself are rheumatoid arthritis, lupus, hypothyroidism, Crohn's disease, Sjogren's syndrome, and ulcerative colitis.

Do you think our Creator would design our body in such a way that would allow it to go haywire–for no particular reason–and launch an attack on *itself*? Or actually start consuming itself? Poppycock! God doesn't make mistakes. Something else is going on here–right under our noses. I'll bet it's that yeast/beast again.

Here is a scenario for the development of Type 1 diabetes that makes much more sense. In this scenario the immune system functions the way God intended it to, and the implausible theory of "autoimmunity" falls by the wayside.

1.  Yeast gains a foothold in the body through breathing air in a moldy home, school, or workplace or through antibiotics or vaccines, or ingesting it through food such as moldy grain, corn, bleu cheese, etc. If a woman is pregnant she can pass yeast on to her unborn child (especially from flu vaccines ingredients) and chances are high the child will develop diabetes at a young age.

2.  Fungal mycotoxins from the invading fungus infect the beta cells and alter their DNA, thereby fooling the body's immune system into thinking they are foreign matter. (If the yeast-free diet and anti-fungals are introduced at this point before all the beta cells are infected, diabetes may be averted.)

3.  The immune system spots the interlopers (the infected beta cells) and creates antibodies to destroy them in order to stop the fungi from inflicting any further damage to the body. Unfortunately the damaged and dying beta cell cannot manufacture insulin, but the immune system, at least, has stopped fungi from spreading throughout the body and killing the patient. The patient must live with diabetes, but at least he

lived. The immune system did not attack its own tissue, but actually saved the day–the way it was designed to.

But why would fungi go after beta cells? Because as beta cells are disabled and destroyed, insulin production falls to rock bottom. With insulin out of the way, blood sugar skyrockets, creating a veritable feast for the wily fungi waiting in the wings. Pretty slick, huh? Time and time again we can see how fungi and their mycotoxins, in a creepy and diabolical way, can alter our body chemistries to ensure their needed food sources!

Both types of diabetes are caused by sugar in the bloodstream not being absorbed and getting to cells that need it. However, Type II diabetes is not classified as an autoimmune disease since beta cells are not destroyed. Instead it is defined by its primary symptom: lack of response to circulating insulin. Scientists theorize that cells gradually lose their sensitivity to insulin, and get lethargic and lazy. They have dubbed this condition "insulin resistance," or Syndrome X, blaming most of the problem on the fact that most of Type II diabetics are overweight and have simply worn out the pancreas from eating too much.

A close study of the yeast/beast reveals quite a different picture.

All of the symptoms for both types of diabetes can be attributed to the activities of fungi and their mycotoxins. And all of the diseases, conditions, and complications associated with diabetes can be attributed to the activities of fungi and their mycotoxins. There can be only one obvious conclusion:

*Invading hordes of fungi create both Type I and Type II diabetes, and all associated conditions–to ensure their food supply–and thereby their survival.*

We know that yeast and fungi and their mycotoxins can manipulate our hormones to their advantage. They readily convert many of them into steroids such as prednisone. What does that do? It raises the amount of sugar in the bloodstream, and guess who is there with fork and spoon ready, smacking their lips. Doctors know that prescriptive corticosteroids raise blood sugar levels and can lead to type II diabetes. The same is true when the yeast/beast does it. Other mycotoxins can decrease oxygen to cells in order to create conditions more amenable to their survival, and still others can cause apoptosis–a kind of cell death that depletes a hormone called GSH (Growth Stimulating Hormone) that neutralizes toxins. Diabetics routinely test low for this vital hormone, indicating their bodies are continually under assault from fungi throughout the course of the disease. All of these "mycotoxin manipulations" reveal the level of sophistication some species of fungi can achieve.

Another disease that is closely linked to diabetes is Alzheimer's disease. As long as I have known Sylvia she has called it "diabetes of the brain," and is makes sense that if sugar-fueled fungi can create plaque in the coronary arteries it could create plaque in the brain. Fungal "caps" have been found on the brains of many Alzheimer's patients upon autopsy. (Ronald Reagan's addiction to jelly beans may have in part fueled his descent into this dreadful disease.)

Along with your pancreas, your brain also produces insulin. Both insulin and insulin receptors are critical for the formation of memory and learning. In the brain, insulin binds to these insulin receptors at synapses, thereby allowing nerve cells to survive and memories to form.

A recent study confirmed that a toxic protein in the brain of Alzheimer's patients called ADDL (amyloid beta-derived diffusible ligands) removes these insulin receptors from neurons and renders them insulin resistant.[4] (It is known that people with diabetes have a higher risk of developing Alzheimer's.) It appears that when ADDLs accumulate they block memory function, and it makes perfect sense that brain cells resistant to the nourishment they need to function become sluggish and eventually die. Yeast and yeast mycotoxins are the culprits, creating beta amyloid plaque (ADDL), breaking the connection between cells and then blocking them from rebuilding. Dementia, Alzheimer's and other brain disorders are the result.

As we have observed, a burgeoning industry has arisen to serve the growing numbers of diabetics in the U.S. and worldwide. From insulin to test strips, to glucose monitors, to meters and insulin pumps, to screening tests and diabetes medications (two of which are required to carry a black box warning stating they increase the risk of heart failure!), Big Pharma is there. Scientists now are busy working to create an artificial pancreas and searching for ways to transplant new beta cells into existing pancreases. They also are working on a drug to treat PRE-diabetes!

Diabetes drugs are not without risk. As I write this, according to a U.S. Senate report just released, (Feb. 2010) the oral diabetes drug, Avandia®, was linked to 83,000 heart attacks between 1999 and 2007. Avandia®, GlaxoSmithKline's third best-selling drug in 2006, saw its sales plummet from $2.2 billion to $1.2 billion by the end of 2008 after safety concerns were disclosed a year earlier. The chairman of the Committee of Finance, headed by Max Baucus, revealed that GlaxoSmithKline knew of the possible heart attack risks associated with its controversial drug, and recommended Avandia® be "removed from the market."[5] We'll see.

Incredibly, the American Diabetes Association (ADA), which has dedicated itself to helping diabetics manage their disease (they don't recognize that it can be cured), maintains that what we eat has little to do with whether we develop diabetes or not. It claims that genetics and weight gain are the culprits. However, studies of separated twins have shown the exact opposite, demonstrating that twins who were reared in separate households display different levels of vulnerability to developing diabetes, while twins reared together, eating the same food, do not.[6] This illustrates that genetics are not calling the shots here. What is going into the body in the form of food, vaccines, drugs and fungi are!

You would think that the ideal diet for treating diabetes—a disease characterized by high blood sugar levels—would logically be a low sugar and carbohydrate diet, but incredibly the ADA instructs otherwise. Even though it cautions against too many carbohydrates, it says it's okay to eat sugar early in the day if you cut back on it later in the day. In other words, if diabetics eat cupcakes and candy for breakfast, they just cut back on pasta for lunch! The ADA also advises that diabetics can keep eating sugar and junk food as long as they control their blood sugar levels with drugs! Whoa, Nellie. How wrong can you get! All diabetics need to restrict or eliminate refined sugars and carbohydrates for LIFE, and many will find their diabetes is eliminated as well.

At the same time the ADA pushes all the artificial and synthetic sweeteners, which we know are so harmful. It shouldn't come as a surprise that artificial sweetener manufacturers have collaborated with drug companies to market "diabetic" sugar-free cough syrups and other medications to the growing numbers of innocent consumers. Is it any coincidence that the ADA is largely funded and sponsored by Big Pharma/Big Chem? Much of the millions of dollars the ADA raises each year comes directly from such companies. In 2005 the ADA accepted more than $23 million from food manufacturers and drug companies.[7]

It has long been known that the mineral chromium lowers blood sugar (and cholesterol) but you will not find that information mentioned on the ADA website, even though an article on a placebo-controlled study in the journal *Diabetes* in 1997 reported that chromium supplementation had "significant beneficial effects" in lowering both numbers. But chromium isn't sexy enough (it's a mineral that can't be patented), and it's too cheap. Only expensive drugs made in the laboratories of pharmaceutical companies will do.

There has to be a better way. Yeast-free eating and anti-fungals such as caprylic acid, oregano oil, grapefruit seed extract, olive leaf extract, and garlic extract are godsends to a diabetic. Careful supplementation with a multivitamin, B-complex, vanadyl sulfate, alpha lipoic acid, cinnamon, and Gymnema sylvestre will lower blood sugar and guard against the complications of the blood vessels, nerves, eyes, and kidneys. (Some studies have shown Gymnema has the ability to increase beta cells.[8]) Minerals such as chromium and zinc are also necessary. A good exercise program is very helpful as it oxygenates the body. Yeast hates oxygen. I have seen many people able to cut way down on insulin and oral medications and gain new leases on life in just a few weeks. Of course, this should be done with careful monitoring from your doctor.

To date there have been numerous scientific studies that support and verify this safe, natural approach. Yet the majority of physicians continue to ignore the research and cling to the status quo by focusing entirely on lowering blood sugar with drugs–no matter the cost or risks to patients. With  pharmaceutical companies calling the shots in medical research, formulating treatment guidelines, and selling their wares through drug reps and direct-to-consumer advertising, attention is being diverted from these natural and very effective therapies–all of which deal with the yeast/beast.

From now on, when you hear the words "autoimmune disease," **think yeast**.

To me, the most convincing clue that diabetes is a fungus-driven disease is that in order to create diabetes in lab rats (to see how they respond to drugs that treat diabetes) they are injected with mold mycotoxins!  Rats don't get diabetes. **Only ones injected with mold do.**

Wouldn't you think someone might put two and two together?

**Chapter 29**

---

# The True Cause of Most Disease

*"Diseases are crises of purification, of toxic elimination. Symptoms are the natural defenses of the body. We call them diseases, but in fact they are the cure of disease."*

... Hippocrates

If the grand thesis of this book is correct, that most of our major and minor diseases are variations on the yeast/fungal theme, that their clinical names are different but the basic underlying condition is the same–then let's look at some of those diseases and describe what is happening in the body that creates the manifestations that we call dis-ease.

Bear in mind that many of our symptoms do not constitute the disease but really the *cure.* Symptoms are the body's attempt to balance and heal itself. That means in reality, measles is not the disease but the body's attempt to cure. Acne is not the disease but the cure. Cancer is not the disease but the cure. Arthritis is not the disease but the cure, etc. All diseases are the body's defense mechanisms swinging into action in an attempt to heal itself.

To illustrate further, a friend of our son's went to his doctor complaining of *five different conditions*: overweight, psoriasis, colitis, esophageal reflux, and frequent urination. He went on the yeast-free diet and three months later *all five conditions had vanished.* His doctor refused to believe there was any connection to the diet, reaffirming the old adage "there is none so blind as one who *will not* see."

Here is a short and very incomplete list of yeast manifestations that will add to your understanding of how wily and adaptable the yeast/beast is. Edgar Cayce said, "ALL disease is in the bloodstream," meaning the bloodstream is where disease starts. The only true and real disease then is toxemia–poisoning of the blood–out of which symptoms arise.

Fungal spores and their mycotoxins are those poisons. They travel the bloodstream highway to whatever destination they choose – brain, heart, muscles, organs, etc. The diseases that appear depend on where they take up housekeeping.

*All these diseases are directly linked to the activities of yeast, fungi, and their mycotoxins:*

*Acne and rosacea*...yeast living on and in the liver and elsewhere coming out through the skin plus liver malfunction and/or allergy to alcohol.

*AIDS*...AIDS virus perhaps, but mainly fungal

*Alcoholism*...yeasts screaming for a fix.

*All autoimmune diseases*...yeast and fungi rampant in the body. (In 1952 there was one recognized autoimmune disease–celiac disease. Now there are over one hundred!)

*Allergies*...yeast boring holes through intestinal lining allowing allergens and food particles to enter the bloodstream. Adrenals become depressed and cannot produce natural cortisone.

*Alzheimer's disease*..."Diabetes of the brain"...yeast living in the brain creating beta amyloid plaques, a toxic protein. Yeast breaks the connection between cells and doesn't allow them to rebuild. Connected also with aluminum.

*Arthritis*…yeast living in warm moist linings of joints, causing swelling and pain.

*Asperger's Syndrome*…yeast living in the brain and other organs.

*Asthma and lung or respiratory disorders*…yeast living in the lungs and lining of lungs. Inhalers actually create more fungus in the lungs as well as the intestinal tract.

*Athlete's Foot and ringworm*…yeast living on skin.

*Bi-Polar Disease, schizophrenia, hallucinations, and hearing voices*…yeast spores and mycotoxins in the brain affecting thought patterns and behavior.

*Birth defects*…yeast and their mycotoxins damage DNA, causing spina bifida, anencephaly, and other defects.

*Cancer*…is a simple fungal infection, grows by spreading spores and growing new colonies known as metastases.

*Cataracts*…yeast living in the corneas and yeast causing drying of the eye muscle.

*Colitis, Irritable Bowel Syndrome, Crohn's disease, diverticulitis*…yeast living in the intestinal tract creating inflammation, pain and infection.

*Congestive heart failure*…yeast attacking and injuring the heart and valves.

*Cystitis and interstitial cystitis*…yeast living in the bladder or urethra. Body too acid.

*Depression*…yeast and spores in the brain and body.

*Diabetes*…yeast living on the pancreas and mycotoxin damage.

*Epilepsy*…yeast causing lesions in the brain.

***Fatigue and Chronic Fatigue Syndrome***…yeast living in many places, especially the pancreas, thyroid, and adrenals. The brain deprived of oxygen.  Antibiotics destroy B-12, a vitamin critical to energy.

*Fibromyalgia*…yeast living in muscles creating inflammation and pain.

*Glaucoma*…yeast spores in the eyes causing eyes to swell and increase ocular pressure.

***Gluten Intolerance and Celiac Disease***…antigens from grains impregnated with yeast mycotoxins causing "allergic" symptoms.

*Gout*…only yeast and their mycotoxins create uric acid crystals. The human body does not.

***Heart disease, heart attacks, arrhythmias,***…yeast living in the coronary arteries and circulatory system.

***Heartburn and acid indigestion, or GERD***…yeast living in the esophagus.

*High cholesterol*…yeast living in coronary arteries and circulatory system.

***Hypo or hyperthyroidism***…yeast living on the thyroid.

*Infertility*…yeast living on ovaries and/or in fallopian tubes blocking union of ova and sperm, or in the testicles.

*Kidney stones*…oxalic acid made by overgrowths of fungi in the intestines. The body cannot process calcium, especially from milk.

*Leukemia*…yeast spores living in bloodstream. Is a fugal infection of white blood cells. Antibiotics intimately connected. May be preceded by trauma to the tailbone.

*Lupus*…yeast living in the lymphatic system and throughout the body.

*Mitral Valve Prolapse*…yeast living in mitral valve.

*Multiple Sclerosis*… A chronic mycotoxicosis…yeast living on and dissolving nerve sheaths and yeast mycotoxins damaging nerve cells. Candida spores and antigens have been found in the spinal fluid of M.S. patients, as has gliotoxin – a heat stable mycotoxin made by yeast and fungi, known to disrupt the central nervous system.

*Obesity*…yeast eating nutrients and creating cravings for carbohydrates, especially sugar.

*Osteoporosis*…yeast living in the center of the bone and eating its way outward.

*Prostatitis*…yeast living in the prostate causing it to swell. (What makes bread rise?)

*Psoriasis*…yeast living on skin plus liver malfunction.

*Retinitis Pigmentosa*…yeast inflaming the retina. six months to two years on diet and anti-fungals needed before eyesight slowly returns, proving retinitis pigmentosa is not necessarily genetic.

*Rheumatoid Arthritis, or RA*…yeast and mycotoxins living on nerve sheaths, dissolving them. RA is a chronic mycotoxicosis coupled with an allergy to milk and milk products.

*Scerloderma*…yeast consuming connective tissue in skin and organs.

***Sinus infections***…yeast living in the sinus cavities. (In 1999, the Mayo Clinic declared that 97 percent of sinus infections were fungal infections, not bacterial infections.)

***Tics and Tourette's Syndrome***…virus plus yeast living in the nervous system.

Remember that in the plant world fungus is the farmer's number one enemy. I hope I have made a credible case that **fungus is our number one enemy also.** The farmer's nemesis is our nemesis. We share the same planet. We share the same environment. Our lives, health, and futures are intimately intertwined.

Just as our planet has various living ecological systems, so do our bodies. Just as the ecological systems of the planet are dependent upon balance to remain healthy, so do our bodies. Just as plants are vulnerable to attacks by fungi, so are our bodies. Don't forget that the ecological system in our digestive tract is referred to as micro flora. Micro flora means *small plants.* We are mirrors of our environment.

Doug Kaufmann summed it up quite well when he wrote in *The Fungal Link*: **"I believe that fungus, either acting alone or in unison with its metabolites, causes nearly every malady known to man. …There is reason to believe that we remain ignorant as to why these diseases are killing so many because the medical profession has not been properly educated in the field of mycology, the study of fungi."**

When all is said and done, we should ask: If anti-fungals kill cancer cells, what then is cancer? If statins lower cholesterol because they kill fungus, what then is high cholesterol or heart disease? If antifungals cure acne, what then causes acne? If Prozac® relieves depression because it is an antifungal, what then causes depression? If anti-fungals cure gout, bi-polar disease, autoimmune diseases, and a myriad of other diseases, what then *caused* them?

Ask this same question for most diseases, and the only clear answer has to be "the yeast/beast."

We have learned that this tiny organism has enormous power over us. It loves to eat the soft, warm, moist tissue and bone of the human body, yet it can grow on and consume even carpet, wood, leather, and rocks. We have learned that it can disguise itself so well that it can sneak into the body and the immune system won't recognize it. We have learned it can then mutate and morph into viruses, bacteria and back into yeasts again in its efforts to elude our immune systems, thereby creating most of the diseases that plague humanity. We have learned that it can progress from one location in the body to another as it moves around in its search for food, creating various symptoms and/or illnesses as it goes. We have learned of the enormous amounts of money required to treat it and the incalculable amounts of money made because of it. We have learned it is elusive, smart, wily, and difficult to eradicate. We have learned in great numbers it can eat its host alive, and, conversely, when yeast levels are low, the host enjoys good health. We have learned it *is* cancer and can infect our brains and thinking processes. We have learned that it is truly a force to be reckoned with, but can be reckoned with safely–with the right tools of diet and anti-fungals.

So far this "bad actor" in the drama of our lives has been successful in its attempts to fool us with its many disguises, machinations, and sleights of hand. Ever the opportunist, waiting behind the curtain (the disease behind disease) for his cues to dazzle us with his acting talents and magic tricks, yeast waits patiently. But now the time has come to unclothe this impersonator and expose the true villain for the audience to see. The time has come to lower the curtain on the last act.

We recognize it now. How did we miss it? It was there all the time, right under our noses, hiding in plain view. The yeast/beast has been revealed for a waiting audience to see. This performer really is not an artist at all, but a con artist instead. Or better yet, a quick-change artist. *In the final analysis it is simply the same actor masquerading in different costumes.*

The human body was designed to be healthy. So, in the end, the question that goes to the heart of disease is: Who or what is breaking strands of DNA in cells to precipitate disease? Who or what has the power to alter the original design and wreak havoc in something that once was perfect? It has to be the beast.

Disease *is* a crisis of purification and of toxic elimination as Hippocrates told us over two thousand years ago. The diet outlined in this book will empower you to eliminate toxins from your body and pave the way for it to become purified and whole again. Once purified and whole, your body, mind, and spirit will experience the health they were designed to enjoy.

*Recage the Beast.* You now know what to do and how to do it.

The rest is up to you.

**Chapter 30**

# Where Do We Go From Here?

*"All nations are deceived by her sorcerers."*

...Revelation 18:23

So far you have been reading about all the horrors that are associated with overgrowths of *Candida albicans*. No doubt this condition is dangerous and can be fatal. But, there is another side to the coin. Now let's try to look at the yeast/beast as a friend–a true "friend in need," one who has come to wake us up and *warn* us.

The explosion of yeast and yeast-related illnesses is trying to teach us an important lesson for our very *survival*. Like all hard lessons, if we learn from our mistakes and use what we have learned for the good, then the experience of having been ill and then overcoming the illness will have been put to good use.

If we see yeast infection as a "wake-up call," and take the warning seriously, we may have time to regroup and re-fortify our defenses. In the end, we may even thank them for waking us up to our errors and mistakes, and giving us a chance to rectify them.

By alerting us to our weaknesses, yeasts are giving us a second chance. If we can "clean up our act," do a thorough house-cleaning and "throw the bums out," we may have time to turn the looming Candida calamity around. If not, the acceleration of yeast growths will be irreversible, as will be our early demise.

It was interesting to learn while doing the research for this project, that in ancient Israel, ill-health was looked upon with contempt. It was considered a *sin* to get sick. The early Jews both knew and taught that illness was a reflection of the breaking of God's laws. Anyone who "sinned" was seen as "missing the mark" (an archery term), or falling short of Divine Law, or the law of God. Disease was the result of the sinner's own transgressions. The early Jews were well aware of the intimate connection between the mind and the body. This may be the reason Christ said so many times as He healed the sick: "Thy sins be forgiven thee," "Go, and sin no more," "Go, you are healed. Your sins are forgiven."

The quote from the Bible which heads this chapter is one of the most meaningful sentences in this great wise book. The Greek word for sorcery is PHARMEKIA–the science of preparing medicines. Even more astounding is the fact that the English root word for "pharmacy" has to do with the dispensing of drugs, as well as sorcery, witchcraft, and magic. *It literally means drug abuse.* Truly, all nations have been deceived by the use of these drugs. No wonder we get sicker and sicker the longer we use them.

Will we be able to accept responsibility for our own health, to repent (re-think), change our minds, and thereby change our ways? Will we be able to "go and sin no more?" I think there's hope. If we all approach this problem with an attitude of positive optimism and deep faith, then perhaps we can keep yeast from mushrooming completely out of control.

The mushroom is a perfect symbol with which to end this book. To me it has become a symbol of death, like a mushroom cloud after a nuclear detonation. The symbolism is powerful. For our purposes it symbolizes both fungus and death.

As you know, mushrooms are not allowed on the diet. Even the Bible tells us not to eat them. In Genesis, man is told to eat foods "whose seed is in itself," and can reproduce "after its kind." This includes green herbs, nuts, grains, and vegetables. Yeast products and mushrooms do not have "seeds within themselves," but reproduce by spores, and are parasites that live off other organisms and speed up their decay. There is no health in them.

Interestingly, all of our modern hybrid fruits and vegetables, such as tangelos and broccoflower, do not have that "seed" by which they can reproduce themselves. We have even developed "seedless" lines of fruits and vegetables. They are thereby man's creation and do not follow God's instructions. Ultimately they will not bring us health.

It is also interesting to note that leavening and yeast is always *symbolic of sin* in the Bible, and unleavened or yeastless bread was commanded to be used at feasts or during high holy days in order to clean and purify their bodies. "A little yeast leaveneth the whole lump" from 1 Corinthians affirmed that a little yeast, or a small number of people who "sin," infects and affects the whole of society. Like the proverbial rotten apple in a barrel that slowly infects all the apples with mold, a little pornography, a little adultery, a little dishonesty slowly seeps through society, metastasizing and infecting us all.

There are over 100 references to yeast in the Bible. All have a negative connotation.

In Exodus, Moses is told by God how to prepare the Passover feast:

"That same night they are to eat the meat roasted over the fire, along with bitter herbs, and bread made *without yeast.*"[1] (Emphasis added.)

Preparations for the Festival of Unleavened Bread included:

"Celebrate the Feast of Unleavened Bread....In the first month you are to eat bread made without yeast, from the evening of the fourteenth day until the evening of the twenty-first day. For seven days no yeast is to be found in your houses. And whoever eats anything with yeast in it must be cut off from the community of Israel, whether he is alien or native-born. Eat nothing made with yeast. Wherever you live, *you must eat unleavened bread.*"[2] (Emphasis added.)

And concerning sacrifices:

"Do not offer the blood of a sacrifice to me along with *anything containing yeast.*"[3] (Emphasis added.)

In Leviticus there are specific instructions for preparing grain offerings:

"If you bring a grain offering baked in an oven, it is to consist of fine flour: cakes made *without yeast* and mixed with oil, or wafers made *without yeast* and spread with oil. If your grain offering is prepared on a griddle, it is to be made of fine flour mixed with oil, and *without yeast.*"[4] (Emphasis added.)

Even more interesting are the biblical regulations concerning mildew. They are fascinating.

In Leviticus pages of precise instructions for the removal of mildew include:

"If any clothing is contaminated with mildew–any woolen or knitted clothing, any woven or knitted material or wool, any leather or anything made of leather–and the contamination...is greenish or reddish, it is a spreading mildew and must be shown to a priest. The priest is to examine the mildew and isolate the affected article for seven days. On the seventh day he is to examine it, and if the mildew has spread in the clothing, or the woven or knitted material, or the leather, whatever its use, it is a destructive mildew; the article is *unclean.* He must burn up the clothing, or the woven or knitted material of wool or linen, or any leather article that has the contamination in it, because the mildew is destructive; the article must be burned up."[5]

"But if, when the priest examines it, the mildew has not spread...he shall order that the contaminated article be washed. Then he is to isolate it for another seven days. After the affected article has been washed, the priest is to examine it, and if the mildew has not changed it appearance, even though it has not spread, it is *unclean.* Burn it with fire, whether the mildew has affected one side or the other. If, when the priest examines it, the mildew has faded after the article has been washed, he is to tear the contaminated part out...But if it reappears...it is spreading and whatever has the mildew must be burned with fire."[6]

Likewise, the early Jews were warned to watch carefully for anything that resembled mold in their homes. When mildew was found on the walls they were told:

"The priest is to order the house to be emptied before he is to go in to examine the mildew so that nothing in the house would be pronounced *unclean*. After this the priest is to go in and inspect the house. He is to examine the mildew on the walls, and if it has greenish or reddish depressions that appear to be deeper than the surface of the wall, the priest shall go out the doorway of the house and close it up for seven days. On the seventh day, the priest shall return to inspect the house. If the mildew has spread on the walls, he is to order that the contaminated stones be torn out and thrown into an unclean place outside the town. He must have all the inside walls of the house scraped and the material that is scraped off dumped into an unclean place outside the town. Then they are to take other stones to replace these and take new clay and plaster the house."[7]

"If the mildew reappears in the house after the stones have been torn out and the house scraped and plastered, the priest is to go and examine it and, if the mildew has spread in the house, it is a destructive mildew; the house is *unclean*. It must be torn down—its stones, timbers, and all the plaster—taken out of the town to an unclean place."[8]

"Anyone who goes into the house while it is closed up will be unclean until evening. Anyone who sleeps or eats in the house must wash his clothes."[9]

Specific instructions are given for the leveling of homes that have "black stains" on the ceiling that grow and spread. (*Stachybotrys* fungi are black and one of the most virulent strains of fungi.) Eight men must surround the dwelling and destroy it by pushing the walls *inward* so that the fungi-laden debris doesn't spread outward to contaminate new areas. The occupants of the house are then told to burn their clothes before they can go on with their lives.

Why was God so adamant in teaching the Jews the dangers of mildew, mold, and yeast? *Because He knew they were human contagions.* They cause disease, and all the laws, dietary restrictions, spiritual instructions were given with the intention of keeping His chosen people healthy–in body, mind, and spirit.

It does seem the ancient Jews were fixated on fungi, to the point that today we might assign them the label of "obsessive-compulsive disorder!" But when you look deeper at the Jewish faith, you see a people who loved symbolism and ritual in the practice of their faith. If yeast was the symbol of sin for them, then it is very logical that they would do anything and everything to root it out of their daily physical lives as well as their spiritual lives. They considered anything that was contaminated with yeast as unclean, and therefore sinful.

Could it be that that the "house" with mildew is a metaphor for our bodies? We know that "house" and "temple" were used interchangeably to symbolize the body. ("Know ye not that your body is a temple of the Holy Spirit who is in you?"[10]) Physiologists tell us that a whole organism is built cell by cell and destroyed cell by cell. Are the stones, timbers and plasters that were scraped, torn down, and taken to a garbage dump outside of town really alluding to the unhealthy, infected, yeast-laden cells inside us, and God is commanding us to remove and destroy them? The metaphor is powerful.

To the Jews, the act of cleansing and purifying their food, their clothes, their homes, and their bodies, were concrete ways of pleasing God, and at the same time symbolic ways of remaining "whole," "healthy", and "holy" in both body and spirit.

Doctors everywhere are finally recognizing a new disease called "Sick Building Syndrome," or SBS. People who live and work in mold-ridden environments are notorious for developing debilitating and wide-ranging illnesses. The Rayburn Office Building in Washington, D.C. is a classic example. Employees had to evacuate the premises in order to get well. So many of our school buildings with flat roofs that leak and harbor toxic molds are intimately connected with the sick, fidgety, ADD and ADHD children inside. When contaminated buildings are cleaned of all sources of toxic mold and are remediated, people return and illnesses don't recur. Our body temples can be infected with toxic mold also, and thank goodness we have learned how to remediate them as well!

I see this as what ultimately happens to us as we reclaim our bodies from the yeast/beast. As we become "cleaner," the light drives away the darkness, where mold and fungi live. As we become "clean," our self-healing mechanisms are set free to function the way our Creator intended them to function, and health and wholeness will follow. Then, being freed from the pain and distraction of illness and disease, we can become all we were intended to be.

Like the Jews of old, it is now time for the priest (our higher selves) to inspect our body-temples for any sign of the yeast/beast. If it is found, we must begin to eradicate and exorcise it–before it consumes us. Brick by brick, timber by timber, cell by cell it must be removed to an unclean place outside of town. Then, our bodies will "take other stones to replace these, and take new clay and plaster the house." Brick by brick, timber by timber and cell by cell we will rebuild a new and more acceptable residence for our souls. In due time we will be pronounced *clean.*

I pray now that we will be empowered to back the rampaging beast back into its cage and establish order and peace once again. Living in harmony with wholeness of body, mind, and spirit, we can become free to become our highest selves.

Perhaps Candida has come to expose us to ourselves. It is giving us both a challenge–to grow and learn–and an opportunity–to re-create ourselves more in His image, clean and full of light.

The prophet Isaiah pointed forward to a time in the future when these beautiful words would apply to us all:

"And no resident will say 'I am sick'."[11]

*Godspeed!*

# *Epilogue*

---

*"Be sober, be vigilant, because your adversary the devil, as a roaring lion, walketh about, seeking whom he may devour."*

1 Peter: 5:8

For thirty chapters you have been reading and learning about yeast as it pertains to its existence on the physical level. Now let's explore a hypothesis about its possible existence and influence on the metaphysical level–in our minds and spirits.

Just as humans have both physical and spiritual natures, could The Third Kingdom, the kingdom of fungi, have a dual nature also? Is it possible that yeast, fungi, and mold, which "devil" us with so many diseases in our physical bodies, are capable of influencing negatively our thoughts and emotions? If so, could it be that the devil of the Bible is a metaphor for the dangerous form of yeast known as fungi? *Could it be that yeast and the entity known as the devil are one and the same?*

I am not a biblical scholar, and no one would ever call me a wild-eyed, bible-thumping evangelist. There is no way this esoteric "flight-of-fancy" can be proved. However, I do know that the research into its possibility has proved fascinating, rewarding, and fun. What follows is simply my interpretation, and you are welcome to accept it or reject it. I offer this exercise to you now, in hopes it will help you see with more clarity, the true role of fungi in both our bodies and our minds.

Let's look at the similarities between the devil and the activities of yeast/fungi in the Bible, and some of the adjectives that describe them.

The Bible is full of metaphors: some simple, some complex, some inscrutable. One of the strongest recurring metaphors is that of "darkness" versus "light."  Over and over the devil is associated with darkness and God with light.  The devil is called the "Prince of Darkness," the "Power of Darkness", and the "Author of All Evil."  Christians are told to "come out of the darkness and into light," and in the Book of Acts to "turn them from darkness to light and from the power of Satan unto God."  Light means the absence of darkness.  Yeast and the devil occupy the same realm–that of the dark.  It is interesting to note that as we grow in wisdom and understanding we are considered "enlightened" or bathed in the light of God.

We know that yeast, mold, mildew, and fungi all thrive in darkness: in basements, swamps, and in the warm dark recesses of our bodies, hiding from the light.  But when the swamps are drained, the basements aired, the overgrowths are eradicated, and light is returned, God is revealed and health is restored, illustrating the universal principle of *"where light is darkness cannot be."*  This truly shows us that even though Satan may be powerful, *he is not as powerful as God.*  His power and control in our lives can be eliminated through God's light shining into human understanding.  A remarkable analogy.

### *In the book of Job:*

There is a scene in which God asks Satan, "Whence comest thou?"  Satan answers, "From going to and fro in the earth and walking up and down in it."  (Don't forget that earth often is a metaphor for our bodies.)  Soon afterwards, "Satan left the presence of the Lord to smite Job with sore boils from the sole of his foot unto his crown."  What a perfect description of the modus operandi of yeast.  It is always "going to and fro" and "walking up and down", scouring the terrain for something to eat.  Boils are one of the ways the body, in its infinite wisdom, defensively walls off festering infections in an attempt to protect itself from further damage.  The instigator of infections and pus is *yeast!*  Could this part of Job's story be a metaphor for yeast?  Is the infectious pus a metaphor for Satan?

## *In the book of John:*

In this book the devil is referred to as "The Prince of This World" and "Ruler of This Earth." That makes sense if you think of yeasts and molds as having enormous power in the physical world and can indeed be considered "rulers" of the earth (and our bodies). Fungal diseases continue to wipe out huge crops all over the world if the conditions are right. As I write this in 2009, Cornell University is committing a $26.8 million grant to find a way to combat the emergence of deadly new strains of rust disease in hopes of averting a pandemic that could result in catastrophic wheat crop losses worldwide. The Prince and Ruler of this world is powerful indeed. But John reassures us that "now shall the prince of this world be cast out." Surely with Divine understanding we will be able to find ways to eradicate these scourges.

Also in John we read that the devil is referred to as a "trickster" and an unreliable source of information, or a "liar." We know that yeast has the remarkable ability to change its own DNA and morph into fungi, bacteria, viruses, cancer cells and back into its original form. In the twinkling of an eye, it can change disguises like a chameleon to confound and disarm our immune systems. Tricky, wouldn't you say? Fungi bind with immune cells, creating hybrid cells containing human DNA plus fungal DNA. With the fungal DNA masked by the human DNA, the immune system is "lied to" and "tricked" into believing all is well. Fungi remain unscathed to do their dirty work. Liar and trickster to the max. Diabolical, too.

## *In the book of Ephesians:*

Here we find the devil being referred to as the "Prince of the Power of the Air." This is fascinating, as yeast spores are all around us in the air we breathe. Every time we inhale, we inhale yeast spores. The first breath we breathe in at birth contaminates our pure, clean, newborn bodies with fungal spores. When we dig in the garden we stir up fungi living underground and breathe more fungal spores into our lungs. The smoke inhaled from cigarettes contains fungal spores from the aged and cured tobacco. In a sense, we literally breathe in the seeds of our own destruction. The Prince of the power of the Air, ever the opportunist just like yeast, whirls around us continuously, waiting for its chance to find entry and do its dirty work.

### In the book of Matthew:

In this book the devil is described as having and leading "a personal army of *demons*." Fungal colonies (cysts and tumors perhaps?) are masses of millions of cells and can be considered huge armies of demons, banding together and plotting their military moves and methods of attacks on surrounding tissues. "Personal army of demons" could further be a metaphor for mycotoxins–the poisons that yeast give off as they rampage through the body and brain. The damage mycotoxins create could certainly be described as "demonic."

In Greek, the word *daimon,* or devil, means *intelligent.* Indeed, each fungal cell has an intelligence or mind of its own. It seems to be able to decide which form it wants to take (yeast or fungus, bacteria or virus), where it wants to go (digestive system, liver, muscles, brain, pancreas, etc.) and what it wants to do (lie low, attack, or live peacefully). Fungi even communicate among themselves! It looks like intelligent fungi and the devil both have consciousness and decision-making capabilities.

A demon also has the ability to enter into a human body and influence a person's thoughts and behavior. We read in the Bible that the devil "put into Judas' mind the decision to betray Jesus." Yeast spores in the brain can produce deranged and irrational thinking. Was yeast there, tempting Judas with thoughts of silver but giving no thoughts to the consequences? Jesus knew beforehand that Judas would betray him. At the Last Supper, he handed Judas a *sop*, which is a piece of bread soaked in a sauce, wine, or milk. We are told that as soon as Judas ate the sop, "Satan entered into him" and he soon betrayed his Master. By handing him a sop, could Jesus have been illustrating a yeast reaction to Judas' subsequent behavior?

Also in Matthew Jesus admonished his disciples to be careful and be on their guard against the *yeast* of the Pharisees and Sadducees. He wasn't telling them to guard against the yeast in bread but against the *teaching* of the Pharisees and Sadducees that could *infect their minds with untruths and distorted thinking.* Overgrowths of yeast are *infections.*

### In the book of 2 Corinthians:

The devil is described as a spirit "in whom the *god of this world* hath blinded the minds of them that believe." Judas again comes to mind as he was *blinded* by thoughts of thirty pieces of silver, even though he believed in Jesus. So it seems that yeast and the devil can and do influence our thoughts and actions, by "blinding our minds," confusing our thoughts, and enticing us into harmful behaviors in order to control us. Both have the power to place humans in extreme peril.

### In the book of Revelation:

John writes, "and I looked and behold, a pale horse, and its name was death, and hell followed him." Could this be a vivid description of yeast on the warpath? A scene of yeast in locked battle devouring live healthy cells could definitely be described as a scene from hell. Death and destruction, mayhem, littered battlefields–all appear in the wake of war. And the pale horse? All yeast infections, thrush, and cancers are pale and whitish! Truly startling similarities.

In many of the books of the Bible, the devil is referred to as the "tempter." What an apt description of yeast. When a person is battling yeast overgrowths, he is constantly tempted by the yeast to eat food that quickly satisfies the yeast's insistent demand to be fed. Sugar, carbohydrates, alcohol, caffeine, grains, yeast breads, milk products are all definite temptations. And when you eat them, they in turn set up even more cravings. A "devilish" cycle is set as the health of the host breaks down and the devil gets his due.

In Greek, another meaning of the word, "devil" (*diavolos*) is "slanderer." In every sense both yeast and the devil are slanderers. To slander means to assail, assault, attack, injure, and tear down–destructive activities all, and a perfect description of both the devil and yeast.

Other biblical descriptions of Satan are: "the devourer," "a murderer," "father of all lies", and a "seducer." Fungi, indeed, *devour* and *murder* innocent cells in their voracious rampages; *lie* in their tempting promises to "make you feel better if you just heed my urges;" and *seduce* you into foods and activities that benefit them, but harm you. You can almost hear their seductive whispers in your ear: "Here, drink this alcohol–it will make you feel happy." "Here, smoke this cigarette or joint, and take this cocaine–you've had such a stressful day. They'll make you mellow out and help you forget." "Here, take this speed–you'll feel fantastic." "Here, eat this yummy five-layer chocolate cake with triple fudge frosting–you'll love the taste and it will give you energy." "Here, drink this caffeine–you know you can't get started without it." Devourer, seducer, liar, and murderer–the words all fit.

Finally, let's look again at the epigraph for this chapter: "Be sober, be vigilant, because your *adversary*, the devil, as a roaring lion, walketh about, seeking whom he may devour." Here the devil is described as "The Adversary," which means antagonist, challenger, attacker, enemy, foe, competitor, or rival. All these words brilliantly describe many of yeast's and fungi's attributes. They continuously compete for territory and terrain as they challenge and attack our bodies and immune systems. They also constantly antagonize our healthy cells in an endless turf war waged against beneficial bacteria to ensure their survival. An adversarial relationship to the core. The "roaring lion"–the king of the jungle–I believe is the supreme metaphor for the menacing and deadly yeast/beast–on prowl for his prey: you, your body or mind–or both.

Fast forward to August 2010 and let me end with a warning. In recent years rampant fungal infections have been blamed on the precipitous declines of bats (so critical for insect control), amphibians, and honeybees. Now scientists are watching very carefully a strange, previously unknown strain of a deadly airborne fungus that has killed many people in parts of Canada, Oregon, Washington, and Idaho. It is spreading rapidly. It is a new genotype of *Cryptococcus gattii* fungi, normally found in tropical and subtropical locations. Scientists are alarmed and mystified, and can't explain why it is appearing in the Pacific Northwest. There are no known preventions. It has a horrific *10 percent to 25 percent death rate* and is infecting domestic animals as well. The fungus has to be breathed into the lungs, and from there works its way into the spinal fluid and central nervous system and causes fatal meningitis. Symptoms appear 2 to 4 months after exposure and can be treated successfully with anti-fungals if detected early enough. In British Columbia's Vancouver Island alone at least 26 people have died and the fungus has infected and killed dogs, cats, horses, sheep, alpacas, and porpoises. Microbiologists say the mystery fungus has the potential to go anywhere the wind or people take it. It seems that fungus is on a devilish warpath these days.

Keep your eyes on *Cryptococcus gatti.* I hope you know how to protect yourself and your loved ones now. Keep your anti-fungals handy. Remember the lion is always "walking about and seeking whom to devour." He has spotted you. With his eyes riveted on you, slowly and surely he is assuming a crouching position.

Don't put yourself in his path.

\*\*\*\*\*\*\*\*\*\*\*\*\*\*\*\*\*\*\*\*\*\*\*\*\*\*\*\*\*\*\*\*\*\*\*\*\*\*\*\*\*\*\*\*\*\*\*\*\*\*\*\*\*\*\*\*\*\*\*\*\*\*
\*\*\*\*\*\*\*\*\*\*\*\*

## A PERSONAL NOTE

I have had my own "brush with the beast." In January 2005 I was checked into the University of Virginia hospital in Charlottesville, Virginia, to undergo surgery to remove a tumor from my lower left abdomen.

For several months prior to the surgery, I was aware of a small swelling, but attributed it to perhaps a prolapsed bladder (common to many women my age) since I had been experiencing bladder issues. I felt wonderful, had plenty of energy, and saw no cause for alarm. Then the swelling started to get bigger, the scales started climbing, and I began to experience discomfort, fatigue, and loss of appetite. I dragged myself through the Christmas holidays and looked forward to my regular (every eight weeks) appointment with our chiropractor in early January. I showed him the swelling, and he immediately sent me to a clinic to have it x-rayed. A CAT scan soon followed and a week later I was scheduled for surgery.

After a three-and-a-half hour operation, a sixteen pound, fluid-filled, ovarian tumor was removed. Inside there was one small spot of cancer, smaller than the size of a dime. It was identified as a *serous papilloma carcinoma*, and was classified "1–A"–or a pre-stage-one cancer. It had been entirely walled off and encapsulated by my body, and there were no visible signs of metastasis in my abdomen. Eleven biopsies were taken from nearby sites to be certain. After three days I came home and made a speedy and total recovery.

For eight years prior to this, Sylvia and I had been out of touch. My husband and I had moved from Houston to Charlotte, North Carolina, and, sadly, Sylvia and I weren't working together any more. But I always stayed close to the yeast-free diet, and continued to get the yeast-free message to everyone I could.

Fortunately, I had called her on another matter about six months before the swelling was noticed. She said right away, "The number of cancer cells is 'up' in your bloodstream." I was startled but not unnerved as I knew that everyone has cancer cells (fungal spores) in the bloodstream, which are normally eradicated by a healthy immune system. I also had seen so many cancer cures in my years of working with her that I wasn't worried. She sent a box brimming with anti-fungals and immune system stimulators the next day. I stayed on them faithfully.

The night before the surgery I talked to Sylvia on the phone. Miserable and unhappy at the prospects of what was going to happen to me the next morning, I asked her to put on her best medical intuitive cap while I kept pressing her to tell me if she thought the surgeon would find cancer. I was never worried or panicked at the thought, as I knew we could fix whatever it was and I would be fine. Sylvia remained non-committal, which was unusual for her, as she is normally forthright and direct. I asked her again, "Do you think this is cancer?" Finally in exasperation she said, "Jane, if it is I can hardly 'see' it." She then went on to tell me that I would survive the surgery with flying colors, and "there would be no spread" of cancer cells anywhere. Sylvia's clairvoyance gave me peace of mind.

After the surgery, my surgeon, a wonderful and beloved cancer surgeon at UVA, came running into my room, excitedly holding up her thumb and index finger in a pinch configuration. "It was so small we could hardly see it" she bubbled–the very same words Sylvia had used the night before. The surgeon then went on to say that in her twenty-three years of practice she had seen this happen in two, maybe three cases (finding a tumor so small and encapsulated in a tumor so large). She wanted to know what I ate and what supplements I took. "This is nothing but your immune system working the way it should–at peak performance," she said. Of course I attributed my outcome to eating yeast-free, and happily provided her with a copy of *The Yeast-Free Kitchen.* I listed all the supplements I took, especially the Poly–MVA, and told her about Sylvia and what I had seen and learned while working with her. She was genuinely impressed.

In the last five years, all my checkups and routine blood work have been normal. No cancer markers have been found. All the eleven biopsies came back clean, just as Sylvia had predicted. I continue to do the yeast-free diet every three months for twenty-one days, and then stay close to it in the interim. I literally proved my own thesis. I certainly didn't want to develop cancer to do it, but that is what happened. I pray I will be able to continue to illustrate the power of this diet and its ability to heal so many diseases.

I prayed a lot during those dark days of surgery and recovery. I kept remembering a favorite Edgar Cayce quote: "Why worry when you can pray? He (God) is the whole, you are a part. Coordinate your abilities with the Whole."

Cayce was so right. We all *are* a part of God, and God is part of us–each and every one. I truly believe that when we coordinate our abilities with Him, the Whole, we can change ourselves–and the world–for the better.

\*\*\*\*\*\*\*\*\*\*\*\*\*\*\*\*\*\*\*\*\*\*\*\*\*\*\*\*\*\*\*\*\*\*\*\*\*\*\*\*\*\*\*\*\*\*\*\*\*\*\*\*\*\*\*\*\*\*\*\*\*\*
\*\*\*\*

### *Post Script*

Sylvia and I are working together again and I continue to chronicle her work. She comes regularly to see her patients here in Gordonsville, Virginia. She lives in Austin, Texas, and also travels to see patients in Houston, Denver, New York City, and Kingston, New York. You can read about her at her website: SylviaFlesner.com

# *References*

**Foreword (Dr. Buttram)**

1. Sources: Centers for Disease Control and Prevention, California Department of Health and Human Services.
2. Rimland B., The autism epidemic: vaccinations and mercury, Journal of Nutrition and Environmental Medicine, 2000: 261-266.
3. Prevalence of autism spectrum disorders: Autism and developmental disabilities monitoring network, six sites, United States, 2000. Morbidity and Mortality Weekly Report, 2000 - Feb. 9, 2007, 56(No. SS-1):1.
4. Bloom B, Dey AN. Summary health statistics for U.S. children, National health interview survey, 2004. U.S. Centers for Disease Control and prevention, National Center for Health Statistics.
5. Singh, VK, Warren RP, Averett R, Ghaziuddin M, Circulating auto-antibodies to neural and glial filament proteins in autism. Pediatric Neurology, 1997; 17:88-90.
6. Singh VK, Warren RP, Odell JD, Warren WL, Cole P, Antibodies to myelin basic protein in children with autistic behavior. Brain, Behavior, and Immunology. 1993; 7:97-103.
7. Bock, Kenneth and Stauth, Cameron. Healing the New Childhood Epidemics: Autism, ADHD, Asthma, Allergies. New York: Ballantine Books, 2007.
8. Kirby, David, Evidence of Harm, New York, St. Martin Press, 2005.
9. Eibl M, Maannhalter JW, Zblinger G. Abnormal T-lymphocyte subpopulation in healthy subjects after tetanus booster immunization, (letter). New England Journal of Medicine, 1984; 310(3):198-199.
10. Miller NZ, Vaccine Safety Manual, for Concerned Families and Health Practitioners, New Atlantean Press, Sante Fe, New Mexico, 2008: page 202.

## Chapter 2: How Did This Happen

1.     http://www.femmslender.com/articles/beat_candida
2.     http://innovation.edf.org/page=cfm?tagid=31088
3.     http://www.mbschachter.com/dangers_of_flourida.htm
4.     http://www.alive.com/3780a2.php?subject_bread_cramb=658


## Chapter 3: Back in Time

1.     http:// www. biology.ualberta.ca/courses.hp/ent207/lec29–30.htm


## Chapter 7:  What Causes Symptoms

1.     http://cme.medscsape.com/viewarticle/55816
2.     www.acepilots.com /Pioneer/hughes.html


## Chapter 9: The No No's

1.     http://articles.Mercola.com/sites/articles/archive/2009/02/12/Your-Genes-Remember-a-Sugar-Hit.aspx
2.     http://www.muschealth.com/healthyaging/breastcancer_alcohol.htm
3.     http://www.snopes.com/food/warnings/butter.asp


## Chapter 10:  Eating Yeast Free

1.     World Poultry News "Arsenic Compound in Chicken Affecting Americans" June  29, 2009

## Chapter 14: The Body–Mind Connection

1.    Zimmerman, M. (1980) "The nervous system in the context of information theory." In R.F.Schmidt&G.Thews(eds.)*HumanPhysiology*pp.166-173, Berlin,Germany:Springer–Verdag
2.    James 5:16 NIV
3.    http://www.slinxtra.com/healthy_lifestyle_genetic_change.html

## Chapter 15: Tips

1.    http://www.mercola.com/article/microwave/hazards2.htm
2.    chttp://www.globalhealingcenter.com/microwave-ovens-the-proven-dangers
3.    Blaylock Wellness Report "Why Fluoride is Toxic" Sept. 2004, Vol.1, No.4

(Buttram)

1. Multiple Chemical Sensitivities, Washington, D.C., National Research Council, National Academy Press, 1989. pg. 52.
2. Wallace, LA et al, The TEAM study: Personal exposures to toxic substances in air, drinking water, and breath of 400 residents of New Jersey, North Carolina, and North Dakota, Environmental Research, 1987; 43:290-307.
3. Morrow LA et al, PET and neurobehavioral evidence of tetrabromoethane encephalopathy, Journal of Neuropsychiatry, 1990; 2:431-435.
4. Morrow, LA et al, Cacosmia and neurobehavioral dysfunction associated with occupational exposure to mixtures of organic solvents, American Journal of Psychology, 1988; 145:1442-1445.
5. Ryan CM et al, Assessment of neuropsychological dysfunction in the workplace: normative data from the Pittsburgh occupational test battery. Journal Clinical Experimental Neuropsychology, 1987; 9:666-679.

6. Morrow LA, et al, Psychiatric symptomatology in persons with organic solvent exposures, Journal of Consulting Clinical Psychology, 1993; 51:171-174.

7. Morrow LA, Assessment of attention and memory efficiency in persons with solvent neurotoxicity, 1992; Neurophsycologia, 1992; 30(10):911-922.

8. Pesticides in Diets of Infants and Children, Washington D.C., sponsored by the National Research Council, National Academy Press, 1993: pg. 3.

9. Neurotoxicity, Identifying and Controlling Poisons of the Nervous System,
Washington D.C. Superintendent of Documents,   Government Printing Office, April, 1990, 44, GPO Stock #052-003-01184-1.

10. Weiss B, Environmental contaminants and behavioral disorders. Journal of the Development of Pharmacology Therapies, 1967; 10346-353.

11. Chester AC and Levine PH. Concurrent Sick Building Syndrome and Chronic Fatigue Syndrome: Epidemic neuromyasthenia revisited. Clinical Infectious Diseases, 1994; 18:S43-S48.

12. Schubert J, Riley EJ, and Tyler SA, Combined effects in toxicology: A rapid systematic testing procedure: cadmium, mercury, and lead. Journal of Toxicology and Environmental Health, 1978; 4:763-776.

13. Abou-Donia, MB, Wilmarth KR, Ochme F et al, Neurotoxicity resulting from coexposure to Pyridostigmine Bromide, DEET, and Permithrin: Implications of Gulf War chemical exposures. Journal of Toxicology and Environmental Health, 1996; 48:35-56.

14. Arnold SF, Koltz DM, Collins B, et al, Syndergistic activation of estrogten receptor and combinations of environmental chemicals, Science, 1996; 272: 1489-1492.

**Chapter 17:  The Rise of Big Pharma**

1.      www.naturalnews.com/025303.html
2.      www.naturalnews.com/FDA_raids.html

3.      www.healthcaregoesmobile.com/.../AMA-draws-fierce-criticism-
        practicing-physicians
4.      http://articles.mercola.com/sites/articles/archives/2008/09/27/fda-
        announces-20-dangerous-drugs-you-should-not-be-on.aspx
5.      *The New York Times* Brody, Jane "The 'Poisonous Cocktail' by
        Multiple Drugs," Sept. 18, 2007
6.      www.medicine-no.com/DrugPromotion.htm
7.      *Charlottesville Daily Progress* Sept. 3, 2009 "Pfizer Slapped with
        Record Penalty"
8.      Kluger, Jeffry, "Is Drug Company Money Tainting Medical
        Education?"
        http://www.time.com/time/health/article/0,8599,1883449,00,html
        Accessed March 6, 2009
9.      Mercola.com "Drug Companies Still Make Bundle Even When
        They Admit to Lie" Posted Sept.4, 2004
10      Choudhry NK., Stelfox HT., Detsy AS., Relationships between
        authors of clinical practice and the pharmaceutical industry JAMA
        2002;287(5)612–7
11.     http://psychdata.com/2009_04_archive.html

## Chapter 18:  Statins…Cure or Curse?

1.      www.greatplainslaboratory.com/home/eng/cholesterol.asp
2.      Krumholz, HM et al Lack of association between cholesterol and
        coronary artery mortality and morbidity and all-cause mortality in
        persons older than 70 years.
        JAMA 272,1335–40, 1990
3.      JAMA, Feb. 2002;287:612–617.
4.      www.Squidoo.com/dangersof statindrugs
5.      http://archives.mercola.com/sites/article/archive/2008/02/how-
        statin-drugs-wreck-your-muscles.aspx
6.      Am J Med 04;117:823–829
7.      *Alternatives* Williams, David Dr., January 2009 Vol. 12 No. 19
8.      www.westonaprice.org/The-Benefits-of-High-Cholesterol.html

9. http://articlesofhealth.blogspot.com/2010/01/truth-about-heart-disease-and-strokes.html

10. Whitaker, Julian *World's Worst Drugs, World's Best Alternatives Pocket Guide 2008*

11. www.westonaprice.org/The-Benefits-of-High-Cholesterol.html

12. Blaylock, Russell *The Blaylock Wellness Report* March 2009 Vol. 6, No.3

13. Ridker, PM., et al, "C–reactive protein levels and outcomes after statin therapy," New Eng J Med 2005; 352:20–8

14. Blaylock, Russell, *The Blaylock Wellness Report* Vol.6, No.3

15. Sinatra, Stephen *Heart Beat Special Winter Bulletin 2009* "What the Average M.D. Doesn't Know About Heart Disease Could Get You Killed"

16. http://www.natural-cancer-cures.com/high-cholesterol-foods.html

17. www.marksdailyapple.com/nnt-numbers-needed-to-treat/

18. Bloomberg Business Week January 17, 2008 "Do Cholesterol Drugs Do Any Good?'

19. Brownstein, David, M.D. Newsmax.com July 19, 2009

20. *Charlottesville Daily Progress* Nov.16, 2009 "Study deals blow to Merck cholesterol pill."

21. http://www.mercola.com/sites/articles/archive/2008/2/2/cholesterol-has-benefits- too.aspx

22. Colpo A. LDL Cholesterol Bad Cholesterol or Bad Science J Am Phys Surg. 2005:10:83–89

23. *Townsend Letter* Feb/Mar 2008 "Statins and Increased Cancer: The Hidden Story and a New Solution" by Brian Peskin

24. http://www.doctorzebra.com/prez/z_x34mirx_g.htm

25. www.jpands.org/Vol1no3/colp2.pdf

26. http://www.mercola.com/sites/articles/archives/2009/02/21/900-Studies-Show-Statin-Drugs-are-Dangerous.aspx

27. Constantini, H.V. *Fungalbionics:Atherosclerosis* 1994 ISBN # 3–930939–00–2

## Chapter 19:  Vaccines:  Prescriptions for Disaster

1.  *Charlottesville Daily Progress* "Chickenpox It's Party Time" Sept. 23 2008
2.  *Blaylock Wellness Report* "The Trouble with Vaccines" May 2008 Vol.5, No.5
3.  http://www.thinktwice.com/
4.  http://www.detoxmychild.org/what's_in_vaccines.htm
5.  http://vactruth.com/2010/07/15/non-disclosed-hyper-allergenic-vaccine-adjuvant/
6.  http://forum.prisonplanet.com/index.php?topic=28758.0
7.  *Pathways Magazine* Spring 09 "Aluminum and Vaccine Ingredients: What Do We Know? What Don't We Know?" Lawrence B. Palevsky, M.D.
8.  http:/www.whale.to/vaccineadjuvants.html
9.  http://viewzone2.com/sv40x.html
10. http://huffingtonpost.com/david–Kirby/new–study–hepatitis–b–vac_b_289288 html
11. http://www.mombu.com/medicine/t-argentina-investigates-deaths-of-vaccinated-kids-pneumonia-5319-last.html
12. http://danceswithshadows.com/pillscribe/trovan-vaccine-clinical-trial-victims-in-kano-to-get-n26250000-for-death-injury-from-pfizer/
13. http://www.mercola.com/sites/articles/archive/2008/06/21/rebel-scientist-battles-dangerous-vaccines-and-antibiotics.aspx
14. Government of Australia official statistics:
    http://childhealthsafety.wordpress.com/graphs/
    "Vaccinations Did Not Save Us–2 Centuries of Official Statistics

## Chapter 20:  Autism…A Sign of the Times

1.  http://serendip.brynmawr.edu/bb/neuro06/web2/bpeterson.html
2.  www.globalresearch.ca/index.php?context=va&aid=15074
3.  www.wanttoknow.info/060215vaccinesmercurydangers
4.  http://www.whale.to/a/howenstine.html

5.     http://www.emagazine.com/view/?4984
6.     *The Blaylock Wellness Report* March 2009 Vol.6, No.3
7.     http://www.autismboulder.org/pdf/CongressionalFindings.pdf
8.     http://wholisticpeds.com/uploads/Rolling%20%20deadly%20
       Immunity/htm
9.     Ibid
10.    Ibid
11.    Ibid
12.    Ibid
13.    http://www.healthfreedomusa.org/?p=524
14.    www.ncpa.org  "Obama Says Yes to Dr. No." Jeanette Nordstrom
       July 16, 2010 National Center for Policy Analysis
15.    *NewsmaxHealth* "U.S. Concedes Vaccines Cause Autism" Mar.3,
       2008

## Chapter 21: H1N1: The Pandemic That Didn't Pan Out

1.     http://www.selfhealthsystems.com/archiveletter.php?id=339
2.     http://www.sodahead.com/fun/evidence-the-swine-flu-vaccines-are-
       bioweapons/blog-126541/
3.     http://www.infowars.com/forced-vaccinations-quarantine-camps-
       health-care-interrogations-and-mandatory-decontaminations/
4.     *The Charlottesville Daily Progress, July 2, 2010 "$260M of swine
       flu vaccine wasted"* AP
5.     http://www.exactyempire.com/?p+6524
6.     *Time* magazine Oct 19, 2009 "Can Health Care Workers Be Forced
       to Get Flu Shots?" Alice Park

## Chapter 22:  Gardasil–Guarding Whom?

1.	Mercola.com "HPV Vaccine Blamed for Teen's Paralysis" Aug.2, 2008
2.	*NewsmaxHealth* "Gardasil: Oversold, Overhyped, and Risky?" Sept. 13, 2009  Sylvia Booth Hubbard
3.	http://www.cancer.gov/cancertopics/factsheet/Risk/HPV
4.	*NewsmaxHealth* "Gardasil: Oversold, Overhyped, and Risky?" Sept. 13, 2009 Sylvia Booth Hubbard
5.	Mercola.com "HPV Vaccine Blamed for Teen's Paralysis" Aug. 2, 2008
6.	*New England Journal of Medicine* "Condom Use and the Risk of Genital Human Papillomavirus Infection in Young Women" Vol. 345:2645–2654 June 22, 2006 No. 25
7.	AFP news report "Spain withdraws cervical cancer shot after illnesses" Feb. 10, 2009
8.	Newsmaxhealth "Gardasil: Oversold, Overhyped, and Risky?" Sept. 13, 2009 Sylvia Booth Hubbard

## Chapter 23:  Antibiotics and Their Legacy

1.	http://www.cas.muohio.edu/~stevenjr/mbi131/studyguide131a.html
2.	http://worstpills.org//public/page.cfm?op_id=3
3.	*INT J Cancer* 08; 123:2152–2155
4.	*JAMA* 04;291:827–835
5.	http://www.thefreelibrary.com/
6.	http://content.nejm.org/cgi/content/full/351/11/1089
7.	http://www.orthomolecular.org/resources/omns/V04n14.shtml

## Chapter 24: The Demise of Big P(harm)a

1.    *Los Angeles Times* April 27, 2009 Swine Flu 'debacle' is recalled Shari Roan
2.    http://articles.mercola.com/sites/articles/archive/2008/03/15/tamiflu-s-effects-on-your-brain.aspx
3.    http://www.mercola.com/sites/articles/archive/2004/05/15/drug-companies-evil-aspx
4.    http://articles.mercola.com/sites/articles/archive/2005/04//23/mercury-poison.aspx
5.    http://www.royalrife.com/flu_shots.html
6.    *Blaylock Wellness Report* "Vaccinations: The Hidden Dangers" May 2004 Vol.1, No.1
7.    *Newsmax Magazine* Sept. 2008 "RX for Death" Sherry Baker
8.    *Charlottesville Daily Progress* Sept. 20, 2009 "Researchers: hormone therapy nearly doubles lung cancer risk"
9.    Null, Gary et al *Death by Medicine* Oct. 2003
10.   Charlottesville Daily Progress Oct. 11, 2009 "U.S health system bankrupts families"
11.   http://www.laleva.cc/petizone/english/ronlaw_eng.html
12.   www.naturalnews.com/023430_adhd_disease_drugs.html
13.   Balch, James *Prescriptions for Healthy Living Special Report*
14.   AP April 12 2004 "Fosamax can cause rotting of jawbone" Theresa Agovino
15.   Mercola.com Oct. 8, 2009 "Is Your Doctor Saying No to Drug Companies' 'Free Lunch' Deception"
16.   Ibid
17.   Mercola.com Sept.4, 2004 "Drug Companies Still Make Bundle Even When They Admit to Lie"

## Chapter 25: The Future of Food

1.    http://articles.mecola.com/sites/articles/archive/2008/07/08/tthe-most-evil-company-on-the-planet-monsanto.aspx?source=nl
2.    Ibid

3.  http://artices.Mercola.com/sites/archive/2009/03/07/monsantos-many-attempts-to-destroy-all-seeds-but-their-own.aspx
4.  *Well Being Journal* "The Politics of Food" Vol.12, No.3 May/June 2003
5.  *Well Being Journal* "GM Foods Are Not Safe" Vol. 17, No.4 July/August 2008
6.  http://organicconsumers.org/articles/article_15573cfm
7.  www.seedsof deception.com/utility/showArticle/object/?objectID=1078
8.  http:healthyandliving.org/featured–news/128/Recent–study–shows–toxicity–in–labrats%E2%80%99–livers–in–connection–to–GM–food
9.  www.saynotogmos.org/ud2005/unovO5.html
10. http://www.healthfreedomusa.org/?p=599
11. http://www.commondreams.org/views02/0209-01.htm
12. http://www.commondreams.org/view/2009/03/21-5
13. www.globalresearch.ca/index.php?context=va&aid=8148
14. Ecclesiastes 11:15 NIV with permission

**Chapter 26: *Codex Alimentarius***

1.  http://baltimorechronicle.com/2009/082409Lendman.html
2.  http://preventdisease.com/tips103.shtmlwww.healthfreedomusa.org/docs/ codex_fer.pdf
3.  http://www.healthfreedomusa.org/docs/codex_flyer.pdf
4.  http://www.knowthelies.com?q=node/5020
5.  http://preventdisease.com/home/tips103.shtml
6.  http:// www.albionmonitor.com/free/codexthreat.html
7.  *Newsmax* Maxlife July, 2009 "Supplements at Risk of Disappearing"
8.  http://http://blogs.wsj.com/health/2009/05/12/fda-warns-general-mills-cheerios-is-a-drug

## Chapter 27: The Answer to Cancer

1. Simoncini, Tullio, M. D. *Cancer is a Fungus* p.19
2. Abramson, John, M.D. *Overdosed America* p.50
3. Whitaker, Julian, M. D. *Health and Healing Newsletter* Nov. 2009 Vol. 19, No.11 "Cancer Treatment: The Dawn of Enlightenment"
4. Ibid
5. Simoncini, Tullio, M. D. *Cancer is a Fungus* p.56
6. Morgan G, Ward R, Barton M, ClinOncol (R.Coll Radiol) 2004, Dec; 16(8) 549–60
7. http://www.distance-healer.com/4.html
8. Goffman, John, M. D. *Radiation from Medical Procedures in the Pathogenesis of Cancer and Ischemic Heart Disease* http://www.burtongoldberg.com/healthcare-freedom/medical-xrays-a-cause-of-cancer-and-heart-disease.php
9. *Journal of the National Cancer Institute* Sept. 20, 2009; 92: 1490–1499
10. *The Blaylock Wellness Report* Oct. 8, 2008 "The Great Cancer Lie" Vol.5 No.10
11. Shim, H & Dang, C. *Proceedings of the National Academy of Sciences* Vol. 95, pp. 1511–16.
12. White, M.W. *Medical Hypotheses* 1996: 47, 35–38

## Chapter 28: Diabetes: A Feast for Yeast

1. *Health and Healing Newsletter* Aug. 2009 Dr. Julian Whitaker
2. Schatz, DA et al, Prevention of insulin-dependent diabetes mellitus: an overview of three trials. *Cleveland Clinic Journal of Medicine* 63(5):270–274, 1996
3. http://21daybodymakover.com/blog/100-the-war-on-fat-may-be-making-us-sicker.html
4. Zhoa, Wei–Qin et al *The FASEB Journal* "Amyloid beta oligomers induce impairment of neuronal insulin receptors" Aug. 24, 2007

5.    *Washington Post* AP Feb. 21, 2010 "Senate report ties
      GlaxoSmitKline diabetes drug Avandia to heart attack risks"
6.    Kaufmann, Doug A. *Infectious Diabetes* Ch. 2 p. 25
7.    http://www.naturalnews.com/021183.html
8.    http://intelegen.com/nutrients/gymnema_sylvestre_for_diabetes.htm

**Chapter 30:  Where Do We Go From Here?**

1.    Exodus 12:08 Taken from the Holy Bible, New International
      Version© 1978 by the New York International Society, with
      permission.
2.    Exodus 12:17–21 NIV as above
3.    Exodus 23:18 NIV as above
4.    Leviticus 2:4–6 NIV as above
5.    Leviticus 13:47–53 NIV as above
6.    Leviticus 13:53–58 NIV as above
7.    Leviticus 14:36–43 NIV as above
8.    Leviticus 14: 43–46 NIV as above
9.    Leviticus 14: 46–48 NIV as above
10.   1 Corinthians 6:19 NIV as above
11.   Isaiah 33:24 Scripture taken from the NEW AMERICAN
      STANDARD BIBLE ®, © 1960, 1962, 1963, 1968, 1971, 1972,
      1973, 1975, 1977, 1995 by the Lockman Foundation Used by
      permission. (www.Lockman.org)

## *Bibliography and Recommended Reading*

Abramson, John, M.D. 2004. *Overdo$ed America* Harper-Collins Publishers
ISBN 0–06–056853–4

Allen, Christian B., PhD. Wolfgang Lutz, M.D. 2000. *Life Without Bread* McGraw–Hill ISBN 10:0658001701.

Baroody, Theodore N.D., D.C., PHD. Nutrition, C.N.C. 1991. *Alkalyze or Die* Holographic Health Press ISBN 0–9619595–3–3.

Batmanghelidj, F., M.D. 1997. *Your Body's Many Cries For Water* Global Health Solutions, Inc. ISBN 0–9629942–3–5.

Beattie, Greg. 1997. *Vaccinations A Parent's Dilemma* Oracle Press
ISBN 1–876308–00–1.

Berger, Stuart M. M.D. 1990. *What Your Doctor Didn't Learn in Medical School* William Morrow & Co. ISBN 9780688065539.

Bigelsen, Harvey, M.D. 2010. *Doctors Are More Harmful Than Germs* Bolger ISBN 9780982477809.

Blaylock, Russell, M.D. 1996. *Excitotoxins: The Taste That Kills* Health Press ISBN 10:0929173252.

Bryson, Christopher. 2004. *The Fluoride Deception* Seven
Stories Press
ISBN l–58322–526–9.

Cave, Stephanie. M.D. 2001. *What Your Doctor May Not Tell
You about Children's Vaccines* Warner Books ISBN 0–446–
67707–8.

Cherniske, Stephen. 1998. *Caffeine Blues* Warner Books
ISBN 0–446–67391–9.

Chopra, Deepak, M.D. 1990. *Quantum Healing* Bantam ISBN
10:0553348698

Constantini, A.V. 1998. *Prevention of Breast Cancer – Hope at
Last* Freiburg, Germany: Johan Friedrick Obverlin Verlas
Publishers ISBN 3930939029.

Coulter, Harris.L., Barbara Loe Fisher 1991. *A Shot in the Dark*
Avery ISBN 0–89529–463–x.

Crook, William G. M.D. 1992. *Chronic Fatigue Syndrome and
the Yeast Connection* Professional Books ISBH 0933478–20–8.

Crook, William G., M.D. 1986 *The Yeast Connection* Vintage
Books
ISBN 0–394–74700–3

Duffy, William. 1986. *Sugar Blues* Grand Central Publishing
ISBN 10:0446343129.

Frompovich, Catherine J. 2009. *Our Chemical Lives and the Hijacking of our DNA* Book Surge ISBN 978–1–4392–5536–0.

Galland, Leo, M.D. 1997. *The Four Pillars of Healing* Random House
ISBN 0–679–44888–8.

Gerber, Richard, M.D. 1988. *Vibrational Medicine* Bear & Company
ISBN 0–939–680–46–7.

Hay, Louise L. 1984. *You Can Heal Your Life* Hay House
ISBN 0–937611–01–8.

Honenberger, Sarah Collins. 2006. *White Lies* Cedar Creek Publishing
ISBN 13:978–0–9790205–1–3.

Ingram, Cass, M.D. 2001. *The Cure is in the Cupboard* Knowledge House
ISBN 091111974–4.

Jaffee, Richard. 2008. *Gallileo's Lawyer* Thumbs Up Press
ISBN 10:0980118301.

Kaufmann, Doug A. 2000. *The Fungal Link Vol.1* Media Trition Inc.
ISBN 0–9703418–0–6

Kaufmann, Doug A. 2003. *The Fungus Link Vol. 2*
MediaTrition Inc.
ISBN 0–9703418–4–9

Kaufmann, Doug. A. 2003. The *Fungal Link to Diabetes*
MediaTrition Inc.
ISBN 0–9703418–2–2

Kaufmann, Doug A. 2004. *The Germ That Causes Cancer*
MediaTrition Inc. ISBN 0–9703418–1–4

Kaufmann, Doug, A. 2005. *The Fungus Link Vol. 3*
MediaTrition Inc.
ISBN 0–9703418–7–3

Kaufmann, Doug. A. 2004. *What Makes Bread Rise?*
MediaTrition Inc.
ISBN 0–9703418–3–0

Kirby, David. 2005. *Evidence of Harm* St. Martin's Press
ISBN 10:03123326440.

McMillen, S.I., M.D. & David E. Stern, M.D. 2000. *None of These Diseases* Fleming H. Revell ISBN 10: 0–8007–5719–x

Mendelsohn, Robert, M.D. 1987. *How to Raise a Healthy Child in Spite of Your Doctor* Ballantine Books ISBN 10:0345342763.

Mercola, Joseph, D.O. 2006. *Sweet Deception* Nelson Books
ISBN 10:0785221791.

Miller, Neil., Russell Blaylock, M.D. 2008. *Vaccine Safety Manual* New Atlantean Press ASIN:Boo1tk6078.

Null, Gary. 2010. *Death by Medicine* Praktikos Books ISBN 10:1607660026.

Pollan, Michael. 2006. *The Omnivore's Dilemma* Penguin Press 10:1594200823.

Pringle, Peter. 2009. *Food, Inc.* Public Affairs ISBN 10:1586486942.

Ravnskov, U. M.D., PHD. 2000. *The Cholesterol Myths: Exposing the Fallacy That Saturated Fat And Cholesterol Cause Heart Disease* New Trends Publishing ISBN 10–0967089700.

Remington, Dennis W., M.D. 1989. *Back to Health* Vitality House International, Inc. ISBN0–912547–03–0.

Rollins, James. 2009. *The Doomsday Key* William Morrow ISBN 10:0061231401.

Schmidt, Michael A., M.D., Keith Sehnert, M.D. Lendon Smith, M.D. 1994. *Beyond Antibiotics* North Atlantic Books ISBN 1–55643–1805.

Shoemaker, Ritchie, M.D. 2005. *Mold Warriors* Gateway Press, Inc.
ISBN 0–9665535–3–5.

Simoncini, Tullio M.D. 2007. *Cancer is a Fungus* Edizioni Lampis
ISBN 88–87241–08–2

Smith, Jeffrey. 2003. *Seeds of Deception* Yes! Books ISBN 10:0972966587.

Smith, Jeffrey. 2007. *Genetic Roulette* Chelsea Green ISBN 10:0972966528.

Sykes, Lisa. 2009. *Sacred Spark* Fourth Lord Productions ISBN 10:0971780641.

Trowbridge, John Parks, M.D. 1986. *The Yeast Syndrome* Bantam Books
ISBN 0–553–26269–6.

Trudeau, Kevin. 2006. *More Natural "Cures" Revealed* Alliance Publishing Group, Inc. ISBN 13 978–0–9755995–4–9

Trudeau, Kevin 2006 *Natural Cures "They" Don't Want You to Know About* Alliance Publishing Group, Inc. ISBN 0–9755995–0–x

Truman, Karol K. 1998. *Feelings Buried Alive Never Die* Olympus Distributing ISBN 0–911207–02–3.

Wakefield, Andrew, M.D. 2010. *Callous Disregard: Autism and Vaccines* Skyhorse Publishing ISBN–10:1616081694

Young, Robert O. PhD., Shelley Redford Young. 2002. *The pH Miracle* Warner Books ISBN 0–446–69049–x.

# INDEX

# A

# B

# H

Made in the USA
Middletown, DE
22 September 2017